Bailey's

# Research & Evidence-Based Practice for the Health Professional

Fourth Edition

# BAILEY'S Research & Evidence-Based Practice for the Health Professional

FOURTH EDITION

**Jennifer E. Lape, OTD, MOT, OTR/L**
Program Director, Occupational Therapy Programs
Associate Professor of Occupational Therapy
Chatham University
Pittsburgh, Pennsylvania

**Angela N. Hissong, DEd, OTR/L, CMCP, CMMT, RYT-200**
Professor-in-Charge
Occupational Therapy & Science
The Pennsylvania State University
Mont Alto, Pennsylvania

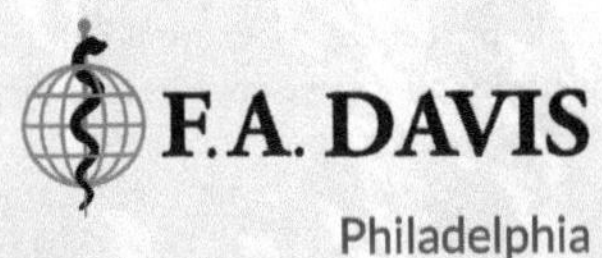


Philadelphia

F. A. Davis Company
Philadelphia
F. A. Davis Company
1915 Arch Street
Philadelphia, PA 19103
www.fadavis.com



Printed in the United States of America

Last digit indicates print number: 10 9 8 7 6 5 4 3 2 1

*Editor-in-Chief:* Margaret M. Biblis
*Publisher, Health Professions:* Christa A. Fratantoro
*Director of Content Development:* George W. Lang
*Senior Developmental Editor:* Jill Rembetski
*Content Project Manager:* Elizabeth Stepchin
*Art and Design Manager:* Carolyn O'Brien



**Library of Congress Cataloging-in-Publication Data**

Names: Lape, Jennifer E., author. | Hissong, Angela N., author. | Bailey, Diana M., 1942- Bailey's research for the health professional.
Title: Bailey's research & evidence-based practice for the health professional / Jennifer E. Lape, Angela N. Hissong.
Other titles: Bailey's research and evidence-based practice for the health professional
Description: Fourth edition. | Philadelphia : F.A. Davis Company, [2025] | Preceded by Bailey's research for the health professional / Angela N. Hissong, Jennifer E. Lape, Diana M. Bailey. Third edition. [2015]. | Includes bibliographical references and index.
Identifiers: LCCN 2024045870 (print) | LCCN 2024045871 (ebook) | ISBN 9781719648684 (paperback) | ISBN 9781719654326 (epub) | ISBN 9781719654333 (pdf)
Subjects: MESH: Research Design | Data Collection--methods | Data Interpretation, Statistical | Writing | Publishing
Classification: LCC R850 (print) | LCC R850 (ebook) | NLM W 20.5 | DDC 610.72--dc23/eng/20241120
LC record available at https://lccn.loc.gov/2024045870
LC ebook record available at https://lccn.loc.gov/2024045871

Standing on a rocky cliff with panoramic views, you see endless possibilities to explore. Your eyes shift between where you stand and a distant point where you hope to be someday. It's not just about getting there, but about learning and enjoying the journey. There's a great big, beautiful tomorrow. With compass in hand, you are ready to begin.

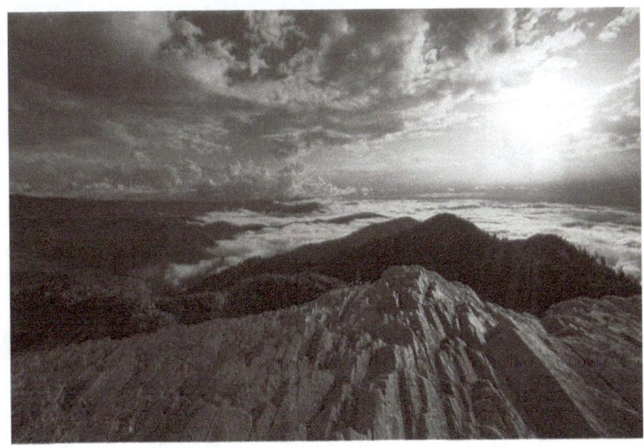

Cover image: Sunset on Mt. LeConte, Great Smoky Mountain National Park.

# Preface

*Research and Evidence-Based Practice for the Health Professional*, Fourth Edition, is an informative and practical guide to support allied healthcare students and practitioners in learning about and engaging in research or evidence-based practice projects. The text will assist you to:

1. Differentiate features of research studies and evidence-based practice projects.
2. Describe design features and technical aspects of quantitative, qualitative, and mixed methods research methodologies.
3. Access and critically evaluate literature on a topic of interest.
4. Design, implement, and evaluate meaningful research studies or innovative, evidence-based practice projects.
5. Explore funding opportunities and strategies for successful grant writing.
6. Disseminate research and evidence-based practice project outcomes through presentations and publications.
7. Engage in self-directed and collaborative learning activities to hone your research, evidence-based practice, and leadership skills.

## Philosophy of New Edition

This text emphasizes a straightforward, learner-centered approach to understanding and engaging in research and evidence-based practice. This approach is drawn from teaching and mentoring hundreds of students from associate to doctoral levels. The philosophy of this new edition is to get you excited about research and evidence-based practice, inspire you to learn these processes through doing, and help you envision your future success and impact on your profession and others. You will master this content through learner-friendly explanations, examples, application assignments, discussions, and collaboration with others.

In teaching this content, I often use the metaphor of a journey, which may initially convey a well-plotted path with sequential steps from start to finish and arrival at a final destination. In reality, engaging in research or completing a formal evidence-based practice project seldom takes this form. In the beginning, you contemplate possible destinations (topics, outcomes, and ideas) and commit to one, though your final destination will be further shaped by people, knowledge, and experiences along the way. Your journey is bound to have twists and turns, including some that further inspire you and others that test your limits. Shifts in your journey may be necessary to navigate barriers, acclimate to new conditions, and reenergize and refocus yourself. You may arrive at an unexpected peak compared to your intended destination, yet the views will still be awe-inspiring. At this point, you may feel relief, excitement, and pride in your accomplishment, but do not be fooled into thinking you have arrived. There is always something new to explore. I intend for this text to serve as a compass for your journey, whether you are learning the foundations of research and evidence-based practice or engaging in your own study or project.

A special note to faculty who will use this text to guide and teach your students: I have developed an updated set of instructor ancillaries available on fadavis.com. These include PowerPoints, test questions, an image bank, and an instructor's guide that offers a map to structure a syllabus, classroom discussions, and learning activities.

## What's New?

This compass (the text) is packed with new information and features to support you on your journey.

- The new title and content organization signal one of the most significant changes—the integration of research and evidence-based practice content. These processes are interdependent, so they are no longer presented separately in the text.
- New content related to mixed methods research designs and systematic reviews (Chapter 10) and pilot and feasibility studies (Chapter 11) supports you in understanding existing research and designing new inquiries.
- Three new chapters walk you through critically appraising quantitative (Chapter 6), qualitative (Chapter 9), mixed methods, and systematic review research (Chapter 10), including templates for appraisal of each of these designs.
- Expanded and reorganized content on completing a literature search (Chapter 3) better guides this process and includes how to assess the credibility of sources; identify search terms, criteria, and strategies; and track and organize your search with tracking log and literature matrix templates.
- Expanded chapters on quantitative (Chapters 4 and 5) and qualitative research (Chapters 7 and 8) include more study designs, explanations of data analysis methods, and current literature examples.
- Chapter 11, Developing Your Inquiry Plan, incorporates enhanced and reorganized content on choosing an inquiry design, creating a survey, and drafting your inquiry procedures.
- Expanded content on protecting human subjects or participants (Chapter 12) includes components of an Institutional Review Board proposal, levels of review, new templates, examples, and guidelines for constructing recruitment materials, informed consent, assent forms, and volunteer agreements, plus a brief history of the protection of human subjects.
- Chapter 13, Funding Your Inquiry, notably expands on types of grants, grant sources, components of a grant proposal, and practical grant writing tips to help you identify and pursue funding sources.
- New content on program development (Chapter 13) and completing a needs assessment (Chapters 2 and 13) further support grant writing and evidence-based practice.
- Knowledge translation has a greater presence in the text to emphasize the connection between research and evidence-based practice and the value of disseminating outcomes.
- Chapter 15, Presenting Your Inquiry, now includes more information on the advantages, disadvantages, and etiquette for virtual presentations.
- Finally, new content supporting publication (Chapter 16) emphasizes defining your publishing goals, outlining your key argument, evaluating potential journals, and responding to requests for revisions or rejections.

## Organization of the Text

The text is organized into four sections, representing key phases of the research and evidence-based practice journey. **Section 1—Embarking on Your Journey** (Chapters 1–3) will help you differentiate research and evidence-based practice, identify and refine a topic to explore, and complete a comprehensive literature search. **Section 2—Understanding and Appraising Research** (Chapters 4–10) provides straightforward explanations and examples of quantitative, qualitative, mixed methods, and systematic review research designs. Sampling, data collection tools, and analysis methods relative to each design are carefully explained. Finally, templates and detailed instructions walk you through how to critically appraise each design. If you plan to complete a study or project of your own, **Section 3—Designing Your Inquiry** (Chapters 11–13) will assist you in developing your inquiry plan, designing a survey, drafting an Institutional Review Board proposal, and identifying and securing funding for your plan. Finally, **Section 4—Disseminating Your Outcomes** (Chapters 14–16) focuses on sharing your outcomes through various outlets, including formal reports, presentations, and publications.

I have found the chronological review of the chapters most effective for understanding key features and steps of research and evidence-based practice, with later content building on earlier chapters. However, if you plan to complete your own research study or evidence-based practice project, reviewing some chapters concurrently or in an altered order may be necessary. For example, tasks discussed in Chapters 2 and 3 are interconnected, so collective review may help you fully grasp the concepts and hone your inquiry ideas. Similarly, if you are completing a research study or formal evidence-based practice project as part of academic coursework, you may be required to complete a formal inquiry report. Writing this report typically begins as you work through phases of the inquiry rather than waiting until the end, so you may need to skip ahead to scope out Chapter 14. The chapter titles and organization of the text should allow you to easily locate important information when needed.

## Chapter Features

Each chapter contains several features to support your learning, including the following:

- **Learning Outcomes:** Each chapter begins with specific learning outcomes to let you know what you can expect to learn as you review the chapter content.
- **Tips & Inspiration:** This new feature, purposefully placed throughout each chapter, includes practical hints for understanding and applying chapter content and inspiration to keep you going. These tips have been accumulated through my experiences conducting research and evidence-based practice projects and teaching and mentoring others in these endeavors. They should motivate you and help you avoid unnecessary bumps along the way.
- **Chapter Summary:** A bulleted outline of the chapter's main concepts, organized by learning outcomes, helps you review key points once you have read the chapter.
- **Test Your Knowledge:** This new feature, located at the end of each chapter, includes a series of closed-ended questions with fixed response choices for you to assess your learning after reviewing the chapter. Some questions test your recall of basic chapter content, while others require you to apply the content. The correct answers are provided in the back of the text so you can confirm your understanding.
- **Next Steps:** Each chapter concludes with a list of recommended learning activities or *Next Steps* to help you reflect on the chapter content and begin to apply it. These activities can serve as a foundation for engaging in your own inquiry by allowing you to consider chapter content from the perspective of your topic, setting, or situation.
- **Resources and Templates:** These are available within the chapters and appendices to guide you on your journey. In addition, various examples from multiple disciplines have been included throughout the chapters to demystify more complex concepts.
- **Inspirational Photos:** The chapter images and cover photo represent the importance of finding time to enjoy life's simple pleasures, even in the face of difficult situations, tasks, and experiences. While research and evidence-based practice can be challenging and time-consuming, I have found these processes transformative, exciting, and fun with proper life balance. I frequently remind my students that breaks are needed and that there is joy in the journey—not just in the final destination. These photos were taken throughout my writing journey for this text as I tried to stay true to my own philosophy. I hope they serve as a reminder to you to enjoy your journey. Don't be so focused on the destination that you miss the good stuff along the way!

*Jennifer E. Lape*

# Reviewers

**Jana Cason, DHSc, OTR/L, FAOTA**
Professor
Occupational Therapy
Hawai'i Pacific University
Honolulu, HI

**Amanda Urowsky Davis, OTD, OTR/L**
Assistant Professor
Occupational Therapy
Pfeiffer University
Misenheimer, NC

**Shruti Gadkari, OTD, OTR/L**
Assistant Professor
Occupational Therapy
Pacific University
Hillsboro, OR

**Karen D. Giddens, MS, MLS(ASCP)**
Program Director
Medical Laboratory Science
Philadelphia College of Osteopathic Medicine
Suwanee, GA

**Rachel Ellison, PhD**
Associate Professor
Health Sciences
University of Louisiana at Lafayette
Lafayette, LA

**Kelly Erickson, PhD, OTR/L**
Professor, Department Chair
Occupational Therapy
The College of St. Scholastica
Duluth, MN

**Julie Marie Nagle, OTD, OTR/L**
Assistant Professor
Occupational Therapy
Saint Francis University
Loretto, PA

**Debora Oliveira, PhS, OTR/L**
Professor, Program Director
Occupational Therapy
Florida A&M University
Tallahassee, FL

**Ellen Berger Rainville, OTD, MS, OT, FAOTA**
Professor and Site Coordinator
Occupational Therapy
MCPHS University of Worcester
Worcester, MA

**Adrine Reganian, RDHAP, MSDH, MSHS-HPE**
Assistant Professor
Health Sciences
Pasadena City College
Pasadena, CA

**Mary E. Smith, EdD, OTR/L**
Associate Professor
Occupational Therapy
College of Saint Mary
Omaha, NE

# Acknowledgments

My deepest gratitude goes to:

Joe, for supporting me no matter what, taking me along on your photography adventures, and sharing your amazing images for this text. You've helped me see the beauty in the journey, and I couldn't have done this without you.

My family, friends, and colleagues, for checking on me and knowing just when I needed a night out or some chocolate chip cookies.

Christa, Jill, and Elizabeth, for believing I could handle this solo project, being open to my vision for this edition, and talking me through the challenges.

Finally, to my students—past and present—who inspired me through their research and evidence-based practice to be a better therapist and educator, and to write a sensible and light-hearted book to inspire others.

# Brief Contents

# Contents

# Section 1

# Embarking on Your Journey

Section 1 (Chapters 1–3) of this text introduces research and evidence-based practice and reviews foundational steps for embarking on your journey. This journey may include understanding research and evidence-based practice, learning all there is to know about a topic of interest, using research to inform your clinical practice, or conducting a research study or evidence-based practice project of your own. Specifically, Chapter 1 differentiates research and evidence-based practice and explains the steps and potential challenges with each. Chapters 2 and 3 provide guidance for choosing a topic, developing a research or evidence-based practice question, establishing a need and rationale for a study or project, and conducting an effective literature search. These tasks may seem daunting, but this section includes helpful hints, strategies, and examples to support you through the process. Take a deep breath, and let's dive in!

## Chapter 1

# Differentiating Research and Evidence-Based Practice

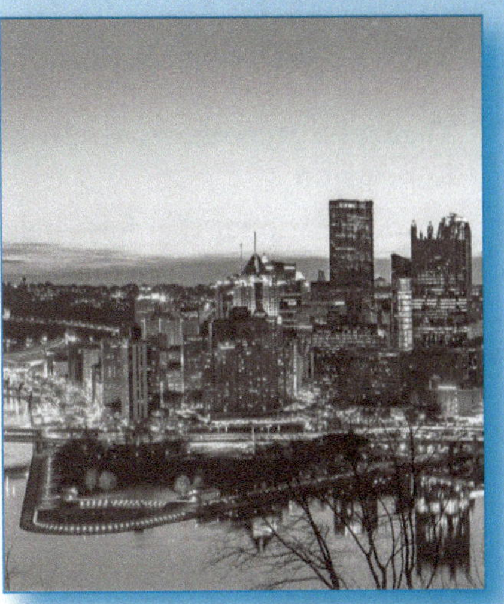

LEARNING OUTCOMES

*The information provided in this chapter will assist you to:*

1.1 Define research.
1.2 Recall the steps for conducting a research study.
1.3 Identify potential challenges in engaging in research.
1.4 Define evidence-based practice.
1.5 Recall the steps for conducting an evidence-based practice project.
1.6 Identify potential challenges in engaging in evidence-based practice.
1.7 Differentiate key features of a research study and an evidence-based practice project.

## Getting Started

Conducting a research study or an evidence-based practice project can be an enjoyable, stimulating, and transformative activity in your professional journey. It is typical to feel a bit overwhelmed as you prepare to embark on this complex and time-consuming work. However, *YOU* have the potential to expand your skills as a student and practitioner, establish yourself as an expert in your chosen topic, and positively impact the clients you serve through this process. You are right where you need to be right now. This text aims to help you understand the features of research and evidence-based practice and guide you through the required steps for conducting a research study or evidence-based practice project when you are ready to embark on your journey. Research and evidence-based practice are distinct yet interrelated processes, so we will address each separately and then compare them.

## What Is Research?

**Research** is the systematic investigation of a problem, issue, or question to produce *new* knowledge that can be generalized to similar groups or populations. This investigation includes reviewing literature on a given topic and drawing new conclusions about that topic, manipulating certain variables to see what happens to other variables, or searching for the meaningfulness of a variable to an individual or group.

Systematic investigation involves the process of logic, often called **deductive** and **inductive** reasoning. Deductive reasoning starts with a general theory and ends with a specific conclusion; this can be referred to as a top-down approach. For example, the researcher begins with a general theory, forms a hypothesis based on the theory, tests the hypothesis, assesses the results, and forms a conclusion (Box 1-1).

Golden Triangle, Pittsburgh, Pennsylvania.

### BOX 1-1 ■ Deductive Reasoning

**Theory → Hypothesis → Observations → Conclusion**

An occupational therapist believes positive encouragement improves client outcomes (**general theory**) and **hypothesizes** that positive reinforcement will decrease stroke recovery time. The therapist conducts a research study to test the hypothesis on 100 clients and finds that stroke recovery time decreased by 50% (**observations**) when positive reinforcement was incorporated. The therapist concludes that positive reinforcement decreases stroke recovery time (**conclusion**), confirming the original theory.

### BOX 1-2 ■ Inductive Reasoning

**Observation → Pattern → Hypothesis → Theory**

An occupational therapist **observes** that a client's ability to climb stairs improves when preceded by a balance task (e.g., standing on one leg with eyes closed). The therapist conducts a research study over the next several months to **look for a pattern** of whether the balance task causes improvements in other areas (cognition, motor skills, etc.). After observing improvements in other areas, the therapist believes that the balance task should be performed at the beginning of every occupational therapy session (**hypothesis**) and implements this as standard protocol for all clients (**theory**).

Inductive reasoning, or a bottom-up approach, starts with a specific observation that eventually forms a general theory. In this type of reasoning, the researcher starts with an interesting observation and then looks for a pattern of similar observations. From this pattern, the researcher develops a hypothesis, which forms the basis of a general theory (Box 1-2).

When using inductive reasoning, one accepts or believes a finding about a situation and then applies that belief to all similar individuals, assuming that the finding will be true for all. For example, suppose a healthcare practitioner finds that having clients complete a specific questionnaire about their health history is beneficial during an initial evaluation. In that case, the practitioner may choose to give all subsequent clients the questionnaire to fill out.

The point of consideration with deductive reasoning is that although the principle is usually true, there may be exceptions. The point of consideration with inductive reasoning is that the individual upon whom you have based the principle may be the exception, so the principle may not apply to all other cases that follow.

## Steps for Conducting a Research Study

Conducting research is a cyclic process, as depicted in Figure 1-1. The researcher starts with a question in mind, goes through the investigative stages, and ends up with an answer to the question. Often, further questions arise during the data analysis and interpretation, leading to more research ideas.

There are different points of entry into the research process. Some people enjoy starting afresh at the question identification stage; others may discover prior study results they question and want to investigate for themselves. Still others begin this process as part of formal coursework to learn the research process or how to interpret and apply existing research. Whatever the entry point, the steps required to complete a research study follow a logical sequence:

1. Identify a problem that needs to be solved or a question that needs to be answered.
2. Review the existing literature related to the problem or question.
3. Formulate a research question or hypothesis about the problem based on the literature.
4. Outline procedures to address the research question or hypothesis and secure Institutional Review Board (IRB) approval to conduct the study (if necessary).
5. Carry out the study and collect data.
6. Analyze the data and interpret the findings.
7. Disseminate your findings as appropriate. This step might involve presenting and publishing your research so that others may benefit from the identified knowledge.

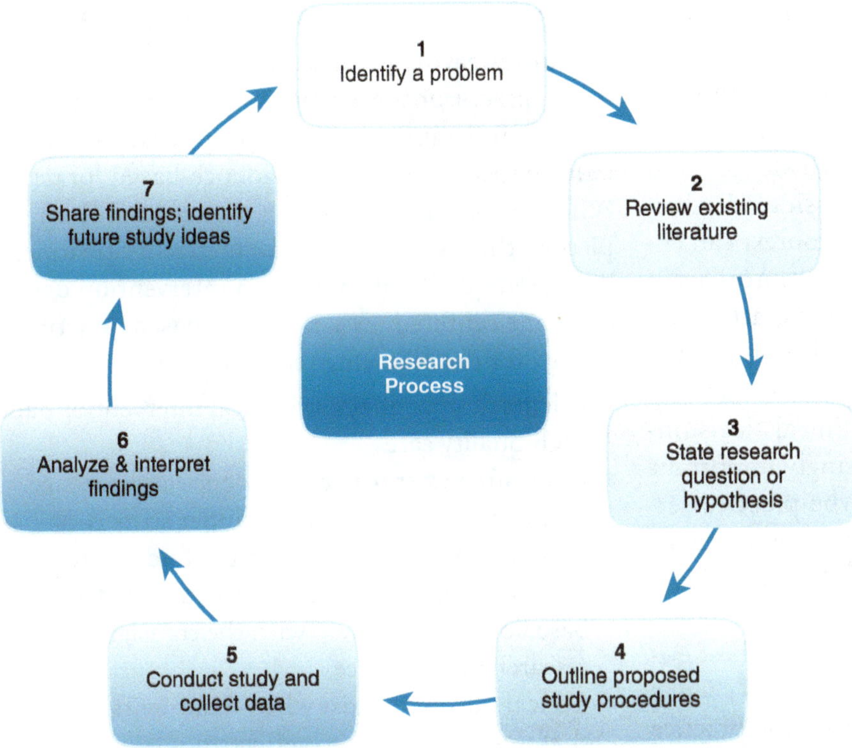


Figure 1-1 Steps for conducting a research study.

## Research Process Challenges

When you begin a research study, decisions must be made regarding your topic, research methodology, and ways to balance your time and integrate the required tasks with your everyday activities. Some common challenges you may encounter in the initial stages of the research process include the following:

- Difficulty balancing time commitments to allow sufficient time to complete all research process steps.
- Underestimating how much assistance or cooperation you need from others involved in the research process.
- Choosing too broad a focus or trying to accomplish too much in an initial research study.
- Lacking relevant experience to get the process started.
- Difficulty selecting the most appropriate research methodology and data analysis methods for your intended purpose.

### TIPS & INSPIRATION

- At this early stage, consider what will help you stay motivated during this scholarly journey. Choose a topic you are passionate about and reward yourself for small successes along the journey to help you stay the course.

## What Is Evidence-Based Practice?

The most popular definition of evidence-based practice originated with the pioneer of evidence-based medicine, David Sackett. His foundational article describes evidence-based practice as "the conscientious, explicit, and judicious use of current best evidence in making decisions about the care of individual patients" (Sackett et al., 1996, p. 71). Although this definition emphasized the importance of using research in clinical decision-making, it failed to acknowledge the significance of the practitioner's knowledge and skills and the client's (or patient's) goals, values, and circumstances. Thus, the definition was expanded to identify **evidence-based practice** as "the integration of best research evidence with our clinical expertise and our patient's unique values and circumstances" (Straus et al., 2011, p. 1). Best research evidence refers to the current applicable research on the efficacy of treatments for a particular diagnosis or condition.

Although research establishing the efficacy of a treatment technique is important, this information cannot be used in isolation. The practitioner's knowledge, skills, and past experiences, as well as each client's goals, values, strengths, challenges, and contexts, must be thoughtfully considered when making practice decisions. A client's context can encompass their physical environment, resources available, social supports and relationships, attitudes, and background, including racial, cultural, gender, and professional identities (American Occupational Therapy Association, 2020). In clinical decision-making, it has also become increasingly important to consider the characteristics of the practice setting, such as the equipment and resources available, reimbursement models, staffing levels, and policies and procedures (Hoffman et al., 2018). Therefore, the integration of these three components—best evidence, practitioner skills and knowledge, and client's goals, values, and circumstances within the practice context—comprise evidence-based practice and is illustrated in Figure 1-2.

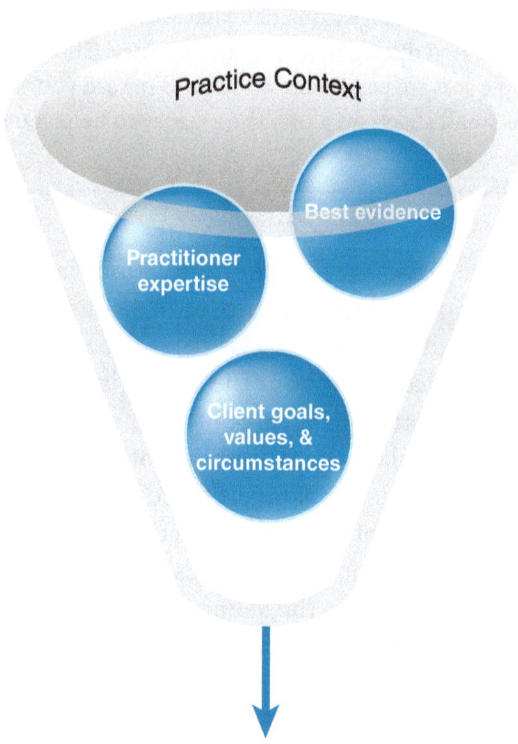


Figure 1-2 Evidence-based practice is the integration of three components.

## Why Is Evidence-Based Practice Needed?

The interweaving of these three elements—best evidence, practitioner expertise, and client goals, values, and circumstances within the practice context—culminates in effective evidence-based practice. When any of these elements are omitted from the picture, the result might be an ineffective treatment, decreased quality of care, or an intervention devoid of client-centeredness. Evidence-based practice is needed for the following reasons:

- Clients deserve effective clinical interventions and high-quality care.
- Gaps often exist between evidence and practice. Some research is completed under strict conditions, making generalizing the findings to real-world practice settings difficult. Evidence-based practice can help with the translation of research into practice.
- Ethical dilemmas exist when treatments are used that were shown to be ineffective.
- Many practitioners are faced with increased caseloads and productivity standards. Evidence-based practice can increase effectiveness and efficiency; time is wasted when interventions not supported by evidence are used, and client outcomes may be poor.
- Today, medical advances and technological changes occur much faster than before. New information is being produced daily, and formerly accepted treatments are now being questioned or refuted.
- Practitioners have an ethical responsibility to remain current on clinical practices. Past practice experiences, clinical judgment, or knowledge gained from initial schooling cannot solely drive practice decisions.
- Practitioners involved in evidence-based practice report a stronger professional identity and the ability to clearly articulate their role and value to others (Sirkka et al., 2014).
- Clients, families, policymakers, and third-party payors demand proof of efficacy for our treatments. Without evidence to support treatments, needed services may no longer be available in facilities, included in legislation, or reimbursed by payment plans.

### Evidence-Based Practice Projects

Healthcare practitioners and students routinely use evidence-based practice to guide clinical decision-making for individual clients, which promotes ethical practice and quality outcomes. However, they may also conduct formal evidence-based practice projects. An **evidence-based practice project** is an initiative focused on designing and implementing an evidence-based intervention, program, protocol, or education to address the needs of a specific population or within a specific setting to improve outcomes or processes. Focusing on groups of clients or populations rather than just one individual may result in clinical practice guidelines or protocols to improve practice. In some healthcare settings, the term **quality improvement project** has also been used to describe evidence-based practice projects that comprehensively address prevalent practice challenges.

### Knowledge Translation

**Knowledge translation** involves implementing existing research, evaluating the outcomes, identifying supports and challenges in applying research to practice, and disseminating the findings to promote better clinical outcomes (Chan et al., 2023; Wensing & Grol, 2019). Knowledge translation goes beyond the mere application of existing evidence to practice (evidence-based practice) to sharing the outcomes with others so that they might also benefit from this information. If you plan to complete an evidence-based practice project, you might consider sharing your results beyond the setting where you implement your project. Sharing your successes and challenges might help others navigate similar challenges and improve their clinical outcomes. Examples of knowledge translation through evidence-based practice are provided in Figure 11-2 and discussed further in Chapter 11.

## Steps for Conducting an Evidence-Based Practice Project

Like research, the evidence-based practice process is cyclic—meaning that after an evidence-based project is completed and the outcomes are fully considered, the evidence-based practice question might be revised, and the cycle is started again. Regardless of the project's scale and scope, most evidence-based practice projects consist of these five basic steps:

1. Identifying a need and an evidence-based practice question
2. Searching the evidence
3. Appraising and synthesizing the evidence
4. Applying the evidence (implementing the project)
5. Evaluating the project (and sharing your outcomes as appropriate)

After identifying a need, evidence-based practice involves searching and appraising available evidence on the treatment being considered or the client's condition. For example, a practitioner might be considering using electrical stimulation to treat a client's lower back pain, or they may search the literature to determine the best treatment(s) for lower back pain because of a specific diagnosis, such as lumbar stenosis. Once the available evidence has been garnered and evaluated, the practitioner must draw on past experiences, knowledge, and skills in treating this condition to determine the research's applicability to the current practice situation. At this point, the practitioner must consult with the client and consider the practice context to make the most effective and appropriate practice decision. In a formal evidence-based practice project, an evidence-based protocol might be established and implemented with all clients with lumbar stenosis who visit the clinic. Client outcome data can be gathered and analyzed to evaluate the impact of the new protocol and inform future practice decisions. For example, should the clinic permanently adopt the protocol, or are revisions necessary? Furthermore, the outcomes, supports, and challenges of implementing this protocol could be disseminated in a conference presentation or a publication to promote knowledge translation.

## Evidence-Based Practice Challenges

Challenges to conducting an evidence-based practice project can be found at the individual and organizational levels. At the individual level, challenges include the following:

- Lack of time to retrieve, appraise, and apply the best evidence to individual clients.

- Lack of confidence or having limited skills to search databases, read and understand research articles, and interpret and apply the results.
- Difficulty applying research to clinical situations. Not all research designs are readily applicable to real-life situations; perhaps a particular intervention was shown to be successful but only under strictly controlled conditions that cannot be replicated in clinical practice (Jette et al., 2003; Salbach et al., 2009) or a client presents with increasing complexities that are not adequately addressed in the research (McArthur et al., 2021).
- Limited motivation or desire to change practice skills or the presence of workplace burnout (McArthur et al., 2021).

Barriers at the organizational level may include the following:

- Lack of access to appropriate resources, including memberships in professional organizations, libraries, research databases, and journals.
- No reimbursement or time allotted for evidence-based continuing education.
- A work culture that emphasizes organizational goals, financial gains, and productivity standards more than evidence-based practice.
- Lack of authority to make decisions about some practice changes.

While these challenges pose threats to evidence-based initiatives, they are not insurmountable. Success is likely when individual practitioners, employers, policymakers, professional organizations, and academics collaborate (Dannapfel et al., 2013; Ilott, 2003). Research also suggests the most effective ways to teach research and evidence-based practice to healthcare students, as well as strategies for successful implementation within clinical settings (Bernhardsson et al., 2017; Hitch et al., 2021; Sirkka et al., 2014). Investment of all parties in the process can lead to more competent practitioners, satisfied clients, and better clinical outcomes.

Employers can support practitioners by providing access to evidence-based resources, time for continuing education and research activities, and additional staffing and financial resources when needed. Strong formal and informal leadership and a culture that values evidenced-based practice can also be advantageous (Dannapfel et al., 2013). Policymakers also need to balance their focus between cost containment and quality of care. Creating local and national systems that support research and its real-life application can benefit practitioners and clients alike. In addition, many resources exist to make applying research easier and less time-consuming for you. These include databases containing preappraised evidence, collections of evidence on specific topics, and systematic reviews. Most professional organizations have subsections, communities of practice, and website resource pages to assist their members in evidence-based practice efforts. Additionally, collaborative relationships among researchers, practitioners, academics, and professional organizations can further bridge the divide between research and clinical practice (Bennett et al., 2018). Evidence-based practice is discussed throughout this text, but Appendix A contains additional evidence-based practice resources by healthcare discipline if you need them.

### TIPS & INSPIRATION

- Trust the process! Conducting a research study or a formal evidence-based practice project requires precise, ordered steps that are thoughtfully laid out in this text. If you are fortunate enough to engage in this scholarly work as part of formal coursework, you likely have instructors, mentors, and peers supporting you and cheering you on. Focus on the required tasks each day or week and try not to worry about things too far into the future. You've got this!

## Research Studies Versus Evidence-Based Practice Projects

As the concept of evidence-based practice has grown, students and practitioners alike have made the mistake of confusing it with research. Research studies are conducted to test hypotheses and generate *new* information on a particular condition, treatment, or phenomenon. Researchers attempt to describe lived experiences, assert connections among study concepts, or suggest cause-and-effect relationships. Conversely, evidence-based practice projects involve reviewing, appraising, and applying *existing* research to practice situations.

Research and evidence-based practice are distinct but intricately connected processes. Quality research guides decision-making for evidence-based clinical practice. Likewise, evidence-based practice promotes the translation of research to real-world practice scenarios. As such, one process can drive the other. For example, you might use existing research on the efficacy of stress management strategies for healthcare professionals to design and implement a new evidence-based stress management program at a healthcare clinic (evidence-based practice project). The data you gather to evaluate the success of the new program (stress scale ratings and surveys to participants) might support revising the program through another evidence-based practice project or justify the need for a research study to explore new concepts or issues that occurred. One process is not more valuable than the other, and the choice will depend on your topic and aims.

Table 1-1 summarizes the key features of a research study versus an evidence-based practice project. Throughout the rest of this text, the term **inquiry** is used to collectively represent research studies and evidence-based practice projects since the information being discussed applies to both in many instances. When it is important to differentiate, individual terms will be employed.

### TIPS & INSPIRATION

- You might be using this text to learn about research and evidence-based practice or as a tool to help you conduct your own research study or evidence-based practice project. In either case, don't get so caught up in the details that you miss the thrill of the journey. Getting there is half the fun!

**TABLE 1-1 ■ Comparison of Research Study and Evidence-Based Practice Project**

| Features | Research Study | Evidence-Based Practice Project |
|---|---|---|
| **Purpose** | To generate *new* knowledge that can be generalized | To apply *existing* research to a clinical practice organization |
| **Procedures** | Systematic, well-planned, *strict* procedures | Systematic search and appraisal of best available evidence; *flexible* procedures in applying evidence to practice |
| **Scope** | Population *beyond* the research setting | Specific patient or patient population *within* a clinical practice organization |
| **Sample Composition and Size** (number of subjects or participants)* | *Varies* based on study purpose; size based on power analysis or saturation | Often *small* convenience samples (large enough to detect changes but feasible to logistically manage) |
| **Approvals Required** | *Always* requires Institutional Review Board (IRB) approval or exemption to initiate study and for dissemination of results | *Sometimes* requires IRB approval or exemption (typically only if results will be disseminated outside the clinical practice organization) |
| **Dissemination Goals and Audience** | **Primary aim:** Presentation and publication with broad national or international audiences<br>**Secondary:** May share results locally or within the study site; students undertaking research may share within their academic institutions | **Primary aim:** Locally/within clinical practice organization; students undertaking these projects may share within their academic institutions<br>**Secondary:** May share results through presentation and publication with broad national or international audiences for knowledge translation |

*The terms "subjects" and "participants" are often used interchangeably to refer to individuals being studied, though the use of "participants" has gained traction in recent years to emphasize the autonomy of these individuals. You may still find both terms in published literature and in IRB applications. The choice of terminology for your own inquiry may be based on your specific discipline, publication or academic requirements, or your preference. You will find both terms in this text.

## CHAPTER SUMMARY

1. Define research.
   - Research is the systematic investigation of a problem, issue, or question to produce *new* knowledge that can be generalized to similar groups or populations.
2. Recall the steps for conducting a research study.
   - Research is a seven-step systematic, strict process.
   - The seven steps are as follows: (1) identify a problem that needs to be solved or a question that needs to be answered, (2) review the existing literature related to the problem or question, (3) formulate a research question or hypothesis about the problem based on the literature, (4) outline procedures to address the research question or hypothesis and secure IRB approval (if necessary), (5) carry out the study and collect data, (6) analyze the data and interpret the findings, and (7) disseminate your findings as appropriate.
3. Identify potential challenges in engaging in research.
   - Common challenges in the research process can include difficulty balancing time commitments, underestimating the help needed from others, choosing too broad a focus, lack of research knowledge and experiences, and difficulty selecting the most appropriate methodology or data analysis methods.
4. Define evidence-based practice.
   - Evidence-based practice is the review, appraisal, and application of *existing* research to clinical practice. This process involves the integration of best evidence, practitioner skills and knowledge, and the client's goals, values, and circumstances within the practice context to make practice decisions.
   - An evidence-based practice project is an initiative focused on designing and implementing an evidence-based intervention, program, protocol, or education to address the needs of a specific population or within a specific setting to improve outcomes or processes.
   - Knowledge translation involves implementing existing research, evaluating the outcomes, identifying supports and challenges in applying research to practice, and disseminating the findings to promote better clinical outcomes.
5. Recall the steps for conducting an evidence-based practice project.
   - Evidence-based practice is a five-step systematic, flexible process.
   - The five steps are (1) identifying a need and an evidence-based practice question, (2) searching the evidence, (3) appraising and synthesizing the evidence, (4) applying the evidence (implementing the project), and (5) evaluating the project (and sharing your outcomes as appropriate).
6. Identify potential challenges in engaging in evidence-based practice.
   - Challenges in the evidence-based practice process can be found at both the individual and organizational levels.
   - Challenges at the individual level can include a lack of time, skills, and confidence to engage in evidence-based practice.
   - Challenges at the organizational level may include a lack of support for evidence-based practice activities.
7. Differentiate key features of a research study and an evidence-based practice project.
   - A research study is conducted to test hypotheses and generate *new* information on a topic for generalization to similar groups or populations. In contrast, an evidence-based practice project involves the review, appraisal, and application of *existing research* to groups of clients or practice situations.
   - Key elements that differ between a research study and an evidence-based practice project include the purpose, procedures, scope, sample size, approval process, and if and where the outcomes are shared.

## TEST YOUR KNOWLEDGE

1. Which of the following BEST describes research?
   a. A process for generating new knowledge that can be generalized to similar populations
   b. A process that involves flexible procedures based on the needs of the participants
   c. A process that can usually be implemented without Institutional Review Board approval
   d. A process that incorporates small samples of participants to pilot clinical interventions
2. Which of the following is the FIRST step in conducting a research study?
   a. Secure approval to conduct the study
   b. Identify a problem to explore
   c. Review existing literature on the topic
   d. Draft the proposed study procedures

3. Which of the following BEST describes evidence-based practice?
   a. A linear process for evaluating clinical programs
   b. A cyclic process for appraising research
   c. A systematic, flexible process for applying existing research to practice
   d. A process used by researchers to determine the feasibility of a study's design
4. Which of the following is the FIRST step in conducting an evidence-based practice project?
   a. Applying the evidence
   b. Identifying a need
   c. Searching the evidence
   d. Evaluating the project
5. Identify whether each inquiry refers to a research study OR an evidence-based practice project.
   a. A nursing facility receives a citation from an inspector due to a high incidence of client falls. In response, the nursing and therapy staff incorporate the best available evidence on effective fall prevention programs to create and implement a multifactorial program to promote decreased incidence of falls.
   b. A home health therapist routinely works with clients with low vision and is interested in exploring their perceptions of the home evaluation process.
   c. A group of faculty wants to explore the impact of virtual class attendance versus in-person class attendance on students' academic performance to inform their future curriculum design.
   d. An occupational therapy student collaborates with a local school district to address concerns about youth mental health. The occupational therapy student incorporates high-quality research into a teacher education series to increase teachers' knowledge and confidence in using social-emotional learning strategies in the classroom.

Answer key appears at the end of this text.

## NEXT STEPS

1. Identify five motivations you have for completing a research study or evidence-based practice project.
2. What challenges and supports to research or evidence-based practice do you anticipate personally and within your setting? Make a list of each and then contemplate how you might use the supports to address each challenge.

## REFERENCES


American Occupational Therapy Association. (2020). Occupational therapy practice framework: Domain and process (4th ed.). *American Journal of Occupational Therapy, 74*(Suppl. 2), 7412410010p1–7412410010p87. https://doi.org/10.5014/ajot.2020.74S2001

Bennett, S., Laver, K., & Clemson, L. (2018). Progressing knowledge translation in occupational therapy. *Australian Journal of Occupational Therapy, 65*, 156–160. https://doi.org/10.1111/1440-1630.12473

Bernhardsson, S., Lynch, E., Dizon, J. M., Fernades, J., Gonzalez-Suarez, C., Lizarondo, L., Luker, J., Wiles, L., & Grimer, K. (2017). Advancing evidence-based practice in physical therapy settings: Multinational perspectives on implementation strategies and interventions. *Physical Therapy, 97*(1), 51–60. https://doi.org/10.2522/ptj.20160141

Chan, R. J., Knowles, R., Hunter, S., Conroy, T., Tieu, M., & Kitson, A. (2023). From evidence-based practice to knowledge translation: What is the difference? What are the roles of nurse leaders? *Seminars in Oncology Nursing, 39*(1), 151363. https://doi.org/10.1016/j.soncn.2022.151363

Dannapfel, T., Peolsson, A., & Nilsen, P. (2013). What supports physiotherapists' use of research in clinical practice? A qualitative study in Sweden. *Implementation Science, 8*, Article 31. https://doi.org/10.1186/1748-5908-8-31

Hitch, D., Nicola-Richmond, K., Richards, K., & Stefaniak, R. (2021). Student perspectives on factors that influence the implementation of evidence-based practice in occupational therapy. *JBI Evidence Implementation, 19*, 409–418. https://doi.org/10.1097/xeb.0000000000000285

Hoffman, T., Bennett, S., & Del Mar, C. B. (2018). *Evidence-based practice across the health professions* (3rd ed.). Elsevier.

Ilott, I. (2003). Challenging the rhetoric and reality: Only an individual and systemic approach will work for evidence-based occupational therapy. *American Journal of Occupational Therapy, 57*(3), 351–354. https://doi.org/10.5014/ajot.57.3.351

Jette, D. U., Bacon, K., Batty, C., Carlson, M., Ferland, A., Hemingway, R. D., Hill, J. C., Ogilvie, L., & Volk, D. (2003). Evidence-based practice: Beliefs, attitudes, knowledge, and behaviors of physical therapists. *Physical Therapy, 83*(9), 786–805. https://doi.org/10.1093/ptj/83.9.786

McArthur, C., Bai, Y., Hewston, P., Giangregorio, L., Straus, S., & Papaioannou, A. (2021). Barriers and facilitators to implementing evidence-based guidelines in long-term care: A qualitative evidence synthesis. *Implementation Science, 16*, Article 70. https://doi.org/10.1186/s13012-021-01140-0

Sackett, D. L., Rosenberg, W. M. C., Gray, J. A. M., Haynes, R. B., & Richardson, W. S. (1996). Evidence based medicine: What it is and what it isn't. *British Medical Journal, 312*, 71–72. https://doi.org/10.1136/bmj.312.7023.71

Salbach, N. M., Guilcher, S. J. T., Jaglal, S. B., & Davis, D. A. (2009). Factors influencing information seeking by physical therapists providing stroke management. *Physical Therapy, 89*(10), 1039–1050. https://doi.org/10.2522/ptj.20090081

Sirkka, M., Zingmark, K., & Larsson-Lund, M. (2014). A process for developing sustainable evidence-based occupational therapy practice. *Scandinavian Journal of Occupational Therapy, 21*(6), 429–437. https://doi.org/10.3109/11038128.2014.952333

Straus, S. E., Glasziou, P., Richardson, W. S., & Haynes, R. B. (2011). *Evidence-based medicine: How to practice and teach it* (4th ed.). Elsevier Churchill Livingstone.

Wensing, M., & Grol, R. (2019). Knowledge translation in health: How implementation science could contribute more. *BMC Medicine, 17*(1), 1–6. https://doi.org/10.1186/s12916-019-1322-9

## Chapter 2

# Identifying and Refining Your Topic

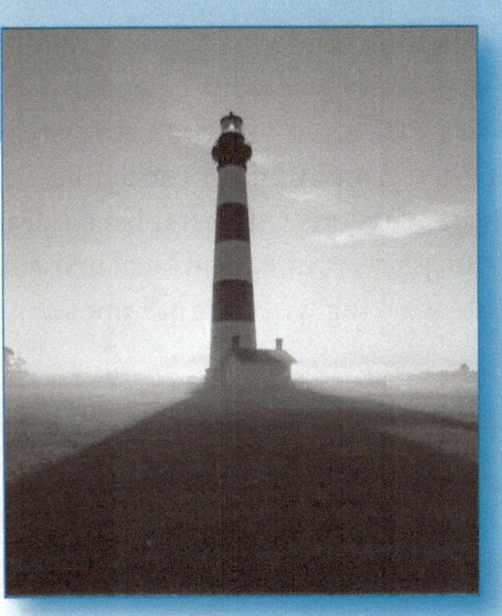

LEARNING OUTCOMES

*The information provided in this chapter will assist you to:*

2.1 Examine the time required to complete an inquiry.
2.2 Differentiate preliminary and comprehensive literature searches.
2.3 Identify a topic for your research study or evidence-based practice project.
2.4 State the elements of a quality research or evidence-based practice question.
2.5 Develop a quality PIO or PICO question to guide your inquiry.
2.6 Construct a problem statement for your inquiry.
2.7 Draft a quality rationale for an inquiry, including the need, background, purpose, and significance.
2.8 Explain the components of a needs assessment and how this information is useful in planning an inquiry.

## Time Considerations for an Inquiry

If you plan to conduct a formal research study or evidence-based practice project, you may wonder about the time commitment for such an endeavor. If you are doing so within the context of formal education, your overall time frame is likely dictated by the curriculum or course sequence. If you are conducting an inquiry as a practitioner in a clinical setting, you may be bound by time constraints within your site. Regardless of the context, formal inquiries usually take a minimum of 6 to 12 months but may span 1 to 2 years, depending on the scope of the inquiry. These time frames account for all the activities in the process, including identifying the topic, conducting the inquiry, and writing the final report or manuscript.

Of course, the time commitment for different phases of an inquiry can also vary. For example, some inquiries may require more time during the implementation phase if the procedures or assessments are more detailed and time-consuming. Other inquiries may require more time up front during the literature review and planning phases but have more straightforward procedures, lending to less time spent in that phase. The length of time for data analysis can also vary greatly based on the volume of data collected and the inquiry purpose. Suffice it to say that conducting any inquiry will require dedication and consistent focus on the work.

Those who are more successful tend to "touch" their work every day or at least several times a week, ensuring they do not need to spend extended time reorienting to the work after lengthy breaks. During

Bodie Island Lighthouse, Nags Head, North Carolina.

this time of identifying and refining your topic, it is wise to look at your calendar and determine where you can carve out time consistently for this work. When examining your schedule, be sure to align your work sessions with established deadlines that the inquiry site, your educational institution, or others you are working with might impose.

## Preliminary Versus Comprehensive Literature Searches

This chapter reviews the initial steps of an inquiry, including how to identify and refine your inquiry topic, write an inquiry question, construct a problem statement, and develop a rationale for your inquiry. These steps can occur sequentially as they are discussed here, but they might also happen simultaneously or in a slightly altered order. For example, you might concurrently identify your inquiry topic and construct the problem statement or draft the problem statement before writing your inquiry question.

Regardless, these steps usually involve a preliminary search of the literature. A **preliminary literature search** is an initial exploration of the literature on a topic to gain a broad understanding of the relevant research and trends, which can help you refine your ideas at this early stage. As the name implies, the preliminary literature search occurs first before the more comprehensive literature search. A **comprehensive literature search**, discussed in detail in Chapter 3, is an exhaustive search of the literature using well-defined search terms, search strategies, and search tracking to fully determine the breadth of information specific to your topic. A comprehensive literature search is used to write your formal literature review and make decisions about your inquiry procedures.

During your preliminary search, it is most important to ensure you are consulting credible sources. **Credible sources** typically include documents from professional, government, and other reputable organization websites, professional journals, and academic texts. Blog posts, personal opinion pieces, and social media posts and videos warrant further scrutiny before relying on them. Chapter 3 provides additional information on assessing the credibility of sources.

Finally, it bears mentioning that the problem statement and rationale, reviewed in this chapter, may be further refined after the later comprehensive literature search. In other words, you will draft these items now based on your preliminary literature search using the best information you have at this moment. Later, after you have firmly committed to a topic and completed the comprehensive literature review, you can revise these elements before submitting your final proposal or manuscript. In reality, many students benefit from reviewing Chapters 2 and 3 in tandem, since these tasks are interconnected.

## Identifying a Topic

The first step in any inquiry is identifying a potential topic for your research study or evidence-based practice project. You likely already have some general ideas based on the professional literature you have read and on your prior coursework, interests, and clinical experiences. Some questions to consider in this process include:

- **What topics or subject areas are you excited about?** Seeing an inquiry through to completion can be demanding, so focusing on a topic that energizes you to keep going is important.
- **What sites/locations and populations do you have access to?** Gaining access to the site and having an adequate number of subjects/participants are vital to any successful inquiry, so you should confirm these details before committing to a topic.
- **What problems or needs exist in the setting where the inquiry will take place?** It will be much easier to garner support from others in the inquiry process if they readily see the need for your work. Inquiries of value address existing problems, extend prior work on the topic, or explore new ideas.
- **What is your baseline knowledge of the topic you are considering?** Prior knowledge or experience with a topic and a desire to expand your skills and knowledge in this area are recommended. If you are starting with a topic completely new to you, you should consider collaborating with someone who has foundational knowledge on the topic already.

- **Will the results be of interest to others?** Exploring a topic that interests others in your profession or practice area is vital if you hope to disseminate your work via professional presentations or scholarly publications.
- **What supports do you need, and what supports are available as you engage in this inquiry?** Consider the presence (or absence) of time, space, money, personnel, and other resources in the process. If you are new to research or evidence-based practice, you may need to collaborate with others with more advanced knowledge of the process. Also, some topics may require more time, financial resources, or equipment for success.
- **What are your career goals?** Whether you are a student engaging in your first inquiry as part of your coursework or an experienced practitioner taking on this work as part of your professional development, considering your career goals will help you align this work with your career trajectory and further development of your professional identity.

Brainstorm by listing potential topics and then consider each topic in light of the prior questions. You will need to balance the need and purpose of the inquiry with your passion for the topic and the available resources to settle on a feasible and exciting topic. If you are in a formal education setting, your research advisor or mentor might also provide support at this point to ensure your general topic is appropriate.

### TIPS & INSPIRATION

- Explore several topics that you are passionate about before you begin the inquiry. Do not settle on a topic just because you can easily find a literature base to support it or because you perceive the topic to be easily addressed. The best topics are often the most challenging ones to pursue, but they hold the greatest potential for impact and will energize you to keep going.

### Refining Your Topic

To further refine your topic, you should consider **keywords** that explain it. Your keywords might describe the client or population of focus (for example, clients who experienced a stroke), a specific intervention you want to focus on (for example, constraint-induced movement therapy), possible outcomes you are interested in (for example, satisfaction with treatment or improved motor control), or specific problems you want to address (for example, shoulder subluxation or frequent payment denials). You can use these keywords to conduct a preliminary literature search to gauge the available literature on your topic and determine the best terminology for explaining your topic. Refinement of your topic may be warranted based on the findings from your preliminary literature search.

You might also try describing your topic in just one sentence and sharing that with others for feedback. Using some prior examples, your statement might be, "I am interested in exploring the most effective interventions for improving motor control of the affected upper extremity in clients with a recent stroke." A simpler example might be, "Recent payment denials for therapy services for clients with stroke have motivated me to explore ways to increase reimbursement." Once you have a general topic of focus, you will craft a specific question to guide your inquiry.

### TIPS & INSPIRATION

- Good places to start your preliminary literature search include your academic institution's library, a professional organization you have access to, or Google Scholar, which is a free search engine for scholarly literature.
- Use some preliminary literature searches to see what information you can find on your topic. Do not be overly concerned with your search process or techniques now. You will learn specific strategies for completing a comprehensive literature search in Chapter 3. Right now, focus on exploring your potential topic and the terminology that best explains it.

## Identifying Your Inquiry Question

A well-constructed research or evidence-based practice question will effectively guide your later comprehensive literature search. The question is commonly drafted using the PICO or PIO format to clearly identify the focus of an inquiry: "P" represents the population, "I" the intervention, "C" the comparison intervention (if applicable), and "O" the anticipated outcome. A comparison (C) is used if the intention is to compare two or more interventions or approaches in the inquiry; the simpler PIO format is employed when this is not necessary or desired.

In theory, formulating just one question seems like a relatively simple task; however, it might take a couple of weeks to narrow your focus and adequately define each element in your question. Sufficiently narrowing your population and intervention of focus will allow you to locate literature that specifically relates to your situation. Conversely, narrowing the topic too much could yield minimal results from your literature search. Conducting a preliminary search of the literature in your area of interest can help you solidify your question or show you where it might need refining. Sharing your ideas with your peers, mentors, supervisors, or instructors can help you determine whether the question is logical, sufficiently specific, and applicable to the current practice situation and aims. Your initial question may continue to evolve as you go through the initial stages of inquiry. Also, remember that at this point, you need not be concerned with what you will *actually* do in your inquiry—you will use your inquiry question to guide your literature search; the information you locate in that search, along with your own experiences, observations, theories, and aims, will help you establish your procedures later on.

Let us consider how a question might evolve. Perhaps you work with clients who recently had a stroke, and you want to improve their independence. This list illustrates how your thoughts might progress:

- An initial PIO question could be, "Does occupational therapy intervention (I) improve independence (O) in clients who had a recent stroke (P)?"
- This question includes all the necessary elements, but some are rather vague. For example, what does improved independence look like? What tasks do you want the clients to be more independent in? Similarly, occupational therapy is a rather broad category of intervention and could involve many strategies and education of the client.
- A preliminary literature search with vague terms would likely result in many articles not aligned with your intentions. You must then revise your terms and be more specific.
- You decide to revise your question based on your practice area (home health) and a focused performance area (self-care tasks). Your revised question is: "Does home health occupational therapy intervention (I) improve independence in self-care tasks (O) in clients with a recent stroke?"
- Another preliminary literature search might prompt you to refine your terms further. For example, you learn that the term "ADLs," or activities of daily living, is commonly used in literature to reference self-care tasks. You also find various studies in home care settings focused on environmental modifications to improve independence, which piques your interest.
- As such, you might further refine your question: "Does environmental modification and education (I) improve independence in ADLs (O) in clients with a recent stroke (P)?"

As an alternative example, imagine you are interested in developing a new program or a resource manual for healthcare professionals related to providing end-of-life care. To design this program or manual, you would need to explore the literature on effective end-of-life care interventions and resources. You might also explore the literature on best educational practices or resource construction for healthcare professionals. Your question might be, "What are the most effective interventions and resources (I) to increase the knowledge and confidence (O) of healthcare professionals working in end-of-life care (P)?" Your preliminary literature search may support refinement of the terminology to best represent the concepts you are interested in. For example, the terms "hospice" and "palliative care" are commonly found in the literature to represent end-of-life care. Incorporating these into your question might yield more useful information. Your final inquiry question will guide your literature search and help you locate the best evidence on the topic to create an evidence-based program or resource. Figure 2-1 includes examples of quality inquiry questions using the PICO or PIO format.

Does the use of touch screen technology (I) increase attention (O) in 6-year-olds with autism spectrum disorder (P)?

Does massage therapy (I) decrease pain and anxiety (O) in patients who underwent cardiac surgery (P)?

What are the most effective handwriting curriculums (I) to promote legibility (O) in first graders (P)?

Does formal interprofessional education (I) improve collaboration (O) among healthcare practitioners in a hospital setting (P)?

Does use of a discharge protocol (I) by nurses (P) decrease patients' rate of return (O)?

What is the average length of stay (O) of patients with a hip replacement (P) who started rehab the same day as surgery (I) versus those who started later (C)?

Is diathermy (I) more effective than ultrasound (C) to decrease upper extremity joint pain (O) in college athletes (P)?

Can implementing a multifactorial fall prevention program (I) increase knowledge and confidence in preventing falls (O) of skilled nursing staff (P)?

Does development and provision of a diabetic skin care manual (I) improve practitioners' (P) perceptions of quality care at their clinic (O)?

Figure 2-1 Examples of inquiry questions.

### TIPS & INSPIRATION

- Remember that the inquiry question you start with will most likely evolve based on your preliminary literature search. The concepts will be similar, but the question may look different. Write down several versions of the same question, contemplate them, and share them with others for feedback.
- A common misconception is that your inquiry question must define what you will actually do in your research study or evidence-based practice project. Since you have not completed a comprehensive literature search yet, this is not a reasonable expectation. Remember that the inquiry question will guide your comprehensive literature search. The literature you uncover relevant to your topic will guide the steps you will actually take. For some, this might be implementing and testing one or more clinical interventions. For others, this might involve developing a new program or protocol, designing and providing structured education, or creating an advocacy campaign.

After you have a solid inquiry question, you will begin "setting the stage" for your inquiry. This includes constructing a problem statement, establishing the need or rationale for the inquiry, sharing any pertinent background information, and outlining the purpose and significance of the inquiry. The following sections will explain each of these elements. It is important to mention that completing these steps often involves recording or writing out this information, which can take several forms. Suppose you are completing an inquiry as part of a formal educational process. In that case, you may be required to share this information in a proposal or within chapters of a thesis or capstone. If an inquiry is being undertaken as a practitioner, you may be required to complete a formal report for administration before the inquiry can proceed. In cases where the aim is to publish the outcomes of the inquiry, you might begin an initial draft of a manuscript aligned with the guidelines of the targeted journal. Further details and suggestions for writing up your inquiry are provided in Chapter 14.

## Constructing a Problem Statement

The heart of any inquiry is the problem statement, from which all other elements will flow. This is the reason for undertaking the inquiry; it is the problem or question that caught your attention in the first place or the issue you want to solve in your clinical practice. An inquiry is usually driven by identifying something wrong or needing attention or by noticing that old ideas or methods are no longer adequate. After a preliminary review of the literature on your topic, you should be ready to construct your problem statement.

The paragraph describing the problem should be brief and to the point. Use objective information, statistics, and credible references to illustrate the problem. It is not enough to share evidence of the problem solely from your experience or at your site; others may not be supportive of or interested in your work if the problem does not extend beyond your immediate practice setting. Start by writing two or three sentences about the problem and read them to a colleague or peer. If they miss the point, try again. Ask clarifying questions about what is missing or does not make sense to them; feedback from others can help solidify your idea. Boxes 2-1 and 2-2 present examples of well-refined problem statements and their guiding inquiry questions. Both examples include existing evidence and statistics from credible sources to illustrate the problem to be addressed. These problem statements are from published literature and the result of multiple revisions; do not be discouraged if it takes you several attempts to write a clear and compelling problem statement. As mentioned previously, your problem statement may be further refined after your comprehensive literature review.

### BOX 2-1 ■ Example 1 Problem Statement

Newbury and Lape (2021), both occupational therapists, identified challenges in their practice related to helping older adults successfully age in place. This prompted the development of their inquiry question: **Does education on aging in place with the Kawa model (I) improve well-being (O) in community-dwelling older adults (P)?**

The authors cite prior literature from credible sources indicating that older adults want to age in place, but that their knowledge, skills, and readiness to do so varies, to illustrate the problem addressed in their study:

> *Although the overwhelming majority of U.S. older adults prefer and expect to age in place (Khalfani-Cox, 2017), recent studies have shown variation in their knowledge and perception of available resources and their preparation for aging in place (Johansson et al., 2009; Peek et al., 2016; Tang & Pickard, 2008). Older adults have shown varied levels of readiness to use compensatory strategies, such as environmental and behavioral modifications, to improve their chances of successfully aging in place (Rose et al., 2010). (Newbury & Lape, 2021, p. 16)*

## Drafting the Rationale for Your Inquiry

Once you are satisfied with your problem statement, you are ready to delve into the rationale or need for the inquiry. As noted previously, the rationale is drafted in conjunction with the preliminary literature search but is often refined after the later comprehensive literature search. The rationale should build on your problem statement and include the following:

- Further evidence of why the inquiry is necessary
- **Background** information to situate the proposed inquiry within the setting and existing evidence
- The **significance** or importance of the inquiry
- The **purpose** of the inquiry

Justifying your ideas will be necessary for getting buy-in from other stakeholders, including clients, team members, and administration; gaining approval to conduct your inquiry (if required); and eventually disseminating your work. Your rationale should be supported with references from multiple credible sources. A needs assessment, which is discussed later, might also be completed in this phase. The elements of a quality rationale are consistent, but the sequencing of information and length may vary based on journal or institutional guidelines or at the author's discretion. Whatever order you choose to present your ideas, ensure that your rationale proceeds logically and the reader can easily connect one idea to the next. Use strong topic sentences to identify the main ideas of each paragraph in your rationale and strong transitions to connect your ideas. The rationale for your inquiry should leave others agreeing unequivocally that the problem is worthy of investigation.

**BOX 2-2 ■ Example 2 Problem Statement**

Raj et al. (2022) were interested in exploring the development and feasibility of an evidence-based occupational therapy program. A potential PIO question for their inquiry might be: **What is the feasibility (O) of a home-based occupational therapy program (I) for clients with Down syndrome and dementia (P)?**

They used prior literature and statistics from credible sources to describe the problem of focus in their study:

> *Early-onset dementia is a major health problem for adults with Down syndrome (DS) causing progressive loss of skills (disability) (Fonseca et al., 2020), and increasing care dependency on their significant others (Coppus et al., 2006; Janicki et al., 2010). Coppus et al. (2006) reported that dementia among people with DS is observed after 40 years of age with prevalence increasing with age (40–49 years = 8.9%; 50–54 years = 17.7%; 55–59 years = 32.1%). In addition, these individuals experience premature ageing-associated health issues such as visual and auditory impairments (Coppus et al., 2006) and musculoskeletal problems (Carr & Collins, 2014) affecting their participation and performance in daily occupations, and escalating caregiving demands on their informal caregivers (Janicki et al., 2010). (Raj et al., 2022, p. 397)*

If readers are not captivated by this section, they may not read further.

Use the following steps to craft a quality rationale for your inquiry:

1. Build on your prior problem statement to fully explain the problem of focus. Include pertinent statistics and objective evidence of the problem.
2. Share relevant **background** information and define key concepts that are not common knowledge.
3. Clearly and concisely summarize relevant literature on the topic.
4. Identify gaps or shortcomings in prior literature or work. When conducting a research study, you should fully explain the gaps or shortcomings in the existing literature you plan to address. If implementing an evidence-based practice project, you should focus on the gaps within the current practice setting. For example, you might describe an unmet need or the misalignment of current practice with existing literature.
5. Explain why exploring the aforementioned gaps or shortcomings is important (**significance**).
6. Clearly state the **purpose** or aim of the inquiry.

Box 2-3 provides an example of a quality rationale, including the background, significance, and purpose components. Each of these important components is discussed individually to help you understand.

## Background

The background helps to establish the context of your inquiry. Within the background, you should fully define or explain any key terms, theories, or ideas that might be unfamiliar to your readers. For example, if you plan to explore falls self-efficacy within your inquiry, you should define this term. If you are approaching your inquiry through a particular viewpoint or theoretical perspective, this information should also be shared. Finally, it might be necessary to share historical information to place the current problem in context—for example, if your inquiry aims to build on prior work.

## Significance

The significance elaborates on why your inquiry is important, what makes it worth pursuing, and the potential impact and relevance of the outcomes to the profession or field of study. This information should answer the question, "So what?" The significance is typically stated in just one or two sentences as part of your rationale and revisited at the conclusion of your inquiry. To be explicit, you can use one of the following phrases to draft your significance statement. Using other terminology embedded within the rationale is also acceptable.

- "The findings of this study may ..."
- "This inquiry may contribute to ..."
- "This work is important because ..."

See Boxes 2-4 and 2-5 for examples of significance statements.

### BOX 2-3 ■ Example of a Quality Rationale

Hamilton et al. (2023) wanted to explore the use of adaptive climbing to improve social skills in children with developmental delays. They began their rationale with statistics on how many children are diagnosed with developmental delay each year and defined developmental delay:

> *In the United States, one in six children is diagnosed with a developmental delay each year.*[1] *The Centers for Disease Control states that "developmental disabilities are a group of conditions due to an impairment in physical, learning, language, or behavior areas. These conditions begin during the developmental period, may impact day-to-day functioning, and usually last throughout a person's lifetime."*[1] *(p. 1).*

Next, they described why development of social skills is important and the impact of limited social skills:

> *Acquiring social skills is a necessary component of a child's growth and development.*[2] *... "Between 9.5 and 14.2 percent of children ages birth to five years old experience social-emotional problems which negatively impact their daily functioning, development, and readiness for school."*[4] *(p. 1).*

Next, they discussed low sports participation rates for children with developmental delays and the benefits of sports participation related to social skills development:

> *Sports participation rates are lower for children with developmental delays when compared to typically developing children.*[5] *... Sports participation in a structured environment can provide opportunities to all children for increasing social skills, and building peer relationships.*[9,10] *(p. 1).*

Finally, after summarizing existing literature on adaptive sports programming, they described the gaps in prior research that they plan to address and end with the purpose:

> *No studies to date have specifically explored the use of adaptive climbing to promote social skill development, and improvements in self-efficacy have not been associated with improvements in social skills in these prior studies. Climbing may offer opportunities for children to engage in social situations and practice social skills including following directions related to safety and use of equipment, waiting turns to climb, asking appropriate questions related to safety and asking for help, and initiating and maintaining conversations during the experience. Therefore, the purpose of this study was to investigate if participation in an adaptive climbing program could positively impact the social skills of children with developmental delays, as well as to assess the feasibility of such a program. (p. 1).*

### BOX 2-4 ■ Example 1 Significance Statement

Elliott et al. (2023) provide two statements of significance within the *Introduction* of their article on burnout and adverse outcomes in athletic training students:

*"Continued use of this model to explore relationships between academic workload, burnout, and adverse outcomes and other samples of healthcare students could further solidify the predicted relationships between these variables" (p. 1).*

*"Further testing of this model and its proposed relationships would help educators further understand if academic workload is an antecedent of burnout and if the presence of burnout predicts adverse outcomes in other healthcare students" (p. 2).*

### BOX 2-5 ■ Example 2 Significance Statement

Wozniak et al. (2023) provide this significance statement for their study on the experiences and routines of caregivers of children with Type 1 diabetes:

> *"Occupational therapists may use this information to provide family-centered care to improve the caregiver's performance and competence in providing their child's T1D health management routines" (p. 2).*

## Purpose

The rationale should include a clear statement of the inquiry's purpose. In published literature, you might also see the purpose identified as the aim or objective.

**TABLE 2-1 ■ Purpose Statements for Research Studies and Evidence-Based Practice Projects**

| Research Studies | Evidence-Based Practice Projects |
|---|---|
| The purpose of this study is to determine if massage or pressure garments are more effective in reducing swelling in the affected upper extremity after a stroke. | The purpose of this evidence-based practice project is to develop and implement a handwriting curriculum based on current evidence for kindergarten and first-grade students to promote improved handwriting legibility. |
| The aim of this study is to describe the factors that impact satisfaction with inpatient rehabilitation services after joint replacement surgery. | The purpose of this evidence-based practice project is to apply existing evidence regarding effective maternal wellness interventions to the creation of online programming for new mothers after labor and delivery to improve their well-being. |
| The objective of this study is to evaluate the relationship between sleep duration and quality on students' academic achievement. | The purpose of this evidence-based practice project is to apply existing evidence on effective adult learning educational practices to revise an existing course for improved student outcomes. |
| This study aimed to evaluate the effects of isometric resistance training on muscle strength, range of motion, and pain in adults with musculoskeletal injuries. | The aim of this evidence-based practice project is to revise existing employee policies and procedures based on current evidence of the factors impacting employee satisfaction to improve employee retention. |

The purpose should clearly and concisely identify what you hope to accomplish by conducting your inquiry. Start your purpose with this phrase: "The purpose of this inquiry (research study or evidence-based practice project) is to ..." Also, recall from Chapter 1 that the purpose of a research study and an evidence-based practice project differs. The purpose of a research study is to generate *new* knowledge that can be generalized, while the purpose of an evidence-based practice project is to apply *existing* evidence to clinical practice. Table 2-1 lists examples of purpose statements for both research studies and evidence-based practice projects to illustrate the difference.

## TIPS & INSPIRATION

- As you develop your rationale for your inquiry, imagine this section as your marketing pitch. What would you say if you had only 2 or 3 minutes to convince someone that your inquiry was needed and important? Delivering this information verbally to someone else will help you identify whether the crux of your argument is effective or where you might need to place greater focus.
- Find at least five topic-related abstracts before you begin writing your rationale. The abstracts typically list the problem, background, purpose, and significance of the inquiry and can be invaluable in helping you hone your own work. Reviewing abstracts from other studies is a quick way to grasp what was done in those studies; this can help guide the initial steps of your inquiry without the burden of reading entire manuscripts.

## Needs Assessment

A **needs assessment** is a systematic process for identifying existing supports, challenges, and opportunities for improvement within an organization, setting, or group to guide future decision-making, programming, and resource allocation. You may be required to conduct a needs assessment as part of your initial proposal for your research study or evidence-based practice project. In clinical settings, practitioners often conduct needs assessments before program development; this process is discussed in greater detail in Chapter 13.

A needs assessment can take various forms but commonly involves these components:

- **Scope of the assessment:** Outline the focus of the assessment. Multiple challenges or issues may exist within a site or organization, but choosing just one specific issue will improve the ability to identify feasible future actions. Imagine that you have chosen to focus your assessment on the issue of increased client falls within the facility where you work.
- **Analysis of existing data:** Study existing information, reports, or other data from the site that is relevant to the scope of the assessment. Using the prior example, this might include examining fall incident reports, current fall prevention policies, staffing levels and training logs, medical records of clients who have fallen, and the physical environment where falls commonly occurred.
- **Stakeholder involvement:** Collect additional data from relevant stakeholders through interviews, focus groups, observations, or surveys. In the current example, this might include conducting a focus group with staff who were working when the falls occurred, surveying clients who have fallen, and interviewing facility administration who can provide insight regarding training practices, regulatory standards, and available resources.
- **Identification of needs and assets:** Analyze data gathered from existing sources and stakeholders to identify gaps or opportunities for improvement as well as existing supports and assets that might be leveraged to address the needs. For example, data may indicate the need for policy revision and a consistent, evidence-based staff training program to prevent falls. Identified supports could include adequate staffing levels, financial resources, and administration's commitment to change.
- **Recommendations for future action:** Prioritize action steps and make recommendations to address the identified needs. Sequential recommendations in the current example might include conducting a focused literature review to identify best practices in fall prevention, revision of the fall risk screening policy, creation of a new evidence-based fall prevention staff training program, structured education of all staff on the new program, and later analysis of fall incident reports to evaluate the success of the new programming.

### SWOT Analysis

Another specific needs assessment format you might encounter is a SWOT analysis. A **SWOT analysis**, which stands for strengths, weaknesses, opportunities, and threats, is a strategic planning tool to evaluate these factors within an organization, setting, or group to develop strategies for viability and improvement. Strengths and weaknesses are considered to be internal aspects of the organization or setting. Reflecting on the financial, physical, and social supports available as well as the potential roadblocks (weaknesses) in the inquiry setting can help you identify whether or how supports could be leveraged to circumvent the weaknesses. Envisioning potential problems and devising a backup plan can greatly increase the success of your inquiry. Finally, the opportunities and threats are considered to be aspects external to the organization or setting. For example, information about the current healthcare climate, the state of reimbursement for services, and existing or proposed legislation in healthcare could present as opportunities or threats, depending on the time and situation.

Even if you are not required to complete a formal needs assessment, it can be beneficial to consider available supports and potential roadblocks you may encounter while conducting your inquiry. Reflecting on the available supports and potential roadblocks at this early stage can help you proactively adjust your plan for success. Sharing your list of supports and barriers with others for feedback can also be helpful to ensure you have not missed something important. Additional information on how to plan and conduct a needs assessment is included in Chapter 13.

## TIPS & INSPIRATION

- If you will be conducting an inquiry, identify three or four people to support you in the process. Consider someone who has experience in conducting a research study or evidence-based practice project, someone familiar with the writing style you will be using (for example, APA–American Psychological Association, AMA–American Medical Association, or MLA–Modern Language Association), someone who knows your topic or discipline, and someone who can provide emotional support, encouragement, and a much-needed break now and then. Having someone who will take you out to dinner, bring you a chocolate cupcake, or sign you up for a massage can make all the difference!

## CHAPTER SUMMARY

1. Examine the time required to complete an inquiry.
   - The length of time for an inquiry can vary from 6 months to several years, and the duration of inquiry phases can fluctuate depending on the procedures and aims.
   - Planning to "touch" your work every day or several times a week will increase your chances of success in this journey.
2. Differentiate preliminary and comprehensive literature searches.
   - A preliminary literature search, which occurs before a comprehensive literature search, is an initial exploration of the literature on a topic to gain a broad understanding of the relevant research and trends, which can help you refine your ideas at an early stage.
   - A comprehensive literature search is an exhaustive search of the literature using well-defined search terms, search strategies, and search tracking to fully determine the breadth of information specific to your topic. A comprehensive literature search is used to write your formal literature review and make decisions about your inquiry procedures.
   - All literature searches should rely on credible sources, including documents from professional, government, and other reputable organization websites; professional journals; and academic texts. Blog posts, personal opinion pieces, and social media posts and videos warrant further scrutiny before relying on them.
3. Identify a topic for your research study or evidence-based practice project.
   - To identify a topic, consider what excites you, the sites or populations you have access to, the existing needs or problems, your baseline knowledge and career goals, the supports available to you, and the topics that might interest others.
   - Try to describe your topic in one sentence using keywords to describe the population, intervention, outcomes, or problems of focus.
4. State the elements of a quality research or evidence-based practice question.
   - The elements of a PICO question are population (P), intervention (I), comparison intervention (C), and outcomes (O).
   - PIO represents a simpler format in which a comparison is not necessary or desirable.
5. Develop a quality PIO or PICO question to guide your inquiry.
   - Write a draft of your PIO or PICO question and share it with others for feedback.
   - Conducting a preliminary literature search on your topic can help you refine and solidify your question.
   - Remember that the inquiry question will guide your comprehensive literature search and does not necessarily convey what you will actually do.
6. Construct a problem statement for your inquiry.
   - A problem statement should include objective information and statistics from credible sources to illustrate the problem you hope to address in your inquiry.
7. Draft a quality rationale for an inquiry, including the need, background, purpose, and significance.
   - A quality rationale should:
     - Build on your problem statement.
     - Include relevant background information and define key concepts that are not common knowledge.
     - Summarize relevant literature on the topic.
     - Identify gaps or shortcomings in prior literature or work.
     - Explain the significance and purpose of the inquiry.

*Continued*

8. Explain the components of a needs assessment and how this information is useful in planning an inquiry.
   - A needs assessment is a systematic process for identifying supports, challenges, and opportunities for improvement within an organization, setting, or group to guide future decision-making, programming, or resource allocation.
   - A needs assessment involves these components: scope of the assessment, analysis of existing data, stakeholder involvement, identification of needs and assets, and recommendations for future action.
   - A SWOT (strengths, weaknesses, opportunities, and threats) analysis is a type of needs assessment used for strategic planning.
   - Even if a formal needs assessment is not completed, it is beneficial to consider supports and potential roadblocks as you plan your inquiry.

## TEST YOUR KNOWLEDGE

1. What is the recommended frequency for working on an inquiry to promote success?
   a. Once a week
   b. Several times a week
   c. On the weekends only
   d. Every other week
2. A preliminary literature review should rely on credible sources. Which of the following is MOST LIKELY to be considered a credible source?
   a. A YouTube video of a therapist explaining exercises for hip pain
   b. A blog post on medication adherence written by a nurse practitioner
   c. A Wikipedia page on historical development and application of mindfulness
   d. An article on adaptive sports published in a professional journal
3. Which of the following BEST describes the considerations when identifying your inquiry topic?
   a. Your passion for the topic to keep you motivated
   b. Where you could publish the work and if you have a good mentor
   c. Your passion for the topic, baseline knowledge of the topic, and access to the population of interest
   d. Access to the population of interest and limited research on the topic
4. In the PICO question format, what does "P" represent?
   a. Patients
   b. Participants
   c. Persons of focus
   d. Population
5. Which of the following BEST describes the purpose of a PICO question?
   a. To identify your topic and guide your literature search
   b. To concisely explain what you will do in your inquiry
   c. To summarize key findings of relevant studies
   d. To evaluate the quality of studies related to your topic
6. What should be included in a quality problem statement?
   a. The planned methodology to address the problem
   b. A comprehensive literature review relevant to the problem
   c. Credible objective information and statistics to describe the problem
   d. Potential interventions or other solutions to the problem
7. Which of the following is TRUE about the rationale for an inquiry?
   a. It builds on the hypothesis statement.
   b. It should not exceed two to four sentences in length.
   c. It should identify gaps or shortcomings in prior inquiries or work.
   d. It should include a full literature review.
8. Which of the following BEST describes the purpose of a needs assessment?
   a. To identify supports, challenges, and opportunities in a setting to guide decision-making
   b. To determine the quality of prior research on a topic to justify an inquiry
   c. To assess stakeholder involvement and willingness to change within an organization
   d. To determine if you need specific skills to successfully complete an inquiry

Answer key appears at the end of this text.

## NEXT STEPS

1. List no more than five ideas you have for an inquiry. Rank these ideas based on your interest or passion for each topic. Next, rank these ideas based on feasibility (available supports, baseline knowledge, need). Do the rankings align or vary? Select the two BEST options based on your rankings, and then offer your 2- to 3-minute marketing pitch on both topics to someone else for feedback before you make your decision.
2. Draft your inquiry question using the PIO or PICO format. Practice writing several versions of the question to broaden or narrow the scope of your inquiry.
3. Write at least three reasons why your inquiry is important/significant to you, your site, your profession, and society. Consider the following in drafting your significance statement:
   - How does this inquiry align with your interests and career goals?
   - Who will benefit from the findings?
   - What might happen if the inquiry is not completed?
4. Find three pieces of evidence of the problem you hope to address in your inquiry. Be sure you use objective information and statistics from credible sources. Use this information to construct a quality problem statement.
5. Compose a rationale for your inquiry, including the background, purpose, and significance.

## REFERENCES


Elliott, A. P., Gallucci, A., Oglesby, L., Funderburk, L., Lanning, B. A., & Tomek, S. (2023). Burnout and adverse reactions in athletic training students: Why all healthcare educators should be concerned. *The Internet Journal of Allied Health Sciences and Practice, 21*(1), Article 16. https://doi.org/10.46743/1540-580X/2023.2264

Hamilton, J., Lape, J. E., & Lee, A. L. (2023). Use of an adaptive climbing program to improve social skills in children with developmental delays: A feasibility study. *The Internet Journal of Allied Health Sciences and Practice, 21*(1), Article 6. https://doi.org/10.46743/1540-580X/2023.2253

Newbury, R. S., & Lape, J. E. (2021). Well-being, aging in place, and use of the Kawa Model: A pilot study. *Annals of Occupational Therapy, 4*(1), 15–25. https://doi.org/10.3928/24761222-20200413-02

Raj, S. E., Mackintosh, S., Kernot, J., Fryer, C., & Stanley, M. (2022). Development and feasibility testing of an evidence-based occupational therapy program for adults with both Down syndrome and dementia. *Journal of Policy and Practice in Intellectual Disabilities, 19,* 396–407. https://doi.org/10.1111/jppi.12435

Wozniak, E., Cover, L., Qi, Y., & Jewell, V. D. (2023). Mixed-method study of the experiences and routines of caregivers of children with Type 1 diabetes. *The Open Journal of Occupational Therapy, 11*(1), 1–14. https://doi.org/10.15453/2168-6408.1956

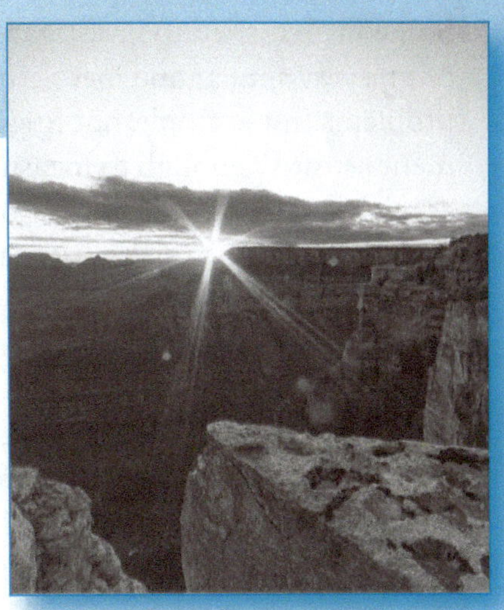

Chapter 3

# Completing a Comprehensive Literature Search

LEARNING OUTCOMES

*The information provided in this chapter will assist you to:*

3.1 Recall reasons for conducting a comprehensive and exhaustive literature search.

3.2 Recognize where to search for literature and how to assess the credibility of sources.

3.3 Identify appropriate search terms, criteria, and strategies for a literature search.

3.4 Explain the benefits and method of tracking a literature search.

3.5 Organize and synthesize research on a topic of focus.

3.6 Construct an outline of a literature review on a focused topic.

## Why You Need to Review the Literature

Now that you have explored some inquiry questions and settled on the one you want to pursue, the next step is conducting a comprehensive literature search to fully determine the breadth of information on your topic and the extent to which your question has been addressed in prior studies. This comprehensive literature search will be used to write your literature review and make decisions about your inquiry procedures. The body of literature you gather related to your topic can be referred to collectively as your **literature portfolio**. The amount of literature in your portfolio will vary based on the topic and aim of your inquiry and the volume of relevant literature. If you aim to conduct a research study, you need to know what research has already been done on your topic so that you can design your study procedures to address something new or in a different way. If you plan to complete an evidence-based practice project, you need to explore the best available evidence on your topic. You will use this evidence along with your skills, knowledge, and experiences and the aims and circumstances of your clients or inquiry site to make practice decisions. At this point, you have likely already conducted a preliminary literature search. So, you may be asking yourself why additional searching of the literature is necessary before planning and beginning an inquiry. There are several reasons:

- If you are planning a research study, someone may have already researched your question and published the answer. You would not want to waste your time and that of your subjects by repeating what has already been reasonably well researched. In this case, the published literature may provide recommendations for future inquiries to build on what has already been discovered; shifting your focus slightly would allow you to pursue a connected yet meaningful topic.

South Rim, Grand Canyon National Park, Arizona.

- Someone has tried to investigate your question or one very similar and met with insurmountable problems (for example, not finding a test instrument sensitive enough to measure one of the crucial variables or inability to recruit sufficient participants due to strict criteria or cumbersome procedures). You should proactively design your procedures to avoid difficulties experienced by others.
- Someone has investigated your question or a similar one, but in a slightly different way than you intend to. For example, you may plan to use slightly different methods or another population as subjects. Prior research methods, strategies, or features could be applied to your inquiry.
- Someone may have already studied one component of your topic, and you can build on that research, thus saving yourself time and energy.
- If prior research has been done on your topic, it will be essential to place your inquiry within that context so readers can fully grasp the scope and importance of your work. You likely explored this idea to some extent in drafting your initial rationale for the inquiry.
- You must identify the theoretical base that is relevant to and will guide your inquiry. The **theoretical base** can include existing concepts and theories that provide insight into your problem (for example, biomechanical, cognitive behavioral, or adult learning theory). Understanding the theoretical base of prior research is important as you consider those results and what they mean for your proposed inquiry.
- If you plan to complete an evidence-based practice project, finding literature to support effective solutions to the problem you aim to solve is vital. You will use this literature to outline your project steps.

## Where to Search for Literature

You will likely find literature in scholarly journals, books, magazines or newsletters, and government, organizational, or professional websites relevant to your topic. Literature within scholarly journals and textbooks is **peer-reviewed**, meaning this content was evaluated for quality by topic experts before publication. Magazines or newsletters are usually non-peer-reviewed and written in layperson's terms for greater understanding by practitioners and the public. Websites associated with discipline-specific organizations (for example, the American Physical Therapy Association [APTA]), cause-specific organizations (for example, the Alzheimer's Association), or government organizations (for example, Centers for Disease Control and Prevention [CDC]) can also be good sources for research, current statistics, and reports. The final place you might locate valuable information is within grey literature. **Grey literature** is most simply defined as unpublished literature—meaning literature that is neither peer-reviewed nor commercially published. Some common examples are unpublished dissertations or theses, conference proceedings, legal documents, and policy statements (Bonato, 2022). Grey literature can be located via some databases that archive dissertations or conference proceedings and through government or organizational websites where reports, policy statements, and other documents are shared.

Today, literature is primarily accessed via electronic databases. A **database** is a searchable, electronic collection of information, including citations, abstracts, and, in many cases, full-text articles. These databases can be discipline-specific (containing only literature from a specific field) or interdisciplinary. Search options within each database allow you to search by keywords, author, title, journal, and publication dates.

So, where do you find and access these databases? Some databases are publicly accessible and offer free access, while others are subscription-based. Some might offer free searching but require a subscription to access full-text articles. Professional organizations, like the American Occupational Therapy Association (AOTA), offer subscription-based access to published literature and resources for its members. Academic institutions and clinical teaching facilities usually have subscriptions to a wide variety of databases that you can search simultaneously through their library site. Students, faculty, employees, and sometimes alumni of these institutions enjoy access to

**TABLE 3-1 ■ Common Allied Health Databases**

| Database | Focus |
|---|---|
| ClinicalTrials.gov | *Free* registry of funded clinical trials, including those in progress. Some trials may have results available. |
| Cochrane Library | *Free* collection of databases of rigorous research in healthcare. One component of this collection is Cochrane Reviews, a systematic review database. |
| CINAHL (Cumulative Index of Nursing and Allied Health Literature) | *Subscription-based* database that indexes more than 3,000 top nursing and allied health journals. |
| ERIC (Education Resources Information Center) | *Free* database of education-related research. This database is useful for health-care practitioners and students involved in academics, policymaking, research, and education-based inquiries. |
| Google Scholar | *Free*, web-based search tool for scholarly literature and resources. Limited search features and more frequently cited works are more likely to appear in search results. |
| MEDLINE | *Free* database of the National Library of Medicine (NLM) that indexes more than 29 million life science and biomedical works. MEDLINE is commonly accessed through PubMed, a free comprehensive search engine for biomedical and life sciences research retrieval. |
| OT Search | *Subscription-based* database of occupational therapy literature and related topics. |
| OTSeeker | *Free* database of abstracts of systematic reviews, randomized controlled trials, and other occupational therapy resources. Some trials have been critically appraised to increase the ease of research translation. |
| PEDro | *Free* database of over 57,000 clinical trials, practice guidelines, and reviews related to physiotherapy. |
| ProQuest | *Subscription-based* collection of multidisciplinary databases, with several focused on the health sciences and one exclusively for dissertations and theses. |
| PsycINFO | *Subscription-based* database of the American Psychological Association with more than 5 million indexed works within the behavioral and social sciences. |
| SPORTDiscus | *Subscription-based* database for physical activity, fitness, and sports medicine research. |

these resources as part of their affiliation. Table 3-1 identifies some of the most common databases accessed by allied health professionals. Choosing the databases most applicable to your topic is the first step in completing a good literature search.

### Credibility of Sources

All sources should be carefully evaluated for credibility before using them. **Credible sources** typically include documents from professional, government, and other reputable organization websites, professional journals, and academic texts. With so much online information, you may be tempted to use blog posts, personal opinion pieces, social media posts and videos, or information from other online sites. However, these warrant further scrutiny before relying on them. Box 3-1 lists questions to help you assess the credibility of online sources.

## Identifying Your Search Terms, Criteria, and Strategies

After identifying the databases and websites most relevant to your topic, you must consider the search terms, criteria, and strategies that you will use to extract pertinent literature from the databases or websites. Each element is discussed separately to help you understand how to maximize your search efforts.

**BOX 3-1 ■ Questions to Assess the Credibility of Online Sources**

- **Who produces the site?** Sites with domain names ending in "gov" (government), "edu" (educational), or "org" (organizational) are usually credible sources. Those that end in "com" (commercial) might be sound but will require further scrutiny.
- **Who authored the work?** Works by appropriately credentialed authors is another sign of trustworthiness. An author with a degree related to the field of study or other published work on the topic is preferred. You may need to do additional searching to confirm this.
- **When was the work created?** Reviewing the date of the report, post, video, or copyright at the bottom of the website lets you know how old the information is and how frequently it might be updated. Sites with limited recent activity may be outdated and should be avoided.
- **What content is included?** Quality content typically links to or references other credible sources, such as peer-reviewed articles. Sources that rely on opinions or unsupported information should be avoided.

## Search Terms

After determining the databases most relevant to your topic, you should identify your search terms. The **search terms** are the keywords representing your topic that you enter into the databases to retrieve relevant articles. The search terms are initially derived from your well-constructed inquiry question. Consider the terminology you selected to identify your population, intervention, outcome, and comparison (if applicable). Were other terms used to represent these components in your preliminary literature searches? Can you think of other terms that might be used, or does a thesaurus reveal other plausible terms? See Table 3-2 for an example inquiry question and potential search terms. This list is not exhaustive but is intended to illustrate that there are usually many possibilities.

### *MeSH Terms*

**MeSH terms**, or Medical Subject Headings, are standardized words or phrases used to index articles by topic; similar words are grouped under the same MeSH term to create a hierarchy of terms ranging from very broad terms on a topic to more specific ones. An example of MeSH terms for mental health is illustrated in Figure 3-1; a definition, synonymous terms, and a hierarchical outline of related terms are provided. When an article is published, qualified indexers hand-assign the appropriate MeSH terms to allow others interested in the topic to locate it easily. The MeSH classification system originated with MEDLINE, the National Library of Medicine database, but is now used in many other databases. Using the search terms you generated from your question and the relevant medical subject headings can improve the quality of your search.

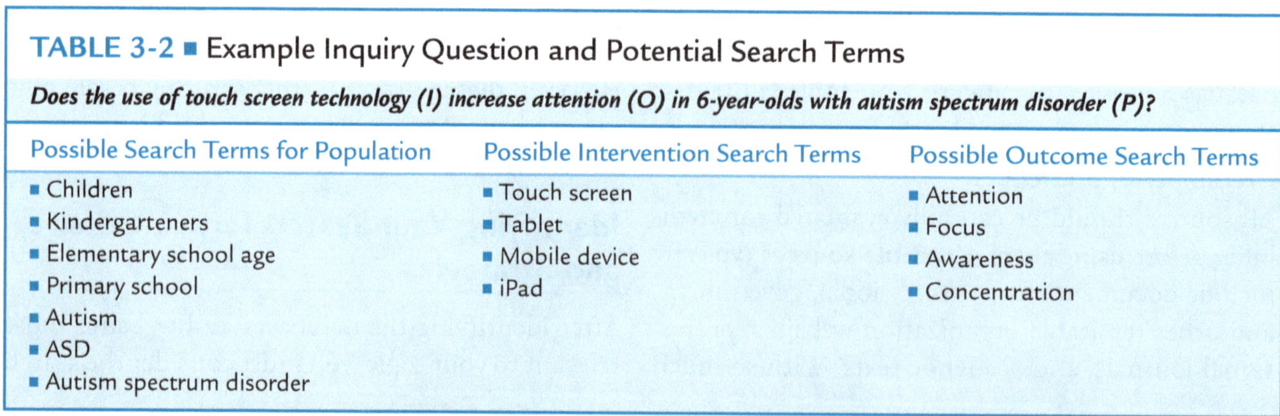

**TABLE 3-2 ■ Example Inquiry Question and Potential Search Terms**

***Does the use of touch screen technology (I) increase attention (O) in 6-year-olds with autism spectrum disorder (P)?***

| Possible Search Terms for Population | Possible Intervention Search Terms | Possible Outcome Search Terms |
|---|---|---|
| ■ Children | ■ Touch screen | ■ Attention |
| ■ Kindergarteners | ■ Tablet | ■ Focus |
| ■ Elementary school age | ■ Mobile device | ■ Awareness |
| ■ Primary school | ■ iPad | ■ Concentration |
| ■ Autism | | |
| ■ ASD | | |
| ■ Autism spectrum disorder | | |

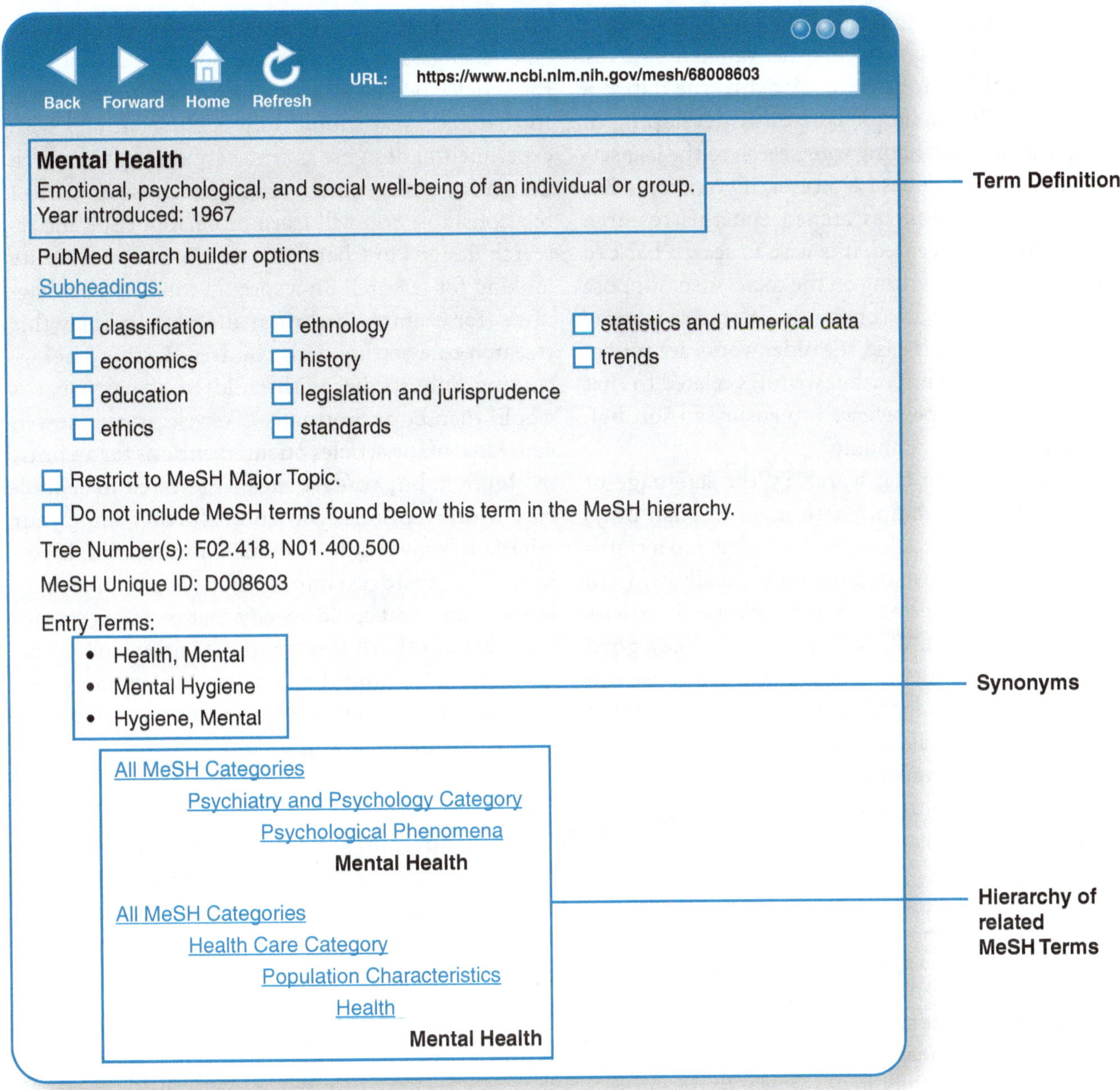


Figure 3-1 Example of MeSH terms; this example is from the National Library of Medicine searched on February 2, 2023.

## Search Criteria

After finalizing your search terms, you should determine your search criteria. The **search criteria** are the other parameters defining the research characteristics you are looking for. In addition to the keywords you select, most databases allow you to search for literature based on several other criteria, including the author's name, title, journal, publication dates, the language of publication, and availability in full text. You might initially conduct your search without any of these parameters and later use one or more parameters to narrow the field. Once your search terms and criteria are entered, the database will scan for literature aligning with the specified conditions.

Limiting by the author's name, title, or journal might be more useful if, for example, you are aware of respected authors in your topic, you are directed to a specific article from another source, or you have found a particular journal to be highly related to your topic and likely to yield other valuable sources. Several considerations exist related to the dates of publication. If your topic is recently developing or changing, then restricting your search to the last several years might be best. However, if your topic has been previously well researched and this research remains widely accepted, it is wise to search back to the most plentiful writing on the topic. Also, suppose several older works are constantly referred to in more recent works. In this case, the older works are probably the classic and important writings related to that topic and should be reviewed to ensure a thorough foundational understanding.

Next, narrowing the search by the language of publication (for example, articles in English only) might be necessary unless you have access to a translator or quality translation software. Finally, you will have to weigh the option of searching for only articles available in full text. While this may seem like a good idea initially, consider that doing so might cause you to miss worthwhile information about your topic. If an article is unavailable in the databases you have access to, it may be available through interlibrary loan or via a peer or colleague who has access to different databases or libraries than you.

### TIPS & INSPIRATION

- As you find articles applicable to your topic, review them more closely. What are the keywords? Who are the authors? What journals or databases did they yield from? This analysis should help you further narrow the terms and criteria that will produce other valuable sources.

## Search Strategies

Using the most appropriate keywords, medical subject headings, and other search features discussed so far will likely leave you with too many articles to reasonably review. At this point, you should consider other criteria that will help you to narrow the pool of articles to those most appropriate for your literature portfolio. Your potential inclusion criteria might focus on the methodology of the research, specific participant characteristics, comparison of various interventions, or studies taking place in specific settings. For example, suppose you are looking for articles on the effectiveness of an intervention. In that case, you should only include studies with experimental designs, as these are the only research designs rigorous enough to suggest cause-and-effect relationships. You will learn more about specific research designs in Chapters 4 and 7. Perhaps you are looking for research on a specific condition or diagnosis (for example, arthritis) and plan to apply this research to a setting with children. In this case, including only studies with children as participants would then be appropriate. Likewise, if your search generated many articles on interventions for arthritis in children, but you are most interested in school-based interventions, you could further limit your criteria to only studies conducted in schools. If you want to compare two interventions or combine them in some way, you could specify that included studies must contain both interventions within the procedures. Keep in mind that you can incorporate some of these inclusion criteria into your search terms to further narrow the results.

### *Boolean Operators*

**Boolean operators** are words that allow you to broaden or narrow a literature search within most databases. The three basic Boolean operators are AND, OR, and NOT. Your search terms can be combined using the connector AND so that you receive only those articles that include both terms. You could connect several words with AND, but you will likely get very few responses when being this specific since the resulting articles would need to include *all* the words in your search. Using the connector OR will broaden your search since the result will be articles that include *any* of the search terms. The OR connector is most effective when searching synonymous terms (for example, stroke and cerebrovascular accident). If your search terms yield articles that match your purpose as well as articles that are related but undesired, the NOT connector will be most effective. Also, using more than one Boolean operator within a single search is sometimes valuable. The purpose of each Boolean operator is further outlined with examples in Table 3-3.

**TABLE 3-3 ■ Boolean Operators and Their Purpose**

| Boolean Operator | Purpose | Examples |
|---|---|---|
| AND | To combine two or more keywords. This operator *narrows* the search by only including articles with all connected words. | arthritis AND joint protection<br>arthritis AND joint protection AND occupational therapy |
| OR | To combine two or more keywords. This operator *broadens* the search by including articles with any of the connected words. | arthritis OR rheumatism<br>arthritis OR rheumatism OR occupational therapy |
| NOT | To exclude one or more keywords. This operator *narrows* the focus by excluding articles with the stated keyword. | arthritis NOT joint protection<br>arthritis AND joint protection NOT energy conservation |

**TABLE 3-4 ■ Additional Search Strategies**

| Search Technique | Purpose | Example |
|---|---|---|
| Truncation | Uses a special symbol (often an asterisk[*]) to search for all words with the same root. *Check the individual database to verify the symbol used.* | Child* (would retrieve articles with child, children, childhood, childcare, childbirth, etc.) |
| Wildcards | Uses a special symbol (often a question mark [?] or hashtag [#]) to search words with different spellings or versions. The symbol is inserted where the spelling may differ. *Check the individual database to verify the symbol used.* | Wom?n (would retrieve articles with woman or women)<br>Lab?r (would retrieve articles with labour or labor) |
| Phrase searching | Uses quotation marks to search for phrases. | "Physical activity" (would retrieve articles that specifically use these two words together) |
| Citation tracking | Also referred to as reference mining or snowballing. Involves scouting through the reference lists of previously located quality articles for additional leads. Prior literature highlights the benefits of this search technique and suggests it should be standard practice (Heath et al., 2020). | Using the reference list of a systematic review on your topic to locate additional topic-related articles. |

### *Other Search Strategies*

Various other search strategies can help you find the most applicable sources on your topic. These strategies include truncation, wildcards, phrase searching, and citation tracking. Table 3-4 explains these strategies with examples.

### *Screening Abstracts*

Even with using carefully selected search terms, search criteria, and search strategies, you will get to a point where you need to scan the abstracts of articles to determine their applicability to your topic. An **abstract** is a short synopsis of a scholarly paper or research study, usually 250 words or less, that summarizes the key points, including the purpose, procedures, and salient outcomes and conclusions of the work. The abstract is placed at the beginning of the paper and can be reviewed first to determine if reading further is warranted. If you review the abstract and the content applies to or aligns with your topic of interest, you will likely read the full article. If the abstract deviates from your topic, you can abandon it and move to the next article for consideration.

### TIPS & INSPIRATION

- When conducting your comprehensive literature search, it is easy to lose sight of your primary topic and get sidetracked into other interesting areas. Keep your inquiry question in a place of high visibility and frequently reorient yourself to it to maintain your focus. If you encounter information of interest but not directly related to your topic, quickly store it for later review and move on.

## Tracking Your Search

Doing a literature search is a time-consuming process that requires patience, skill, and a bit of trial and error. Tracking your literature search involves keeping a record of where and when you searched; the search terms, criteria, and strategies used; and the results generated. Tracking is important for several reasons:

- Tracking allows you to see what searches were successful so that you can hone your terms and criteria.
- Tracking can save you time. With good records, you can easily replicate a prior search if necessary and avoid prior unsuccessful searches.
- Tracking serves as a record of your efforts. Depending on the topic and purpose of your inquiry, it might be necessary to share your search methodology with others to illustrate that you have adequately researched the topic or to support gaps or shortcomings in the existing literature that you plan to address.

A spreadsheet like the one in Table 3-5 can be used to track your search. Some information has been provided in the table for example purposes. An additional blank Literature Search Tracking Log is provided in Appendix B to help you track your own literature search.

### TIPS & INSPIRATION

- Begin tracking your search immediately, even if you are not completely settled on your search terms and criteria. Recall that one of the purposes of tracking is to help you determine what searches are successful.

## Organizing and Synthesizing Your Literature

While gathering appropriate literature for your inquiry, an organizational system will allow you to archive your literature in one place, easily format reference lists, avoid plagiarism, make notes, and quickly locate sources when you need them. While many researchers use reference management software, such as EndNote, Mendeley, and Zotero, a good electronic filing system and a spreadsheet can be equally effective if you are new to this process or do not have access to software specific to this purpose. Whatever method you use, devise your system early on to ensure you can efficiently manage the large amount of information you will gather. Being organized will also be helpful when it comes time to draft the comprehensive literature review for your inquiry.

### TIPS & INSPIRATION

- Before you start searching the literature, establish a system for storing the literature you locate.

Another tool to help you organize your literature is a literature matrix. A **literature matrix** is a comprehensive table used to compare all studies in your literature portfolio by various components, including author, date of publication, study purpose, study design or level of evidence, participants, variables, results, as well as any important points, implications, or themes you want to discuss in your written literature review. Section 2 of this text discusses specific research study components (for example, variables). However, the focus here is to understand the utility of a literature matrix in organizing your literature. Table 3-6 provides an example of a literature matrix, and column headings can be adjusted to best meet your needs.

As you select articles for your portfolio and begin to organize them, it is essential to consider the *quality* of the research you located. Not all research is created equal. Study designs vary in rigor, and many factors could impact or bias study results. This scrutiny of a research study is termed **critical appraisal**, which is discussed in Section 2 of this text. It bears mentioning here because it is irresponsible to reference or apply research without proper appraisal first.

**TABLE 3-5 ■ Sample Literature Search Tracking Log**

***PIO or PICO Question:*** Does structured exercise training and joint protection techniques (I) increase participation in sports activities (O) in children with juvenile arthritis (P)?

| Database Searched | Date | Search Terms Used | Limiters or Additional Criteria Set | No. of Results | Notes/Comments | No. of Articles Selected | Citations for Selected Articles |
|---|---|---|---|---|---|---|---|
| MEDLINE | 12-8-22 | Joint protection AND arthritis | None | 231 | Too broad; many unrelated articles | 0 | |
| MEDLINE | 12-8-22 | Joint protection AND juvenile arthritis | None | 1 | Too narrow; no articles related to sports participation | 0 | |
| MEDLINE | 12-8-22 | Juvenile arthritis AND sports | None | 88 | Many more applicable articles, but still too broad; yielding studies focused on perceptions; searching another database may help improve the search | 0 | |
| MEDLINE, CINAHL, SPORTDiscus | 12-8-22 | Juvenile arthritis AND sports | English language only | 40 | Still a bit too broad; noted some articles using the term "physical activity" or "physical fitness" instead of sports; also many articles still not focused on actual interventions | 1 | Philpott et al., 2010 |
| MEDLINE, CINAHL, SPORTDiscus | 12-8-22 | Juvenile arthritis AND physical activity AND intervention | English language only, full text only, 2018–present, limited age 6–18 years | 16 | Many application articles; scanning abstracts | 3 so far | Iversen et al., 2022; Kattackal et al., 2020; Klepper et al., 2019 |

**TABLE 3-6 ■ Literature Review Matrix**

| Authors (Date) | Purpose | Study Design/ Level of Evidence | No. of Subjects or Participants (or Articles for Systematic Review) | Independent Variable(s) | Dependent Variable(s) | Results | Important Features or Implications for Practice | Themes Identified |
|---|---|---|---|---|---|---|---|---|
| | | | | | | | | |
| | | | | | | | | |
| | | | | | | | | |
| | | | | | | | | |
| | | | | | | | | |
| | | | | | | | | |

You should spend some time thinking about your literature review and start conceptualizing the sections or themes in your mind. **Themes** are central concepts or findings occurring in two or more studies. When multiple studies have the same or similar findings, this adds strength to the conclusions and increases the likelihood that results can be generalized to similar situations and populations with the same outcome. A quality literature review should synthesize findings from multiple studies. **Synthesis** involves integrating and collectively summarizing the findings from multiple studies rather than discussing each study individually. As you review each article, complete the following steps:

1. Add the article to your literature matrix.
2. Identify and record important themes or points you want to emphasize.
3. Make notations, including highlighting quotations and statistics corresponding to the resultant themes.

**BOX 3-2 ■ Example Outline to Guide Writing of a Literature Review**

1. Define dementia
2. Review the incidence of dementia
3. Explain the most common symptoms of dementia
   a. Mood and behavior changes
4. Impact of mood and behavior changes
   a. Impact to patient
   b. Impact to caregivers
5. Common interventions for mood and behavior changes
   a. Medication
   b. Nonpharmacological interventions
      i. Multisensory environments
         (a) Research to date
         (b) Gaps in literature or practice to address

After your literature matrix is complete, organize your themes into a progressive outline that will guide the writing of your literature review. See Box 3-2 for an example outline to guide the writing of a literature review for an inquiry on using multisensory environments to impact negative behaviors in the dementia population. Your literature review should include a detailed description of the various themes, with multiple citations from the referenced articles to support each point. You might also consider using subheadings within the literature review to identify topic transitions. Table 3-7 addresses

**TABLE 3-7 ■ Frequently Asked Questions About the Literature Review**

| Question | Guidance |
|---|---|
| Am I restricted to including research articles published within the last 5–10 years? | Generally, no. Limiting your search to articles published within the last 5–10 years may be best for evidence on the efficacy of interventions. However, searching back further in time may be appropriate if the focus is a well-researched intervention that has been shown to stand the test of time. Determining the appropriate age of applicable research is a judgment call based on your topic, setting, skills and knowledge, and the purpose of your inquiry. |
| How many articles do I need? | There is no definitive answer. The number of articles in your portfolio will vary based on the topic and the volume and quality of literature available. You need literature to adequately explain the context of your inquiry and to summarize the current research on your topic. The portfolio will be smaller for topics having relatively sparse research; for well researched topics, more articles might be included to justify the inquiry. |
| Am I restricted to including only higher-quality research? | There are seldom restrictions on the quality of evidence acceptable for a literature review. A primary criterion in determining the quality of an article is the rigor of the study design or methodology. The researchers select the study design based on the topic and objectives of their inquiry. Some topics lend themselves more easily to rigorous study, while others cannot be studied under such strict conditions. For example, suppose you are looking for research on a rare neurological disorder. In that case, you might find case studies or accounts from experts who have treated clients with this disorder (which represent less rigorous study designs). Conversely, practitioners interested in more commonly occurring diagnoses or treatments might find larger-scale studies in many settings (representing more rigorous study designs). The quality of the evidence available is directly related to the topic and aims of the proposed inquiry. |
| Should my articles all come from journals within my discipline? | It is unnecessary and unlikely that *all* of your research will come from publications specific to your discipline. Searching beyond your discipline is good practice to ensure the inclusion of current literature. Also, remember that researchers within your discipline can publish in journals outside the discipline. For example, it will be essential to look beyond your healthcare discipline for topics related to management, leadership, interprofessional collaboration, or education. Business, psychology, and educational journals can be good sources for research applicable to some healthcare inquiries. |
| What if I cannot find enough literature on my topic? | The answer depends on the purpose of your inquiry. If you plan to conduct a research study, this illustrates a gap in the existing literature and supports the need for your inquiry. (This is great news!) If you plan to conduct an evidence-based practice project, here are some recommendations:<br>1. Revise your search terms and criteria or your topic to improve your search results.<br>2. Locate separate articles supporting components of your focus. For example, if you are looking for articles on a comprehensive program to address anxiety in patients with cancer, locating individual articles that support different interventions (for example, mindfulness, education, sleep hygiene) can support the comprehensive program you hope to create.<br>3. If you still cannot locate sufficient evidence, but there is a definite need for your project, combine the best available relevant evidence with your skills and knowledge. For example, if you cannot locate evidence on interventions for a rare neurological disorder, consider strong evidence on other more common neurological disorders that present with similar symptoms. |
| How long should the literature review be? | The length of your literature review depends on the document being produced. Literature reviews as part of a thesis or capstone may be extensive, ranging from several pages to an entire chapter. Literature reviews for a journal article tend to be brief and to the point, as most journals have space constraints. |

other frequently asked questions about completing a literature review. If you are completing an inquiry as part of a formal educational process, you should always check with your instructor to determine any other course- or discipline-specific requirements.

## TIPS & INSPIRATION

- Do not be discouraged by the time it takes to search, locate, and review the literature on your topic. A good rule of thumb is that you will spend about 70% of your time searching and reading and the other 30% writing the literature review.
- Review two or three well-written literature reviews (likely within articles you select for your portfolio) to understand how information should flow from one topic to the next. Using these to guide your literature review can help you get started.
- If you are overwhelmed with the volume of literature on your topic, focus on only citing works pertinent to your topic, not works of tangential or general significance. If you summarize earlier works, avoid nonessential details; instead, emphasize pertinent findings, relevant methodological issues, and major conclusions. Prioritize comprehensive large-scale studies and more rigorous designs over smaller, weaker ones.
- Once you begin writing your literature review, do not feel pressured to write everything perfectly the first time. Focus on getting your thoughts down; you can polish the writing later after the central ideas are present.
- The literature review is a big task on your journey but is really just composed of many small steps. Focus on the small steps and before you know it, you will shift from beginner to expert on your topic!

## CHAPTER SUMMARY

1. Recall reasons for conducting a comprehensive and exhaustive literature search.
   - A comprehensive literature search allows you to understand the breadth of literature on your topic. This information is used to write your literature review and make decisions about your inquiry procedures.
   - Prior literature can help you save time, avoid problems encountered in prior research, place your inquiry in context, identify solutions to existing problems, and ensure your inquiry is meaningful.
2. Recognize where to search for literature and how to assess the credibility of sources.
   - Literature can be found in electronic databases; scholarly journals; books; magazines; professional, organizational, and government websites; and grey (or unpublished) literature.
   - All sources must be evaluated for credibility before using them. Scrutinizing the source site, author, posting or publication date, and content can help determine whether the source is credible.
3. Identify appropriate search terms, criteria, and strategies for a literature search.
   - Search terms, typically derived from your inquiry question, are the keywords representing your topic that you enter into databases to retrieve relevant articles.
   - MeSH headings are standard words or phrases used to index articles by topic, and these words should also be incorporated into your search terms.
   - Search criteria are the other parameters defining the research characteristics you are looking for, such as the author's name, title, journal, publication dates, the language of publication, and availability in full text.
   - Use of Boolean operators, truncation, wildcards, phrase searching, and citation tracking are additional strategies for a successful search.
4. Explain the benefits and method of tracking a literature search.
   - Tracking helps you identify what search terms and criteria were successful, saves time by allowing replication of a search if necessary, and can verify a quality search.
   - To track a search, clearly document the date, databases, search terms, limiters set, number of results, conclusions or comments about the search, and selected articles.
5. Organize and synthesize research on a topic of focus.
   - Tools to organize your literature include reference management software, an electronic filing system and spreadsheet, and a literature matrix.
   - A literature matrix is a comprehensive table for comparison of all studies in your portfolio by

various components, including author, date of publication, study purpose, study design or level of evidence, subjects/participants, variables, results, and points or themes of importance.
- Synthesis is the integration of findings from all the individual studies into an organized literature review that progresses logically to help the reader understand the topic and why your inquiry is necessary.

6. Construct an outline of a literature review on a focused topic.
   - Identify themes or central concepts or findings occurring in two or more studies within your portfolio. Multiple citations should support each theme when writing the literature review.
   - Consider how the themes logically connect and draft an outline to guide the writing of the literature review.
   - Table 3-7: Frequently Asked Questions About the Literature Review can further guide the writing of your literature review.

## TEST YOUR KNOWLEDGE

1. Why is conducting a comprehensive literature review important before initiating an inquiry?
   a. To understand existing literature on the topic for effective design of your inquiry
   b. To gain a broad understanding of the topic and refine your ideas
   c. To determine if you are passionate about your topic and have sufficient support
   d. To evaluate the credibility of online sources on your topic
2. A source from which of the following would MOST LIKELY require further evaluation to determine credibility?
   a. A peer-reviewed journal
   b. A website that sells the equipment
   c. The MEDLINE database
   d. The National Multiple Sclerosis Society
3. Which Boolean operator is used to broaden your search?
   a. AND
   b. OR
   c. NOT
   d. BUT
4. What is citation tracking?
   a. Looking for a source where you have not looked before
   b. Using a special symbol after your search terms to find articles with different versions of the term
   c. Looking through a reference list of an article to find additional sources
   d. Tracking your literature search so someone can replicate it
5. Why is it important to track and document your literature search?
   a. To ensure you meet the length requirements for the literature review
   b. To maximize efforts in retrieving relevant literature
   c. To keep the details of your search confidential
   d. To demonstrate your organizational skills to your advisor or colleagues
6. A literature matrix is an effective tool for organizing your literature before writing your literature review. True or false?
7. What characterizes a well-constructed literature review?
   a. Synthesizing findings from multiple studies
   b. Summarizing each study individually
   c. Discussing only the most recent studies on the topic
   d. Avoiding citations to streamline the paragraphs

Answer key appears at the end of this text.

## NEXT STEPS

1. Brainstorm applicable search terms for each element of your inquiry question and list them using Table 3-2 as an example. Identify one database most applicable to your inquiry topic and determine if there are additional MeSH terms you should include. Using these terms, conduct and track four or five preliminary searches. Did you find any research that is useful for your purposes? Were the searches too broad or too narrow? Consider the additional search strategies within the chapter to identify your next step.
2. Draft your "wish list" for the research you want to locate. What do you want? And what would you prefer not to have? This is another way of

*Continued*

conceptualizing your inclusion criteria (research you want) and exclusion criteria (research you are not interested in). Making a list of your ideal research can be useful as you quickly scan references and abstracts to determine if they fit your purposes.

3. Find one article that aligns with your search terms and criteria. Mine the reference list of this article for other valuable sources. What did you find?
4. Complete a literature matrix for a topic of interest. Include at least six articles to explore some synthesis of the research on the topic.
5. Draft an outline for your literature review. Share with someone else for feedback. Do the topics lead logically from one to another? Is something missing?
6. Compose a literature review that aligns with your purposes. Recall that the length and format of your literature review depend on the type of document being produced.

## REFERENCES

Bonato, S. (2022). Grey literature searching. In M. J. Foster & S. T. Jewell (Eds.), *Piecing together systematic reviews and other evidence synthesis* (pp. 111–128). The Medical Library Association.

Heath, A., Levay, P., & Tuvey, D. (2020). Literature searching methods or guidance and their application to public health topics: A narrative review. *Health Information & Libraries Journal, 39*(1), 6–21. https://doi.org/10.1111/hir.12414

# Section 2

# Understanding and Appraising Research

Section 2 of this text (Chapters 4–10) reviews the most common research designs, their methodological features, and how to effectively appraise existing research. Specifically, Chapters 4 to 6 address quantitative research designs and appraisal; Chapters 7 to 9 cover qualitative research designs and appraisal; and Chapter 10 considers some additional designs, including mixed methods and systematic reviews. A **research design** is a general plan or overall structure of an inquiry; designs can be quantitative, qualitative, or mixed-methods, and the decision is based on the topic and aims of the inquiry. The **methodology** concerns the specific details of an inquiry plan, such as when and how participants will be recruited, what procedures will be used with participants, and what outcome measures will be used. It is essential to have a foundational knowledge of research designs and methodologies, whether you intend to design and conduct your own inquiry or if you are a consumer of research and plan to apply existing research to your practice. Let's begin with quantitative research.

# Chapter 4

# Quantitative Research Design and Methods

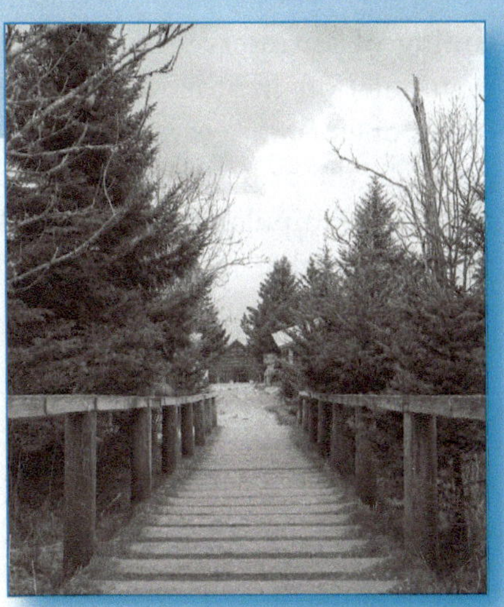

LEARNING OUTCOMES

*The information provided in this chapter will assist you to:*

4.1 Define quantitative research.
4.2 Describe the prominent features of quantitative research, including manipulation, control, and randomization.
4.3 Describe five common experimental designs.
4.4 Describe four common quasi-experimental designs.
4.5 Describe five common nonexperimental designs.

## What Is Quantitative Research?

**Quantitative research** is "a formal, objective, systematic study process implemented to obtain numerical data to answer a research question" (Gray & Grove, 2021, p. 29). Quantitative research designs are most often employed "to describe variables, examine relationships among variables, and determine cause-and-effect interactions between variables" (Gray & Grove, 2021, p. 29). This chapter describes the major quantitative research designs and their advantages and disadvantages. Of course, there are many more designs than those presented here, but these should get you started. The broad categories of quantitative research designs discussed are experimental, quasi-experimental, and nonexperimental designs.

LeConte Lodge, Great Smoky Mountain National Park, Tennessee.

## Features of Quantitative Research

Within quantitative research, several features can impact experimental rigor. These three concepts are explored in the following sections:

1. Manipulation
2. Control
3. Randomization

### Manipulation

**Manipulation** merely means doing something to one or more variables in the study. A **variable** is anything that can vary or change and, therefore, can be measured. For example, if a researcher offers a group of patients with schizophrenia a daily program of self-care activities to determine whether their appearance can be improved, manipulation is provided in the form of daily self-care activities. Generally, any treatment or intervention offered to participants in the hope that they will show improvement or change is manipulation. Changing the environment or the timing of an intervention can also be considered manipulation. In other words, the researcher manipulates one or more variables concerning the participants. In the prior example, the variable of self-care is being manipulated or given as treatment to determine whether it will influence another variable, namely, the patient's appearance.

### *Dependent and Independent Variables*

The **independent variable** is the variable that is being manipulated, which could affect the outcome (or dependent variable). Conversely, the **dependent variable** is typically the variable being measured. In the previous example, the independent variable (self-care) is manipulated to determine the effect on the dependent variable (the patients' appearance). The independent variable is sometimes called the experimental or treatment variable. The dependent variable (appearance) determines the effectiveness of the manipulation or treatment and is the outcome observed and measured at the beginning and end of the study.

Manipulation must be part of the design if the study is to qualify as a true experimental design. Thus, if the researcher does not actually manipulate a variable pertaining to the participants, a study cannot be termed *experimental*. For example, a study in which participants are asked to complete a questionnaire and the researcher merely examines answers or variables after the fact is not experimental.

## Control

The second concept that needs defining to understand quantitative research designs is control. **Control** refers to the researcher's ability to minimize or eliminate interfering and irrelevant influences in a study's design. This allows the researcher to say that the results are caused by manipulation of the variables and not by chance interferences of other variables. In the earlier example, if there were no control, it is possible that instead of the program of self-care skills, some other event in the patients' lives (such as a volunteer taking them to the store to buy new clothes) might have caused improvement in their appearance. Examples of variables a researcher may be able to control include:

- Environmental influences (e.g., the amount of noise or the aesthetics of the surroundings)
- Change of healthcare practitioner providing the treatment (it might be important to the study that the practitioner remain consistent so that patients become accustomed to them, or it might be equally important that different practitioners be used to eliminate the influence of certain practitioners' styles)
- Certain events in the patients' lives (such as obtaining a physician's cooperation in maintaining patients' medications during the period of the study)

However, controlling all variables that may affect the study results is impossible. Thus, it is important to have a control group of participants who experience the same day-to-day occurrences and influences as the experimental group yet do not receive the study treatment. By including a control group, a researcher is attempting to ensure that any helpful or detrimental event influencing the amount of change in the dependent variable (the one being measured) will happen to both groups of participants. At the end of the study, when the dependent variable is measured for both groups, if there is greater improvement in the experimental group, the researcher can say that this was likely due to the manipulation or treatment.

In certain situations, it is not ethical to withhold treatment from a group of patients for them to serve as a control group. There are generally three ways to deal with these circumstances. For example, a researcher might want to know whether a new treatment is more effective for a specific condition than a traditional one. One option to test this question is to have the control group receive the traditional treatment and the experimental group receive the new treatment, holding all other conditions constant. This design satisfies the need for a control group as well as the ethical concern. Another option might involve collecting data on the experimental group before initiating the new treatment. The experimental group functions as its own control by comparing data before and after the new treatment. A third option is to use two distinct groups—an experimental and a control group, with the control group being offered the experimental treatment following the initial phase of the study. This allows the researcher to draw conclusions regarding the experimental treatment and to satisfy ethical concerns by permitting both groups to undergo the same treatment. The concept of control embraces elements of the third concept to be discussed—randomization.

### Randomization

**Systematic bias** refers to inherent flaws in a study's design that can influence or skew results. For example, using faulty equipment, untrained study personnel, or biased sampling methods can all decrease the accuracy of study results. **Randomization** is one method to reduce the risk of this bias creeping into a study. In addition, randomization increases the study's **external validity**, which is the chance that the results found in the participants can be generalized to others who are similar. It also increases the study's **internal validity**, which is the chance that observed changes are due to the intervention or treatment being provided and not attributed to other possible causes. (See Chapter 6 to learn more about validity in quantitative research.) Randomization involves two components—random selection and random assignment.

**Random selection** means that every participant in the population being studied has an equal chance of being selected for the study sample. Researchers carefully consider whom they wish to study and then set criteria for the participants. For example, inclusion criteria might consist of people diagnosed with chronic schizophrenia who have had multiple hospital admissions totaling at least 5 years and who have one or more family members available for support. For the same study, the researchers might determine exclusion criteria as patients younger than 18 and those living more than 25 miles from the research site. Once the inclusion and exclusion criteria are determined, the researchers must choose a method to select a group of individuals (sample) to be in the study from among those who meet the criteria.

In research, the population of interest refers to the entire group of people or items that meet the subject or participant inclusion criteria set by the researcher. The population comprises all such participants, whereas the subpopulation is a researcher-defined population subgroup. A sample is selected from the population or the subpopulation (Box 4-1). A population does not necessarily refer to people; it may also refer to things such as records or events that are being studied (Box 4-2).

For true random selection, every participant in the population of interest must have an equal opportunity of being selected. Therefore, merely using patients who come through your door or client records that happen to land on your desk would mean that not all participants had the same chance of inclusion in the study because all those who did not walk through your door or whose records did not land on your desk had no chance of being selected.

#### BOX 4-1 ■ Example of Participant Selection

In Sahraei et al.'s (2022) study of the effects of Swedish massage on pain, the population of interest included all the patients with pain due to rheumatoid arthritis. However, the subpopulation included all the patients with rheumatoid arthritis pain treated at a rheumatology clinic in Iran. The sample for the study was selected from this subpopulation. Participants were randomly assigned to the experimental group, which received Swedish massage for 8 weeks, or to the control group, which received routine care for their condition.

#### BOX 4-2 ■ Example of Study of Records or Events as Population

In a study investigating whether clients' race or ethnicity impacted healthcare practitioners' use of negative client descriptors, Sun et al. (2022) analyzed electronic medical records from one academic medical facility in Chicago, Illinois. The data examined included medical records for all clients treated in the facility's emergency room, inpatient units, or outpatient clinics during a specific period in 2020.

Instead, a complete list of people or items in the population or subpopulation of interest must be available to the researcher, and a random selection must be made from that list. In the study by Sahraei et al. (2022; see Box 4-1), they would have needed a complete list of all the patients in Iran who met the research criteria, namely, all those with pain due to rheumatoid arthritis. Then, they could have placed all the names in a hat and picked out the required number for the study, or assigned a number to each patient and used a random number chart to select patients for the study sample. Either is an acceptable random selection method, but the latter is probably more practical. Although true random selection is ideal, the ability to access and randomly choose participants from everyone who meets your participant inclusion criteria within an entire population is not usually realistic.

A random number chart, found online or in a statistics text, lists numbers randomly generated by a computer. The chart may be read in any direction (up or down, side to side, diagonally), starting at any point, to produce a list of random numbers. This method is commonly used when researchers mail questionnaires and have access to a complete mailing list of potential participants who meet their criteria—a population. It is simple enough to assign a number to each name, then pick a series of numbers from the chart and include the people with corresponding numbers in the study. If a spreadsheet of names already exists, programs and online tools can assist with random selection, saving the researcher much time. Some examples include *Research Randomizer* (Urbaniak & Plous, 2013) and *Microsoft Excel* (Microsoft Corporation, 2021).

To clarify further, random selection ensures that the sample is as much like the larger population from which it was drawn as possible and improves external validity—that is, the likelihood that similar findings would occur if another portion of this population were studied. Thus, the results of a study can be more readily generalized to the entire population of interest and are more useful to other healthcare practitioners who would like to use the same treatment method with similar patients. Remember, if random selection has not been used, the results of a study may not be easily generalized to other people in the population of interest.

**Random assignment**, the second component of randomization, means that those in the selected sample have an equal chance of being assigned to the experimental or control groups. A complete participant sample should be selected first, and then a similar process should be used to assign participants randomly to the two groups. Random assignment is done primarily to ensure that the participants in each group will be as alike (or as unalike) as possible; it also ensures that a researcher will not be tempted to assign a "good" participant to the experimental group because it looks as if the participant may show a lot of improvement. This technique helps to minimize researcher bias, which can impact study results. Random assignment improves internal validity and specifically helps ensure that the experimental treatment made a difference rather than something else within the study design. It will also "even out" the effect on the study of such things as **attrition** (participants dropping out of the study), developmental maturation (changes or improvements because of natural aging or development), practice effects (changes because of new learning or repeated testing and training), or regression (patients getting sicker over time).

The point of randomization is to ensure that the sample is as representative of the population of interest as possible and that the experimental and control groups are as similar as possible. This enables the researcher to state more confidently that the results are due to the treatment given rather than a difference in characteristics between the two groups. It also minimizes the chance that the sample members were not typical of the population and improved because of some uncontrolled trait they held in common. Remember that some variations in samples are usually expected and preferred, for eliminating all variation among a sample would greatly decrease external validity or limit the ability to generalize results to groups with dissimilar attributes. For example, the results of a study examining the effects of an afterschool recreation program on white female

### BOX 4-3 ■ Example of Poor Randomization

A classic example of poor methodology occurred in the 1969 selection of men to be drafted into the army. A slip of paper with each man's name and month of birth was put into an urn and drawn out, but the slips were not well mixed. The last slips put into the urn were of men whose birthdays fell in October, November, and December, and disproportionately more of these men's names were drawn than others. This was a case in which poor methodology had serious consequences.

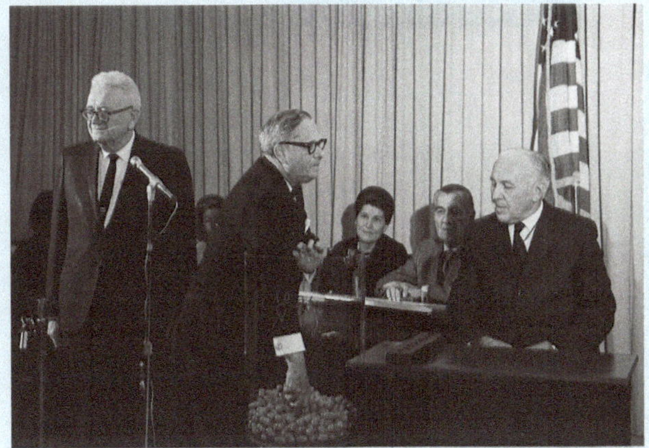

Congressman Alexander Pirnie (R-NY) drawing the first capsule for the Selective Service draft on December 1, 1969.

kindergartners with obesity in the rural Midwestern United States might not be easily generalized to older children, males, those of other ethnicities, or those residing in urban communities. Although the study may yield beneficial information for this select group, application beyond the original study is limited.

Randomization is not perfect. It is based on the laws of probability; however, occasionally the improbable will happen, and a source of bias will appear in a study. For example, one group may end up being composed of patients who are sicker or older than those in the other group. Also, methods must be used correctly for random selection to be effective (Box 4-3). Consider the concepts of manipulation, control, and randomization as three categories of quantitative research designs (experimental, quasi-experimental, and nonexperimental), highlighted in Figure 4-1, are discussed.

## Experimental Designs

True **experimental research designs** involve manipulation of at least one independent variable, control of various other phenomena in the methodology, and random selection and assignment of participants to study groups. These designs are **prospective**, meaning the plans for the study are laid out well in advance, and the participants are followed moving forward in time, as opposed to **retrospective studies**, in which participants or phenomena are examined backward in time concerning an outcome that has already occurred. Experimental designs are most commonly used to determine *cause-and-effect relationships*, thus denoting a strong chance that the manipulation of the independent variable caused a change in the dependent variable. This method allows the researcher to compare different types of treatment and determine which is likely to be the most effective. Designs that are not experimental can show *support* for certain outcomes or suggest an intervention *may* be effective. However, definite conclusions about cause and effect can only be ascertained with an experimental design.

### Basic Experimental Design

In a classic experimental design, the researcher deliberately manipulates the independent variable in the experimental group but not in the control group, and then looks for the differences in the dependent variable. For example, with the rise in the aging population and the increased incidence of

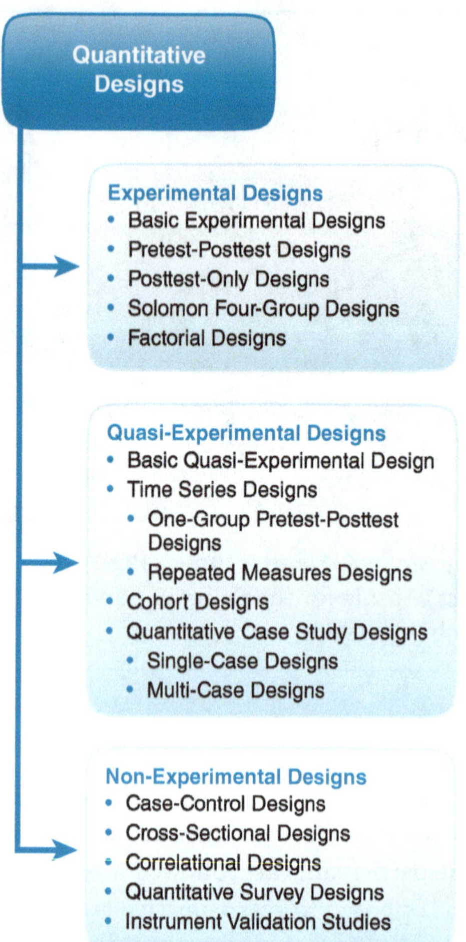


Figure 4-1 Common quantitative designs.

Alzheimer's disease, a researcher might be interested in studying the effects of a formal caregiver training program on the stress level of caregivers of patients with Alzheimer's disease. Caregivers can be randomly selected and assigned to one of two groups—an experimental group that will be provided with formal education on how to care for individuals with Alzheimer's disease and a control group that will not receive this training. The dependent variable, caregiver stress level, is measured for both groups before and after the education so that comparisons can be made on the same group; comparisons between groups can also be made by comparing both "after" tests. The before and after tests are called pretests and posttests.

A variation of the basic research design, a **randomized controlled trial (RCT)** is the most rigorous design, as it has high internal validity and is regarded as the "gold standard" for clinical research (Portney, 2020, p. 193). Internal validity can be further improved if the study is single- or double-blinded, or masked. In a **double-blinded** RCT, the researchers and the participants are unaware of the hypothesis being tested or the assignment of participants to experimental and control groups. This lack of awareness prevents changes in participant performance because of their knowledge of treatment or the researcher's expectations. In a **single-blinded** RCT, only one group, either the participants or the researchers, is blinded to the treatment. Blindness can also be preserved by having different individuals responsible for study design, implementation, data collection, and statistical analysis (Portney, 2020).

For ease of communication with other researchers and to permit the researcher to sketch out designs quickly, a system of shorthand known as research notation was developed by Campbell and Stanley (1969). An "O" represents the observations or measurements that occur at pretesting and posttesting; an "R" represents random assignment; and an "X" represents manipulation or treatment. Each study group is written or represented on a separate line, and time periods are aligned vertically. In research notation, a design consisting of two randomly assigned groups, one with treatment and one without, and both with pretesting and posttesting, would be illustrated as follows:

| R | O | X | O |
|---|---|---|---|
| R | O | | O |

Using this design, the resulting data from the pretests will enable the researcher to see whether the two groups were genuinely similar to begin with. Sometimes, the pretest may be necessary to assist with participant selection. For example, participant inclusion criteria might require participants to be able to remember and follow a short sequence of directions. Pretesting might include a brief cognitive screen to determine that participants fit the study's inclusion criteria. At the end of the study, posttest scores can be compared to see which group shows the greatest change in the dependent variable. Finally, the pretest and posttest of each group can be compared to see how much change occurred for the experimental versus the control group.

If circumstances dictate, the random assignment to groups can be performed after the pretest; however, the pretest results should not influence the assignment. Following random assignment, equivalency between the two groups may be assumed; however, performing a pretest provides a further check on equivalency. This double-check is particularly useful in dealing with small samples (Portney, 2020). Nevertheless, attrition (loss of participants), mainly that which differs between experimental and control groups, is a continuing concern.

### Pretest-Posttest Design With Follow-Up

If you want to determine if the effect of an intervention is long-lasting, the design may be further improved by adding a follow-up observation or posttest ($O_2$ and $O_4$), as shown here:

| R | O | X | $O_1$ | $O_2$ |
|---|---|---|---|---|
| R | O | | $O_3$ | $O_4$ |

This will let you see if any improvements following the treatment are maintained over time. Box 4-4 illustrates the point with a follow-up 26 weeks after the posttest.

### Posttest-Only Design

Sometimes, the treatment results may be influenced by the fact that a pretest has been administered. For example, participants may benefit from practicing a task used in the pretest, thus diminishing the effect of the intervention. In this case, the pretest might be omitted if participants have been randomly selected and assigned to groups. In other cases, the pretest may be excluded when administration is deemed too time-consuming to support its use. A disadvantage of this study design is that the researcher has no way of confirming if the two study groups are equivalent before the intervention, which can impact the ability to draw conclusions about the effectiveness of the intervention (Thomas & Hersen, 2011). Using research notation, this design appears as follows:

| R | X | O |
|---|---|---|
| R | | O |

#### BOX 4-4 ■ Example of a Pretest-Posttest Design With Follow-Up

A study compared the effectiveness of manual therapy, stabilizing exercises, and traditional home exercises (control group) for women with neck pain and postural deficits (Fathollahnejad et al., 2019). The 60 participants were randomly assigned to three groups—one that received manual therapy and stabilizing exercises, one that received only stabilizing exercises, and one that received traditional home exercises. Pain, endurance, and posture were assessed preintervention, postintervention (6 weeks), and at a 1-month follow-up. The group receiving manual therapy and stabilizing exercises demonstrated the most significant improvements in pain and function. This design could be notated as follows:

| R | O | $X_1$ | $O_1$ | $O_2$ |
|---|---|---|---|---|
| R | O | $X_2$ | $O_3$ | $O_4$ |
| R | O | $X_3$ | $O_5$ | $O_6$ |

### Solomon Four-Group Design

If the researcher is unsure if the pretest has an effect or knows it has an effect but feels it provides crucial information, the Solomon four-group design can be employed. Sometimes, pretests could impact outcomes by allowing the participants to practice or learn skills being tested or by raising awareness of the elements being investigated (Portney, 2020). The Solomon four-group design, which involves random assignment to four groups (two experimental and two control groups), can eliminate this design flaw. However, this design requires many participants and a great deal of researcher time. This design is depicted as follows:

| | | | | |
|---|---|---|---|---|
| **Group 1** (receives the pretest, experimental treatment, and the posttest) | R | O | X | $O_1$ |
| **Group 2** (receives the pretest and posttest but undergoes no treatment) | R | O | | $O_2$ |
| **Group 3** (receives the experimental treatment and posttest, but no pretest) | R | | X | $O_3$ |
| **Group 4** (only receives the posttest) | R | | | $O_4$ |

In comparing the posttest results, the researcher can test not only for differences between experimental and control groups but for any interaction between the pretest and experimental treatment by comparing groups 1 and 3 (on $O_1$ and $O_3$) and groups 2 and 4 (on $O_2$ and $O_4$). An example of this study design can be found in Box 4-5.

### Factorial Designs

The experimental designs mentioned so far are designed to cope with one independent variable only; however, researchers may be concerned with more than one variable in the same study. Factorial designs may be used to investigate two or more independent variables and their interaction with the dependent variable. These designs allow the researcher to use the same participants to study the effects of the independent variables on the dependent variable as well as any joint or interaction effects. In factorial designs, each independent variable is called a factor. Box 4-6 provides an example and further explains factorial designs.

**BOX 4-5 ■ Example of Solomon Four-Group Design**

Kumari et al. (2023) used the Solomon four-group design to determine the effect of brief nursing-led psychoeducation on self-stigma for clients with schizophrenia and affective disorders in India.

Participants were randomly assigned to one of two experimental groups (who received individualized education aimed to decrease self-stigma) or one of two control groups (who received brief standard advice). Only one experimental group and one control group underwent pretesting, and all four groups completed posttesting. Results indicate that the completion of the pretest did not impact overall study outcomes, but without use of this study design, researchers would have been unable to confirm this.

**TIPS & INSPIRATION**

- As you consider various quantitative research designs, search the literature for similarly designed studies in your discipline or practice area. Reviewing research studies that employed the designs discussed in this chapter can help you understand each design's purpose and overall process.

## Quasi-Experimental Designs

Like true experimental designs, **basic quasi-experimental designs** contain an independent variable that is manipulated to determine the effect on a dependent variable; however, they typically lack one or more of the following: a control group, random selection, or random assignment. The resulting designs are still very useful for validating treatment methods and techniques. When researchers want to study naturally occurring real-world situations, when there are ethical concerns with use of a control group or withholding treatment from a particular group, or when there are time or financial constraints, quasi-experimental designs may be appropriate. However, caution should be used in generalizing study

## BOX 4-6 ■ Example and Explanation of Factorial Design

Hunt and Bassi (2010) studied the impact of visual acuity and age on cognitive performance; they assessed 124 community-dwelling adults and divided them into six groups as follows:

1. Young adults tested with 20/30 or better visual acuity (control group)
2. Young adults tested with 20/50 visual acuity
3. Young adults tested with 20/100 visual acuity
4. Older adults tested with 20/30 or better visual acuity (control group)
5. Older adults tested with 20/50 visual acuity
6. Older adults tested with 20/100 visual acuity

The two independent variables were visual acuity (20/30 [which served as the control], 20/50, or 20/100) and age (young adult versus older adult). Their study was concerned with the effects of these factors on the dependent variable—performance on common cognitive assessments. This design is depicted as follows:

| Visual Acuity | Young Adult | Older Adult |
|---|---|---|
| 20/30 | Group 1 | Group 4 |
| 20/50 | Group 2 | Group 5 |
| 20/100 | Group 3 | Group 6 |

There are three levels for the independent variable or factor of visual acuity (20/30, 20/50, 20/100) and two levels for the independent variable or factor of age (young adult and older adult). Thus, this is called a 3 × 2 design. If age were expanded to contain a third category, such as middle-aged adult, it would be a 3 × 3 design depicted as follows:

| Visual Acuity | Young Adult | Middle-Aged Adult | Older Adult |
|---|---|---|---|
| 20/30 | Group 1 | Group 4 | Group 7 |
| 20/50 | Group 2 | Group 5 | Group 8 |
| 20/100 | Group 3 | Group 6 | Group 9 |

Finally, a third variable or factor, such as gender, might be added to the original design, with two levels for the gender factor, making it a 3 × 2 × 2 design depicted as follows:

| Young Adult | | | | | | Older Adult | | | | | |
|---|---|---|---|---|---|---|---|---|---|---|---|
| *Male* | | | *Female* | | | *Male* | | | *Female* | | |
| 20/30 | 20/50 | 20/100 | 20/30 | 20/50 | 20/100 | 20/30 | 20/50 | 20/100 | 20/30 | 20/50 | 20/100 |

Age and gender are actually pseudo-independent variables because the researcher is not manipulating them; they are already occurring attributes of the participants. However, in factorial designs, pseudo-independent variables are often treated like true independent variables. As more variables are added, the design's complexity and the number of participants required increases. Specific statistical procedures are used to analyze these designs, and often, the services of a statistician or a statistical software package are required.

### BOX 4-7 ■ Example of a Study Lacking Random Selection and a Control Group

In studying the effects of two treatment approaches on plantar heel pain, Cleland et al. (2009) recruited patients from two outpatient orthopedic clinics—one in New Hampshire, United States, and one in New Zealand. Participants were randomly assigned to one of the two groups, and results of pretesting indicated that the groups were analogous. If they were substantially different at the pretest stage, the researchers could have abandoned the groups and started the study over or used statistical techniques to account for the differences. One group received a series of modalities and an exercise regimen, whereas the other group received manual physical therapy and an exercise regimen. The design looked like this:

| | | | |
|---|---|---|---|
| R | O | $X_1$ | O |
| R | O | $X_2$ | O |

Even though the two groups were found to be equivalent on pretesting, caution must be taken in generalizing results because participants were not randomly selected. Participants were recruited from only two clinics; therefore, they may not represent the broader population of all individuals with plantar heel pain. Outcomes indicate increased success with the manual physical therapy and exercise program versus the program of modalities and exercise. Yet, without a control group (for example, a group that received only the exercise regimen), it is difficult to determine whether it was the combination of these approaches that helped the patients or the manual therapy and modalities alone.

results if randomization or a control group is absent. Box 4-7 includes an example of a study without random selection or a control group.

### BOX 4-8 ■ Example of Time Series Design

Friedman et al. (2021) used a time series design to study the impact of occupational therapy education on students' disability attitudes. Sixty-seven occupational therapy students from three graduate programs were administered a series of outcome measures to assess their implicit and explicit disability attitudes as they progressed through their education. Results indicate more favorable explicit attitudes, but little change to implicit attitudes as they progressed through the curriculum.

## Time Series Designs

**Time series designs**, also referred to as case series or longitudinal studies, are used to study the effects of some treatment or condition over time. These studies can involve multiple measurements (pretests and posttests) before and after treatment, and the study duration can vary from several weeks to decades. For example, Herman et al. (2010) were interested in determining the effect of childhood body mass index (BMI) and physical activity on adult health-related quality of life. Data from a fitness survey in 1981 of 310 participants ages 7 to 18 years were compared to data obtained on follow-up assessments 22 years later. Box 4-8 contains another example of a time series design.

Time series designs *lack a control group*, and the participants in the experimental group act as their own control. Participants receive the treatment but also experience a period of no treatment, which is considered the control period. Participants may be randomly selected to increase the likelihood of representing the population of interest, but random assignment to groups is a moot point since there is only one group. This can be referred to as a **one-group pretest-posttest design**. For example, data on handwriting legibility for second graders might be collected during one semester ($O_1$), and then compared to data on handwriting legibility from this same group obtained in a later semester ($O_2$) after participation in a structured multisensory handwriting curriculum (X). By comparing handwriting legibility in these two semesters, conclusions can be drawn about the potential impact of the multisensory handwriting curriculum on handwriting legibility. This design is depicted here:

| $O_1$ | X | $O_2$ |
|---|---|---|

This design challenges internal and external validity due to the lack of a control group. However, it can be useful if prior research has fully explored the controlled condition, if there are ethical concerns about withholding or deferring treatment, or if the study duration is very brief (Portney, 2020). A pretest-posttest design may also be used to determine the feasibility of a treatment technique or program (Bowen et al., 2009). This design can be strengthened with the use of a repeated measures design.

A **repeated measures design**, another type of time series design, can involve various sequences of treatment and nontreatment alternated with tests for the same group. Some examples are provided here to illustrate the advantages. In one option, a researcher might compare observations at multiple points (for example, at $O_2$, $O_4$, and $O_6$) after interventions (X) to uncover trends in outcomes. The design is notated as follows:

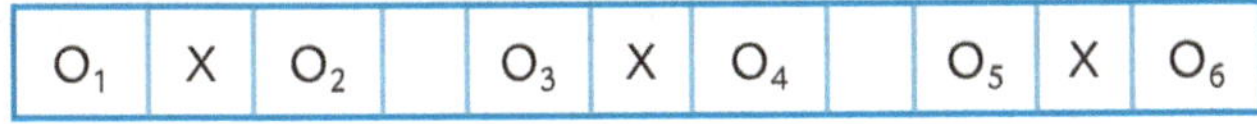

| $O_1$ | X | $O_2$ | | $O_3$ | X | $O_4$ | | $O_5$ | X | $O_6$ |
|---|---|---|---|---|---|---|---|---|---|---|

Another option involves the use of multiple pretests to provide a clearer picture of how participants score on the dependent variable before the experimental treatment, as well as multiple posttests to assess the permanence of change in the dependent variable; this option controls for seasonal or cyclical changes in abilities and eliminates the effect of history:

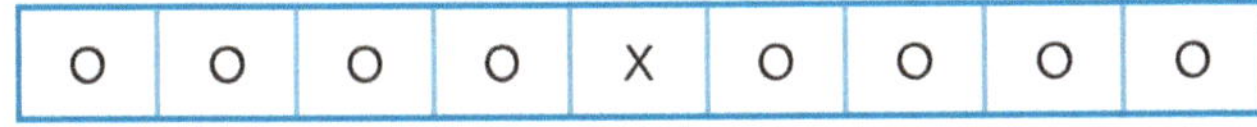

| O | O | O | O | X | O | O | O | O |
|---|---|---|---|---|---|---|---|---|

In a final option, history is controlled for, and the effects of experimental treatment can be viewed on more than one occasion (at $O_1$, $O_2$, and $O_3$), and the permanence of the effect can be measured ($O_3$ through $O_5$). The primary disadvantage of this design is the extended time required to carry out the study:

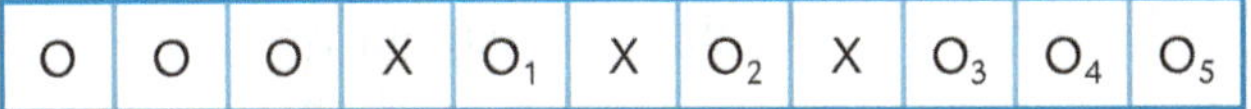

| O | O | O | X | $O_1$ | X | $O_2$ | X | $O_3$ | $O_4$ | $O_5$ |
|---|---|---|---|---|---|---|---|---|---|---|

## Cohort Designs

**Cohort designs** involve naturally occurring groups, or cohorts, of participants followed over time. The groups follow each other through a setting such as cohorts of students moving through a therapist training program. These studies use control and experimental groups, but unlike experimental study designs, the groups are not observed at the same time. One group is selected as the experimental group and subjected to a unique experience, whereas another group acts as the control group and experiences the usual events of the setting. Nonetheless, the two groups may be considered somewhat similar in that they both meet the setting's admission requirements. For further comparison, time series designs lack a control group, but cohort designs lack randomization. A simple cohort design is as follows, where Time 1 and Time 2 represent two distinct time periods:

| **Time 1** | | | **Time 2** | | |
|---|---|---|---|---|---|
| O | X | O | O | | O |

This design has internal validity problems because of the difference in the time of the observations. History (e.g., some global event that influences all participants in the sample) may account for the differences in data from the posttests. The best present-day example is the onset of the COVID-19 pandemic in 2020; social distancing, delayed study procedures, and mental health challenges at the time likely impacted outcomes of clinical trials (Sathian et al., 2020). The cohort design can be improved by employing recurrent institutional cycles, using three different cohorts. The first group receives the experimental treatment followed by a posttest; the second group receives the traditional pretest, treatment, and posttest; and the third group receives only a pretest. The ideal pattern of results from this design would be similar responses on pretests $O_2$ and $O_4$ and on posttests $O_1$ and $O_3$. The effect of the treatment would be evident by comparing scores on pretest $O_2$ and posttest $O_3$. The design is as follows:

| Time 1 | | Time 2 | | | Time 3 |
|---|---|---|---|---|---|
| X | $O_1$ | $O_2$ | X | $O_3$ | $O_4$ |
| | (Posttest) | (Pretest) | | (Posttest) | (Pretest) |

## Quantitative Case Study Designs

In **quantitative case study designs** (also referred to as single-subject, single-case, multiple-case, case series [more than one case], or small-*N* studies), an individual, group, unit, community, institution, or event is studied longitudinally—anywhere from a few weeks to several years. Case study designs are deemed quasi-experimental since variables or interventions are manipulated. A pretest, intervention, and posttest (or some other sequence of observations and interventions, for example, using multiple pretests or altering intervention periods with observations) are conducted with individuals instead of groups. This design examines unique cases or situations in which the participant or intervention is unusual, little understood, or impractical to study under strict experimental conditions (Berg & Latin, 2008).

Case studies in healthcare literature detail responses to treatment techniques and interventions that can support practitioners in clinical decision-making. Practitioners often ask how or why a particular adaptive aid or treatment procedure worked with a specific client, and these questions are best answered with case study designs. In a case study, the researcher's goal is to expand and generalize theories, such as how a phenomenon occurs, changes, or is sustained over time, rather than to determine the frequency or prevalence of the phenomenon. Case studies are useful for practitioners and new researchers to learn the investigation process and to contribute to the body of research in their profession. See Box 4-9 for an example of a case study design.

### BOX 4-9 ■ Example of Case Study Design

Researchers used a single-subject case study design to explore the impact of a therapeutic listening program on sensory processing and language skills (Nwora & Gee, 2009). The program differed from those investigated in prior studies in that it was designed for in-home delivery rather than in a clinic. The case was John, a 5-year-old boy diagnosed with pervasive developmental disorder, who participated in the therapeutic listening program two times per day, for 15 minutes each time, for a total of 20 weeks. As is typical of case studies, data were gathered in several ways. John's medical record was reviewed; standardized assessments were completed, and his in-class performance was videotaped pre- and postintervention. Results indicated he could participate in classroom games and songs, interact more effectively with his peers and siblings, and respond appropriately to directives and questions from his teacher and parents. These results support the need for further research on therapeutic listening interventions with this population.

Case studies can be single-case or multi-case. A **single-case study** involves just one critical, revelatory case and is used when there are limited cases available for the phenomena of interest; when there are many variables to explore, making use of multiple cases impractical; or when the researcher wants to alter the interventions provided to the participant based on data collected as the study progresses. Data can be collected during the intervention period and compared with data collected when the intervention is not provided (using the participant as their own control). Conducting a single-case pilot study to explore a topic and potential study methods is also appropriate before conducting a multi-case study.

A **multi-case study** is appropriate when numerous similar cases are present and the aim is to substantiate experimental outcomes; replicating the same experiment with multiple cases can increase the strength of the evidence and build theory across cases. The original theory should be further contemplated if the findings among multiple cases vary. The number of cases used will depend on the inquiry objectives and the variables being explored.

TIPS & INSPIRATION

- If you are planning to conduct an inquiry, do not feel as if you must choose a design at this point. In the coming chapters, additional aspects of quantitative research are shared, and qualitative research is also covered. You may not be able to decide until you fully consider your topic and all the options.

## Nonexperimental Designs

**Nonexperimental designs**, sometimes referred to as **pre-experimental designs**, are used to describe or characterize phenomena, to examine relationships among variables, or to determine the reliability and validity of evaluations, tests, or equipment, and they often serve as precursors to later experimental or quasi-experimental studies. No variables are manipulated in nonexperimental studies. These designs are commonly used in healthcare where research often focuses on various forms of disability or illness, and the researchers only have access to participants after they have acquired the disability or illness. In these cases, causal relationships cannot be assumed, but insight into the condition and the response to treatments can be explored. The most common nonexperimental designs are reviewed here.

### Case-Control Designs

**Case-control designs** are retrospective studies of two groups of people—one group *with* and one group *without* the condition of interest. Medical history, environmental conditions, and other characteristics of both groups are analyzed to identify risk factors for the condition. See Box 4-10 for an example of a case-control design.

BOX 4-10 ■ Example of Case-Control Design

Currie et al. (2020) used a case-control design to determine factors associated with older adults' participation in balance training classes to prevent falls. The two study groups included older adults who attended the balance classes (experimental case) versus those who did not (control condition). Factors that prompted participation in the experimental cases were increasing age, being female, experiencing "near falls," and receiving targeted social marketing about the trainings (p. 908).

### Cross-Sectional Designs

**Cross-sectional designs** involve a one-time measurement of exposures and outcomes among the participants. For example, a researcher could investigate whether certain environmental factors or living in specific geographic locations (say, living in the Northern Hemisphere where there is less daylight for much of the year) impacts the prevalence of depression. Cross-sectional designs are cost-effective but cannot determine cause and effect or longitudinal changes. See Box 4-11 for an example of a cross-sectional design.

BOX 4-11 ■ Example of a Cross-Sectional Design

A cross-sectional design was used to determine the relationships between physical therapy students' academic and clinical success and a series of noncognitive traits, including grit, resilience, and mindset. Calo et al. (2022) analyzed cross-sectional questionnaires and academic transcripts and found that grit was a predictor of academic and clinical success.

### Correlational Designs

**Correlational designs** are similar to experimental ones in that a hypothesis is being tested; however, they differ in that independent variables are not manipulated, and a cause-effect relationship cannot be established. In correlational research, the researcher compares two or more variables and looks for a relationship between them. Rather than hypothesizing, for instance, that being blind will cause an individual to have heightened tactile sensitivity, one might conjecture that there is simply a relationship between the variables of blindness and heightened tactile sensitivity. Blindness has already occurred by the time the researcher is studying it, making this retrospective, nonexperimental research.

**BOX 4-12 ■ Example of Correlational Design**

A correlational study was conducted to see if there was a relationship between the physical activity level of individuals with spinal cord injury and their levels of pain, fatigue, and depression (Tawashy et al., 2009). High-intensity physical activity was strongly correlated with less fatigue ($r = -0.767$) and pain ($r = -0.612$) and increased self-efficacy ($r = 0.656$). Moreover, mild physical activity was correlated with fewer symptoms of depression ($r = -0.565$; p. 304). For negative $r$ values, the two attributes were inversely proportional, whereas for positive $r$ values, the two attributes were directly proportional.

**BOX 4-13 ■ Example of Quantitative Survey Design**

A survey was used to elicit occupational therapists' and midwives' perceptions of telehealth during the COVID-19 pandemic, including their perceived advantages and disadvantages of care offered via this method. The survey administered to the Switzerland-based practitioners garnered a 22.5% response rate and indicated that occupational therapists were significantly more positive about the use of telehealth than midwives (Klamroth-Marganska et al., 2021, p. 1).

In correlational research, specific statistical tests are used to find an association between two variables. This association, known as a correlation coefficient, yields a value between −1 and +1, where 0 indicates no relationship, and the two extremes indicate a perfect negative (or inverse) relationship (indicated by −1) or a perfect positive (or direct) relationship (indicated by +1). Since this is not experimental research, similar results should be replicated in many studies before healthcare practitioners can claim relationships between variables concerning their patients. Box 4-12 provides an example of a correlational design.

### Quantitative Survey Designs

**Quantitative survey designs** involve data collection via self-reporting from a sample of people to produce numerical data; surveys can be cross-sectional (at one point in time) or longitudinal (surveys of the same sample at multiple points in time). While a survey can be used as an outcome measure in experimental or quasi-experimental designs, the quantitative survey design discussed here involves no intervention, and no variables are manipulated. The purpose of the survey may be to determine the prevalence or distribution of disease or disability, to evaluate the circumstances or needs of a population, or to describe perceptions, values, behaviors, or other characteristics of a population.

This design uses a set of well-developed questions, grounded in literature and systematically evaluated for quality, to collect data via an interview (in-person, video, or phone) or a survey (on paper or electronic). Special attention is given to the sampling methods, mode of distribution, response rate, data analysis, and various quality dimensions, including accessibility, credibility, and relevance (Biemer, 2010; Fowler, 2014). Methods of sampling as well as designing quality survey questions are critically important in survey designs, and these topics are addressed in greater detail in Chapters 5 and 11. Several other texts also provide additional information on these topics (Fink, 2017; Fowler, 2014). Box 4-13 offers an example of a quantitative survey design.

### Instrument Validation Studies

Data collection tools for any of the previously mentioned study designs can include specific equipment (for example, a dynamometer to measure grip strength), tests, or other instruments (for example, a standardized commercially available assessment tool or an author-generated survey). Reasonable care should be taken to use valid and reliable tools to collect study data, because this can increase confidence in the study's results. **Instrument validation studies** are used to develop, test, refine, and validate data collection tools. These studies involve three basic phases:

1. Item development (identifying the primary focus of the tool, developing individual items or questions, using experts and the target population the tool will be used with to assess content validity)

2. Tool development (combining questions, administering the tool to a sample, and using the data to refine the items further)
3. Tool evaluation (completing additional analysis on the tool to further establish validity and reliability). For example, does the tool produce consistent results when repeated? Does the tool produce the expected results? Do results correlate with another test designed to measure the same construct? (Boateng et al., 2018)

The procedures to develop a standardized measure are labor-intensive and rigorous, and tools specific to your phenomenon of interest may not exist. As a result, author-generated instruments are often used to quantify phenomena and determine the impact of experimental interventions. While lack of time and resources may prompt the use of these self-made instruments, care should be taken, at a minimum, to involve experts in the topic and participants from the targeted population in item development and pilot testing. Even these less formal procedures can improve the quality of an author-generated measure. Ultimately, developing, testing, and refining sound standardized measures are critical to producing quality research that can be generalized to broader populations. An example of an instrument validation study appears in Box 4-14.

### BOX 4-14 ■ Example of Instrument Validation Study

Fraser and Precin (2022) conducted a study to validate the *Personal-Professional Development Tool* as a self-rating scale for occupational therapy students to identify professional goals and reflect on skill mastery after community-based service learning. At the time of their study, no validated measures existed for this purpose. The study explains how the items were developed and how the researchers completed initial validation via expert review and statistical analysis. Results indicate that 27 items had excellent content validity, and several other items were further refined related to initially lower content validity.

### TIPS & INSPIRATION

- **Continue** to review the literature on your topic with a critical eye. Did you find studies on your topic that employed various quantitative research designs? If so, those studies may provide insight into possible designs you could use to build on these prior inquiries. Consulting the *Conclusions* or *Future Research* sections of these studies may spark ideas.
- Some of the designs discussed in this chapter (for example, a randomized controlled trial) require large sample sizes, significant resources, and advanced skills to conduct. However, other simpler designs (for example, a one-group pretest-posttest design) can still effectively contribute to the body of knowledge in your areas of interest. Starting small may be the best way to address your topic and develop your inquiry skills.

## CHAPTER SUMMARY

1. Define quantitative research.
   - Quantitative research is a systematic process used to describe variables, examine relationships among variables, and determine cause and effect. Quantitative research results in numerical data.
2. Describe the prominent features of quantitative research, including manipulation, control, and randomization.
   - Manipulation is the varying or changing of a study's independent variable (treatment or intervention) to determine the effect on the dependent variable (the variable being measured).
   - Control is the ability to minimize or eliminate interfering or irrelevant factors that could influence study outcomes. Having both control and experimental groups is one method of control.
   - Randomization involves both random selection (selecting participants randomly so that every participant in a population of interest has an equal opportunity of being selected) and random assignment (assigning participants randomly to study groups). Randomization helps to decrease bias and improves internal and external validity.

*Continued*

3. Describe five common experimental designs.
   - Experimental designs involve manipulating at least one independent variable, a control group or conditions, and random assignment and selection.
   - Cause-and-effect relationships can only be ascertained with an experimental design.
   - The randomized controlled trial (RCT) is the most rigorous experimental design, and it can be used to determine the effectiveness of clinical treatments and interventions.
   - Other variations of experimental designs discussed include pretest-posttest design with follow-up, posttest-only design, Solomon four-group design, and factorial designs.
4. Describe four common quasi-experimental designs.
   - Basic quasi-experimental designs involve manipulating at least one independent variable, but they lack one or more of the following: a control group, random assignment, or random selection.
   - Time series designs, which lack a control group, are used to study the effects of a treatment or condition over time. Two variations of this design are the one-group pretest-posttest design and the repeated measures design.
   - Cohort designs, which include experimental and control groups, involve naturally occurring groups followed over time.
   - Quantitative case study designs (single-subject, single-case, multiple-case, case series [more than one case], or small-*N* studies) examine unique cases or situations in which the participant or intervention is unusual, little understood, or impractical to study under strict experimental conditions. These studies still involve manipulation of one or more variables.
5. Describe five common nonexperimental designs.
   - Nonexperimental designs (pre-experimental designs) are used to describe or characterize phenomena, examine relationships among variables, or determine the reliability and validity of instruments or equipment. No variables are manipulated in these designs.
   - Case-control designs are retrospective studies of two groups of people—one group *with* and one *without* the condition of interest. Data from both groups are analyzed to identify risk factors for the condition.
   - Cross-sectional designs are studies involving a one-time measurement of exposures and outcomes within the participants.
   - Correlational designs compare two or more variables and look for a relationship between them.
   - Quantitative survey designs involve numerical data collection via self-reporting from participants to determine the prevalence or distribution of disease or disability, evaluate the circumstances or needs of a population, or describe perceptions, values, behaviors, or other characteristics of a population.
   - Instrument validation studies are used to develop, test, refine, and validate data collection tools.

## TEST YOUR KNOWLEDGE

1. Which of the following BEST describes the primary purpose of quantitative research?
   a. To understand relationships among study variables
   b. To test hypotheses and describe variables through statistical analysis
   c. To explore the values and experiences of a specific group of people
   d. To gather rich narrative data through rigorous participant interviews
2. Which of the following describes the features of quantitative research that can impact rigor?
   a. Manipulation, randomization, and control
   b. Randomization, blinding, and control
   c. Manipulation, randomization, and analysis
   d. Control, randomization, and generalization
3. Which is the MOST rigorous quantitative research design?
   a. Solomon four-group design
   b. Time series design
   c. Randomized controlled trial
   d. 3 x 2 x 2 factorial design
4. Which of the following is TRUE for quasi-experimental designs?
   a. Quasi-experimental designs only involve one study group.
   b. Quasi-experimental designs have smaller sample sizes than experimental designs.
   c. Quasi-experimental designs can be used when there are ethical concerns with using a control group.
   d. Quasi-experimental designs should be avoided, if possible, due to lower rigor.

5. Which of the following is an example of nonexperimental research?
   a. A case study to explore a rare genetic disorder in children
   b. A study investigating the confidence of healthcare students after an exam prep course
   c. A study to determine the impact of two cardiac rehab programs on heart rates
   d. A study to validate a new data collection tool to assess caregiver burden
6. What is the BEST design to investigate a unique or unusual case?
   a. Case study design
   b. Time series design
   c. Case-control design
   d. Cohort design

Answer key appears at the end of this text.

## NEXT STEPS

1. Locate a randomized controlled trial (RCT) on a topic of interest. Identify the independent and dependent variables. Explain the elements of manipulation, control, and randomization relative to this study.
2. Identify a topic of interest that could be studied via a quantitative research design. Recall that quantitative research designs generate numerical data to determine cause-and-effect relationships, describe variables, or examine relationships among variables. What specific study design best aligns with your topic of interest and why? Consider advantages and disadvantages of this design in your justification.
3. Use the research notation described in this chapter to illustrate a quantitative design you might consider conducting. Identify the specific elements in your notation. For example, X represents what specific intervention?

## REFERENCES


Berg, K. E., & Latin, R. W. (2008). *Essentials of research methods in health, physical education, exercise science, and recreation* (3rd ed.). Lippincott Williams & Wilkins.

Biemer, P. P. (2010). Total survey error: Design, implementation, and evaluation. *Public Opinion Quarterly, 74*(5), 817–848. https://doi.org/10.1093/poq/nfq058

Boateng, G. O., Neilands, T. B., Frongillo, E. A., Melgar-Quiñonez, H. R., & Young, S. L. (2018). Best practices for developing and validating scales for health, social, and behavioral research: A primer. *Frontiers in Public Health, 6*, Article 149. https://doi.org/10.3389/fpubh.2018.00149

Bowen, D. J., Kreuter, M., Spring, B., Cofta-Woerpel, L., Linnan, L., Weiner, D., Bakken, S., Kaplan, C. P., Squiers, L., Fabrizio, C., & Fernandez, M. (2009). How we design feasibility studies. *American Journal of Preventive Medicine, 36*(5), 452–457. https://doi.org/10.1016/j.amepre.2009.02.002

Calo, M., Judd, B., Chipcase, L., Blackstock, F., & Peiris, C. L. (2022). Grit, resilience, mindset, and academic success in physical therapy students: A cross-sectional, multicenter study. *Physical Therapy, 102*(6), pzac038. https://doi.org/10.1093/ptj/pzac038

Campbell, D. T., & Stanley, J. C. (1969). *Experimental and quasi-experimental designs for research*. Rand McNally.

Cleland, J. A., Abbott, J. H., Kidd, M. O., Stockwell, S., Cheney, S., Gerrard, D. F., & Flynn, T. W. (2009). Manual physical therapy & exercise versus electrophysical agents and exercise in the management of plantar heel pain: A multicenter randomized clinical trial. *Journal of Orthopaedic & Sports Physical Therapy, 39*(8), 573–585. https://doi.org/10.2519/jospt.2009.3036

Currie, D. W., Thoreson, S. R., Clark, L., Goss, C. W., Marosits, M. J., & DiGuiseppi, C. G. (2020). Factors associated with older adults' enrollment in balance classes to prevent falls: Case-control study. *Journal of Applied Gerontology, 39*(8), 908–914. https://doi.org/10.1177/0733464818813022

Fathollahnejad, K., Letafatkar, A., & Hadadnezhad, M. (2019). The effect of manual therapy and stabilizing exercises on forward head and rounded shoulder postures: A six-week intervention with a one-month follow-up study. *BMC Musculoskeletal Disorders, 20*, Article 86. https://doi.org/10.1186/s12891-019-2438-y

Fink, A. (2017). *How to conduct surveys: A step-by-step guide* (6th ed.). SAGE Publications.

Fowler, F. J., Jr. (2014). *Survey research methods* (5th ed.). SAGE Publications.

Fraser, M., & Precin, P. (2022). Development and content validity of the Personal-Professional Development Tool for occupational therapy students during community-based service learning. *Journal of Occupational Therapy Education, 6*(4), Article 6. https://doi.org/10.26681/jote.2022.060406

Friedman, C., & VanPuymbrouck, L. (2021). Impact of occupational therapy education on students' disability attitudes: A longitudinal study. *American Journal of Occupational Therapy, 75*(4), 1–11. https://doi.org/10.5014/ajot.2021.047423

Gray, J. R., & Grove, S. K. (2021). *Burns & Grove's the practice of nursing research: Appraisal, synthesis, and generation of evidence* (9th ed.). Elsevier.

Herman, K. M., Hopman, W. M., & Craig, C. L. (2010). Are youth BMI and physical activity associated with better or worse than expected health-related quality of life in adulthood? The physical activity longitudinal study. *Quality of Life Research, 19*(3), 339–349. https://doi.org/10.1007/s11136-010-9586-8

Hunt, L. A., & Bassi, C. J. (2010). Near-vision acuity levels and performance on neuropsychological assessments used in occupational therapy. *American Journal of Occupational Therapy, 64*(1), 105–113. https://doi.org/10.5014/ajot.64.1.105

Klamroth-Marganska, V., Gemperle, M., Ballmer, T., Grylka-Baeschlin, S., Pehlke-Milde, J., & Gantschnig, B. E. (2021). Does therapy always need touch? A cross-sectional study among Switzerland-based occupational therapists and midwives regarding their experiences with health care at a distance during the COVID-19 pandemic in spring 2020. *BMC Health Services Research, 21*, Article 578. https://doi.org/10.1186/s12913-021-06527-9

Kumari, S., Joseph, J., & Singh, B. (2023). Nurse-led brief psychoeducation on self-stigma among clients with schizophrenia and affective disorders: Solomon four-group design. *Applied Nursing Research, 69,* 151657. https://doi.org/10.1016/j.apnr.2022.151657

Microsoft Corporation. (2021). *Microsoft Excel for Microsoft Office 365 MSO* (Version 2212) [Computer software]. https://office.microsoft.com/excel

Nwora, A. J., & Gee, B. M. (2009). A case study of a five-year-old child with pervasive developmental disorder–not otherwise specified using sound-based interventions. *Occupational Therapy International, 16*(1), 25–43. https://doi.org/10.1002/oti.263

Portney, L. G. (2020). *Foundations of clinical research: Applications to evidence-based practice* (4th ed.). F.A. Davis.

Sahraei, F., Rahemi, Z., Sadat, Z., Zamani, B., Ajorpaz, N. M., Afshar, M., & Mianehsaz, E. (2022). The effect of Swedish massage on pain in rheumatoid arthritis patients: A randomized controlled trial. *Complementary Therapies in Clinical Practice, 46,* 101524. https://doi.org/10.1016/j.ctcp.2021.101524

Sathian, B., Asim, M., Banerjee, I., Pizarro, A. B., Roy, B., van Teijlingen, E. R., do Nascimento, I. J. B., & Alhamad, H. K. (2020). Impact of COVID-19 on clinical trials and clinical research: A systematic review. *Nepal Journal of Epidemiology, 10*(3), 878–887. https://doi.org/10.3126/nje.v10i3.31622

Sun, M., Oliwa, T., Peek, M. E., & Tung, E. L. (2022). Negative patient descriptors: Documenting racial bias in the electronic medical record. *Health Affairs, 41*(2), 203–211. https://doi.org/10.1377/hlthaff.2021.01423

Tawashy, A., Eng, J., Lin, K., Tang, P., & Hung, C. (2009). Physical activity is related to lower levels of pain, fatigue and depression in individuals with spinal-cord injury: A correlational study. *Spinal Cord, 47*(4), 301–306. https://doi.org/10.1038/sc.2008.120

Thomas, J., & Hersen, M. (2011). *Understanding research in clinical and counseling psychology* (2nd ed.). Routledge.

Urbaniak, G. C., & Plous, S. (2013). *Research randomizer* (Version 4.0) [Computer software]. http://www.randomizer.org

Chapter 5

# Quantitative Research: Technical Aspects and Data Analysis

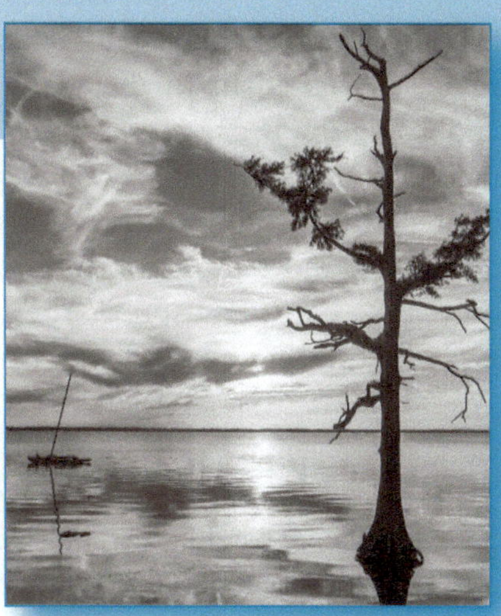

LEARNING OUTCOMES

*The information provided in this chapter will assist you to:*

5.1 Describe the most common sampling methods used in quantitative research.

5.2 Recall factors used to determine sample size in quantitative research.

5.3 Explain the most common data collection tools used in quantitative research.

5.4 Differentiate between descriptive and inferential statistics used in quantitative data analysis.

5.5 Identify the four types of data analyzed in quantitative data analysis.

5.6 Recognize the most common descriptive and inferential statistics.

## Technical Aspects of Quantitative Research

Whether you aim to design and conduct your own quantitative inquiry or to review and understand an existing quantitative research study, you should be familiar with several important technical design elements. These include sampling methods, data collection tools, and data analysis. Each of these topics is covered in greater depth here.

## Sampling Methods

Recall from Chapter 2 how a good inquiry question includes the population, intervention, and outcomes of interest. The **population of interest** is the broader group of people to which you might hope to generalize your results (for example, adults with multiple sclerosis). In an ideal scenario, you would involve all adults with multiple sclerosis worldwide in the inquiry to increase confidence in the results; however, this would be understandably impractical, inefficient, and costly. Therefore, sampling methods are employed. **Sampling** involves selecting a smaller subset of the population of interest to participate in the inquiry.

To begin, you must further specify the participant inclusion and exclusion criteria. **Participant inclusion criteria** consist of characteristics or traits that participants must have to qualify for participation in the inquiry (for example, age 40–60 years and working full time). In contrast, **participant exclusion criteria** consider undesirable features for participants (for example, residing more than 50 miles from the inquiry site or having impaired cognitive abilities that might impact participation in inquiry procedures). Next, you must decide where the participants will be recruited

Currituck Sound, Southern Shores, North Carolina.

from (for example, one large health system). **Recruitment**, discussed in further detail in Chapters 11 and 12, is the process of finding participants who meet the inclusion criteria. Participants could be recruited via flyers, online postings, mailings, or word of mouth, and recruitment decisions can be made only after consideration of the goals, geographic location, funding, and other logistics of the inquiry.

### TIPS & INSPIRATION

- If you plan to conduct an inquiry, ensure that your participant inclusion and exclusion criteria are not overly restrictive. If your criteria are too restrictive, you may not have enough participants for the inquiry or may have to extend the duration of the inquiry. It is important to proactively consider where participants will be recruited from and the projected number of participants that will be available based on the set criteria.

Even after identifying participant inclusion and exclusion criteria and when and how participants will be recruited, the population of interest may still be too large to reasonably manage with the time and resources available. For example, the population of interest might consist of 713 individuals with multiple sclerosis who work full time and were treated at one university hospital system; 200 of those individuals (a sample) could be selected to participate in an inquiry. There are two basic sampling methods—nonprobability sampling and probability sampling.

## Nonprobability Sampling

In **nonprobability sampling**, the participants are selected based on some other phenomena, such as location or convenience access, instead of being selected randomly. **Convenience sampling**, which involves using participants simply because they are available, is the most popular type of nonprobability sampling because it is the easiest and least expensive, and it is utilized when random selection or assignment of participants is unrealistic or unethical. In healthcare, researchers frequently conduct studies on patients they already have on their caseloads or those readily available in their facility. Using volunteers is also a common convenience sampling technique.

Convenience sampling is a practical sampling method if you are a novice researcher, although you should know its limitations. Because participants are not selected or assigned randomly, you cannot assume that the sample will accurately represent the population of interest, and the results may not be generalizable. In a case in which two study groups (experimental and control) are drawn from two different locations (for example, two different nursing facilities), you could match participants from both groups related to attributes important to the study (for example, gender, age, or diagnosis). **Matching** helps to ensure the study groups are similar based on the important attributes before any intervention is offered and therefore helps to decrease bias in the results. See Box 5-1 for an example of convenience sampling. Other types of nonprobability sampling are quota sampling, purposive sampling, and snowball sampling.

**Quota sampling** is the process of dividing the population of interest into two or more subgroups based on some characteristic. You then draw adequate samples from each subgroup to represent the proportion of this characteristic occurring naturally in the population of interest. This technique ensures that the characteristic in question is equally represented in the population and the chosen sample. For example, if you are interested in studying ambulation of seniors in a skilled nursing facility, you would likely want more female participants than male participants because census information reveals more females residing in these facilities. In this case, the desired quota for each subgroup is determined, and

### BOX 5-1 ■ Example of Convenience Sampling

In a study of the effects of educating clients and caregivers on health-promoting behaviors, participants were recruited from two hemodialysis centers in Iran. Even though the sample was one of convenience, the researchers took additional steps to decrease bias. The client-caregiver pairs were randomized to one of four study groups and matched to limit the effects of other characteristics (Hayati et al., 2023).

then participants are selected until the quotas are reached.

**Purposive sampling** involves selecting participants based on specific attributes, such as their diagnoses, motivational level, or perceived compliance. The purpose of the research can dictate selection of a very specific sample, hence the name of this technique. Finally, **snowball sampling**, also known as referral sampling or chain sampling, involves selecting a small number of participants who meet the study criteria; these participants then refer others who also meet the same criteria. The process continues until a sufficient sample is achieved. This technique helps identify participants who might otherwise be inaccessible. Examples include participants with a rare disease, those involved in illicit activity, or members of distinct networks or social groups.

### Probability Sampling

**Probability sampling** is a sampling method that ensures all members of the population of interest have an equal chance of being selected for the sample. **Simple random sampling** is one of the most popular types of probability sampling. Recall from Chapter 4 that random selection involves compiling an exhaustive list of participants that meet the inquiry's inclusion criteria and then randomly selecting the sample from this list. Random sampling increases the likelihood that the inquiry results will be similar to those found if the entire population had been studied.

Other types of probability sampling include stratified random sampling, systematic random sampling, and cluster sampling. **Stratified random sampling** involves dividing the population into homogeneous subgroups and then randomly sampling each subgroup. This technique ensures that each subgroup is adequately represented in the sample. This type of sampling is similar to the quota sampling discussed earlier in that each technique involves dividing the population based on a particular attribute. However, in stratified random sampling, the sample from each subgroup is drawn randomly, but in quota sampling, they are not.

**Systematic random sampling** involves randomly ordering all possible participants and then selecting every *n*th one for participation. You must consider the total number of participants needed for your inquiry (for example, 25) divided by the available participants in your population (say 100). This means you need 25% of the population for your sample. Selecting every fourth participant in the random list of the 100-participant population will accomplish your goal.

**Cluster sampling** is useful when your population is spread out geographically. In this case, it is beneficial to divide the population into smaller clusters, which will then be randomly sampled. This is especially useful if you must be physically present to conduct assessments or interventions with the participants. Finally, **multistage cluster sampling** involves sequential stages of cluster sampling to narrow the final sample further. Portney's (2020) *Foundations of Clinical Research: Applications to Practice* provides further details on the sampling techniques if you need more information.

#### TIPS & INSPIRATION

- To better understand sampling methods in quantitative inquiry, search the literature for quantitative studies in your discipline or practice area. What types of sampling were used, and how might those methods have impacted the results? Reviewing actual studies that employed various probability and nonprobability sampling methods discussed in this chapter can help you understand the process and implications of each.
- You may be drawn to the probability sampling methods because of their increased rigor, but nonprobability sampling is quite common and often appropriate for inquiries in healthcare settings. It is most important to understand the sampling method used, and how it might impact the outcomes and the ability to generalize them.

## Sample Size

Ideally, a sample should accurately represent the population of interest from which it was drawn, thereby allowing you to generalize the results found in the sample to the population. If the sample is too small or is not randomly chosen or assigned, the sample may not reflect the larger population. If the sample is too large, the data collection and analysis could be cumbersome. The sample size can be justified by one or more of the following: purpose of the inquiry, logistics of the inquiry, or a statistical analysis. Although studies with smaller samples may face criticism, using larger samples does not necessarily translate into more accurate results.

Depending on the purpose of an inquiry, drawing a sample may not be necessary; instead, all participants meeting the criteria can be included. For example, if you want to explore the efficacy of practices and policies within a specific health system, you could use all individuals treated there as participants. Although these results may not be generalizable to other health systems, this is not problematic if you only want to gain knowledge on the practices in one system.

Financial resources, the availability of space and equipment, your time and skills, and other logistical circumstances often dictate the sample size; as noted previously, convenience samples are common in healthcare research. How the participants are recruited, sampled, and assigned to inquiry groups must also be considered. Smaller samples may be appropriate, depending on the inquiry's goals, and they are often employed in pilot studies or by novice researchers.

Finally, in quantitative inquiries, two statistical concepts can justify a sample size—the confidence interval and the confidence level. The **confidence interval**, or margin of error, represents a range of values that likely includes the scores or responses of the population. For example, if the margin of error is 5, and 50% of an inquiry sample responds favorably to a new treatment, you can have confidence that if you tested the entire population of interest, 45% to 55% would also respond favorably. The **confidence level** represents the certainty you have that the scores or responses of the population would fall within this range. Confidence levels of 95% or 99% are typically chosen, indicating that you are either 95% or 99% confident that the scores or responses will fall within the margin of error. Once you have determined the size of your population, the confidence interval, and the confidence level, a statistical program or a statistician can help you determine the appropriate sample size.

### TIPS & INSPIRATION

- **Remember** that a larger sample size does not necessarily equate to more accurate, generalizable results. Well-designed inquiries with smaller samples can contribute valuable information to your profession, facility, and clients. If you are new to quantitative inquiry, this may be just the place to start.

## Data Collection Tools

**Data collection** is the process of gathering or measuring inquiry outcomes, and various tools can be used, depending on the inquiry's purpose and design. While this chapter focuses on quantitative inquiry, some of these tools may also be appropriate for qualitative inquiries, and they are discussed further in Chapter 8. Quantitative data collection tools can include the following:

1. Observation
2. Surveys and interviews
3. Record review
4. Equipment
5. Assessments

### Observation

As the name implies, **observation** involves watching human participants or video recordings of participants or events. In quantitative inquiry, the method for recording observations should be formalized in advance, and the raters (or observers) should be well trained. Rather than being asked to observe and record subjective items such as *dependence* or *enjoyment*, raters should be given objective criteria believed to represent those subjective items. For example, *dependence* may be represented by the number of times a participant asks for assistance, and *enjoyment* may be represented by the number of smiles, laughs, or verbal statements that indicate happiness. Raters should be provided with a protocol that defines the items to be observed and the method for recording those items. Observations may be used with any quantitative design and are commonly used with other data collection tools.

You should take additional steps to promote reliability of the observations. Before an inquiry begins, videos are useful to train raters. A rater can record observations from the training video, and you can check the observations until you are satisfied that the rater is making correct and reliable observations. This procedure ensures **intrarater reliability**, or the degree to which a rater is consistent in their ratings. If there are multiple raters in an inquiry, you should confirm **interrater reliability**, which means the raters are checked against one another to ensure that the same observations are made regardless of the rater. Objective observations are made until all raters score similarly and you have confidence, evidenced by statistics, that all raters will rate consistently well. Consistency among raters is critical to protecting the internal validity of the inquiry.

## Surveys and Interviews

Surveys and interviews, discussed together here, involve a set of well-developed questions, grounded in literature and systematically evaluated for quality, used to collect data. Only the data collection method varies; surveys can be completed on paper or electronically, whereas interviews are completed in person, via video, or by phone. When developing survey or interview questions, researchers should give prime consideration to the participants' language style and idiom, which may differ from the researcher's. It is especially important to avoid abbreviations, professional jargon, vaguely worded questions, and those with biased wording or tone (Fowler, 2014). Chapter 11 provides additional guidance on constructing and organizing survey and interview questions.

**Interviewing**, via phone, video, or in person, can be advantageous for clarifying responses to questions and gaining a greater understanding of the topic being studied. Interviews conducted in person or via video are more intimate, allowing the interviewer to physically see the interviewee. This direct interaction helps develop rapport and may be necessary for exploring sensitive issues. Additionally, the interviewer has a chance to "read" the nonverbal cues given by the interviewee. For example, facial expressions may indicate confusion or lack of understanding, so a question can be rephrased. Awareness of cultural norms that impact nonverbal communication is also important. For example, in some cultures, direct eye contact is viewed positively as a sign of connection, but for others, it is disrespectful. One challenge with data obtained from interviews is that it is difficult to know whether participants are telling the truth or trying to impress the interviewer by saying what they think the interviewer wants to hear. Participants may also be embarrassed or ashamed to tell the truth about sensitive issues. Experienced interviewers can learn to read nonverbal cues to determine the degree of truthfulness in answers.

The disadvantage of in-person interviews is the effort required to set up the interview, including contacting participants, arranging mutually convenient times and locations, and traveling. Phone interviewing eliminates these concerns, but the personal contact and the chance to observe nonverbal cues are lost. Also, it is easier for a participant to refuse an interview on the phone. Video interviewing may provide the best of both worlds but could present technological challenges because the interviewer and interviewee must have adequate hardware and software and the skills to operate them effectively.

Interview formats may be structured or unstructured, though structured interviews are much more common in quantitative research. In structured interviews, the same questions are asked in the same order. Although this format may appear stilted and formal, it is less complicated for an inexperienced interviewer or novice researcher; the answers are easier to compare from one participant to another, and data are easily tabulated and analyzed.

**Surveys** are more efficient and cost-effective than interviews for gathering data from larger groups of people. They can be mailed or emailed to respondents, completed electronically via survey software such as SurveyMonkey, Qualtrics, or Microsoft Forms, or hand-delivered to respondents for completion. For example, a survey could be administered immediately after some intervention or education to assess perceptions of the intervention or knowledge gained. For surveys completed without the researcher present, the instructions and questions must be clear and unambiguous because there is no opportunity for clarification.

Another concern with surveys is the **response rate**, defined as the number of surveys returned divided by the total number in the sample. A low response rate may introduce **sampling or nonresponse bias**, meaning that if those who did not respond to the survey are fundamentally different (related to the variables of interest in the inquiry) from those who did respond, the results may be skewed. However, no standard acceptable response rate exists (Fowler, 2014; Morton et al., 2012). Generally, response rates average between 20% and 30%; a response rate below 10% may be considered poor, and those greater than 50% are often deemed very good (Carpenter, 2023; SurveyMonkey, 2023). Some argue that a high response rate does not always equate to high validity. To make a proper assessment of inquiry quality, the method of recruitment, a description of the differences between responders and nonresponders, the strategies used to improve the response rate, and how the response rate was calculated should all be reported in addition to the response rate itself (Morton et al., 2012). Electronic survey distribution is now the most common of all methods, likely due to technological advances. Research indicates greater response rates with electronic surveys compared to other methods of distribution (Holtom et al., 2022).

The type of survey and method of distribution can affect the response rate, but the rate can also be negatively impacted when surveys are returned incomplete and must be removed from the sample being analyzed. Conversely, response rates are likely to be higher if the sample has some vested interest in the topic of the inquiry. Some additional strategies can be used to improve the response rate:

- Clearly outline the purpose of the survey and the expected time to complete it within the survey's introduction or cover letter. Grab the respondent's attention by telling them why it is important that they complete the survey and how the information will be used.
- Offer an incentive for completion. Some examples are a small gift, access to educational content, or entry into a drawing for a gift card.
- Use clear and concise wording for all surveys, including avoiding abbreviations and professional jargon.
- Pilot the survey before the inquiry begins to identify any limitations in the question wording or organization. This will help identify questions that may confuse respondents, increase the accuracy of information gained from the survey, and determine if the delivery method and completion time are appropriate for the inquiry goals.
- Consider the survey's length and the type of questions included. If the survey is too long or requires too many open-ended responses, a participant may not complete the survey. For electronic surveys, including a progress bar to indicate the percentage of the survey remaining can be helpful. Research reveals that the ideal survey length is 10 minutes, and the maximum should be no longer than 20 minutes to ensure quality responses (Revilla & Ochoa, 2017). Other sources estimate that the time respondents will devote to electronic surveys is between 7 and 8 minutes, with respondents abandoning the survey or "satisficing" (speeding) through the survey if it takes longer (Chudoba, 2023).
- Provide a deadline for survey completion and reminders if necessary. Research shows that recipients rarely return surveys via mail after 2 weeks, and approximately 90% of responses for electronic surveys are received within the first 3 days of the invitation (Walonick, 2010).
- Enclose a stamped, self-addressed envelope if the survey is to be mailed back. Respondents may not make an effort to locate and address an envelope and may resent having to pay postage.

### Record Review

Review of written records is an appropriate data collection method for quantitative inquiry. Records can corroborate your observations or what you find during interviews, raise valuable questions, and shape future directions of an inquiry. They can also provide historical, demographic, and sometimes personal information unavailable from other sources.

Written documents may include patients' medical records, minutes of meetings and case conferences, letters, speeches, articles, books, diaries, graffiti, notes, membership lists, newsletters, newspapers, and illustrations. Artifacts may include physical materials such as adaptive equipment, adapted clothing, photographs, audio and video recordings, and films. One way to obtain written materials is to ask participants to keep diaries, journals, or other records. Collaboration with healthcare practitioners might be necessary so that clinical notes simultaneously meet the healthcare facility's and the inquiry's needs. For example, if you are interested in patient satisfaction with healthcare services, you might be able to design a patient satisfaction survey that could simultaneously provide the healthcare facility with useful information and meet the needs of your inquiry.

Records used as inquiry data are divided into primary and secondary sources. **Primary sources** are first-hand accounts about the topic under review, such as autobiographies or eyewitness accounts; **secondary sources** are accounts written on the topic by others that are not based on personal experiences, such as medical records (which are written by clinicians and not by the patients having the experience). It is important to verify both the truth about the writing of the documents (did this person actually write it?) and the truth about the content of the documents (did this actually happen?). Box 4-2 provides an example of medical records for data collection.

### Equipment

Many inquiries performed by healthcare practitioners involve using equipment or testing instruments to measure physiological functions or outcomes. For example, a scale can record weight, or a goniometer can measure joint range of motion. Other examples include fitness trackers, spirometers, electroencephalographs, dynamometers, pinch meters, pedometers, heart rate monitors, digital calipers, volumeters, pulse oximeters, and ultrasound imaging. These objective measures are desirable in experimental inquiries as they are usually valid and reliable for measuring dependent variables. However, you should always review the manufacturer's specifications and settings to ensure the equipment is calibrated and in good working order. Unfortunately, many variables cannot be measured with equipment, and other means must be found to define and quantify them. These other means are assessments, also called tests or measures, which are discussed next.

### Assessments

Assessments can be standardized or non-standardized. **Standardized assessments** have been subject to **normalizing**, a process that establishes validity and reliability in relation to the "normal" population, whereas **non-standardized assessments** have not undergone such rigorous testing. Assessments are routinely used in healthcare to assess and measure patient outcomes and those associated with research or quality improvement. Many standardized assessments exist to measure variables, including psychological factors, functional performance of daily tasks, cognitive abilities, perceptual motor skills, child developmental stages, prevocational skills, vocational interests, personality factors, attitudes, and values. A standardized assessment should always be considered if one is available to measure the phenomenon of interest. A number of authors and organizations have compiled collections of assessments for ease of review and consideration. Some of these collective works appear in Table 5-1. Websites for professional organizations and major assessment publishers are also good resources for lists of assessments. An assessment's purpose, procedures, reliability, and validity should be reviewed to determine possible alignment with your purposes.

If no standardized assessment exists to gather the exact information you are interested in, you will probably need to design your own. Designing valid and reliable assessments is a detailed and time-consuming process beyond this text's scope. For more information on best practices in assessment development, see Boateng et al.'s (2018) article "Best Practices for Developing and Validating Scales for Health, Social, and Behavioral Research: A Primer."

#### TIPS & INSPIRATION

- If you plan to conduct a quantitative inquiry, look at other studies on your topic and outcome of interest. How were the outcomes assessed or measured in the existing literature? Reviewing the data collection tools in existing inquiries can be extremely helpful in choosing a valid and reliable tool for your inquiry. More information about reliability and validity in quantitative inquiries can be found in Chapter 6. Additional considerations in choosing a data collection tool are provided in Chapter 11.

**TABLE 5-1 ■ Collections of Assessments**

| Discipline | Author/Year | Title of Collection | Publication Information |
|---|---|---|---|
| Physical therapy | American Physical Therapy Association (2023) | *Tests and measures* | Available at https://www.apta.org/patient-care/evidence-based-practice-resources/test-measures |
| Occupational therapy | Asher (2014) | *Occupational therapy assessment tools: An annotated index* (4th ed.) | Available from AOTA Press. |
| Recreation therapy and related fields | Burlingame & Blaschko (2009) | *Assessment tools for recreational therapy and related fields* (4th ed.) | Available from Idyll Arbor. |
| Allied health professions | Fischer et al. (2020) | *Measures for clinical practice and research* (6th ed., Vols. 1 and 2) | Available from Oxford University Press. |

## Quantitative Data Analysis

**Data analysis** is the process of organizing and transforming data collected during an inquiry to make meaning of it. This process could allow you to discover new information, draw conclusions, or describe or understand relationships among phenomena of interest. Quantitative analysis involves use of statistical tests and processing of numerical data. Completing data analysis or even understanding the data analysis section of an existing published article can be intimidating. The rest of this chapter offers clear descriptions and examples of the most common statistical tests with the dual aim of helping you understand existing research and determine what statistics you might use if you are completing your own inquiry. Details about specific calculations or how to use statistical software are beyond the scope of this text. Even experienced researchers may solicit help from a statistician, and you may consider this if you are engaging in your own inquiry.

A statistician should be consulted in the design stage of the inquiry while the methodology and data collection measures are being determined. Once you identify your topic of interest, a statistician can ensure selection of the most appropriate inquiry design for your purpose, and can make recommendations regarding sample size, blinding, randomization, structure and timing of the therapeutic interventions, and coding of data (American Statistical Association, 2013). A statistician can also help determine which statistical tests are best suited for data analysis and advise on how many participants are needed to use the chosen tests. Consulting a statistician has a price, but most people who have hired one feel they are worth the cost. You may be fortunate enough to be connected to a university or other facility that employs a statistician willing to help free of charge or for a nominal fee. The *American Statistical Association* (https://www.amstat.org) or the *International Statistical Institute* (https://www.isi-web.org) can provide additional information about hiring a statistician.

### Descriptive Versus Inferential Statistics

Statistics are divided into two categories: descriptive and inferential statistics. **Descriptive statistics** describe, organize, and summarize numerical data. They include frequencies, percentages, measures of central tendency (mean, median, mode), and measures of variation (range, standard deviation). These procedures allow for description of all the individual scores in a sample on one variable by using one or two numbers, such as the mean and standard deviation. They can be used to describe each dependent variable, such as the percentage and mean of each item physical therapists checked off on a list of reasons for moving into supervisory positions and their ages when they moved. Descriptive statistics can also give the variation or spread of scores within each group studied, such as the mean and range of scores for experimental and control groups in a study on a new treatment technique for carpal tunnel syndrome. Descriptive statistics are commonly used by those new to the inquiry process or those undertaking small-scale projects as part of initial research, evidence-based practice, or capstone courses.

**Inferential statistics** are used to test a hypothesis or to make inferences about the population from the sample findings. A sufficient number of participants are needed in the sample to be able to do this; in addition, random selection should be used. If an inquiry involves few participants and lacks randomization, descriptive statistics are probably the best choice. Examples of inferential statistics are the *t* test, the ANOVA, and the Wilcoxon signed rank test; these tests result in probability statements that help you draw conclusions about differences or relationships between groups. For example, if a difference is found between the mean scores of two groups (experimental and control) at the end of an inquiry, inferential statistics can help you determine whether that difference is likely due to the experimental intervention provided or to chance alone. Inferential statistics can also indicate if the results of your inquiry can be reasonably generalized to the population from which your sample was taken. Both descriptive and inferential statistics can be used in the same inquiry, if appropriate. Descriptive statistical methods are the same regardless of the type of data being used; however, inferential statistical methods vary according to the type of data used.

### TIPS & INSPIRATION

- If you find statistics challenging, know that you are not alone. At this point, just focus on understanding the distinct purpose of descriptive versus inferential statistics and the most common types of each. This will be especially important as you read existing literature on your topic and contemplate the implications of the findings.

## Types of Data

Data are classified into four levels or scales of measurement: nominal, ordinal, interval, and ratio. Each data type builds on the characteristics of those previously described.

### Nominal Data

**Nominal data** are the numbers applied to nonnumerical variables; for example, a group of people's disabilities could be coded as follows: right hemiplegia = 1, left hemiplegia = 2, paraplegia = 3, and so on. Each data category must be mutually exclusive, meaning no individual or variable can be assigned to more than one group. There is no ordered relationship between categories, meaning that one category cannot be considered to come before or after another category. This type of data is sometimes referred to as *discrete* as opposed to *continuous*. For discrete data, there is no limit to the number of categories that can be included. In contrast, with continuous data, there are infinite possible values along a continuum. Because there is no numerical value for categories of nominal data, they cannot be meaningfully added, subtracted, multiplied, or divided. One cannot calculate an average (mean) disability, for example. Examples of categories might include male and female; inpatient, outpatient, and day treatment settings; and patients with schizophrenia, bipolar disease, or depression. A nominal scale may also be used to code "yes" or "no" responses on a survey.

### Ordinal Data

**Ordinal data** are numbers that are still discrete but are ordered; however, the intervals between the categories are unknown and cannot be assumed to be equal. In contrast to nominal data, to which numbers are arbitrarily assigned, numbers assigned to groups of ordinal data signify a rank order or meaningful sequence. For instance, a review committee may rank-order a series of program proposals and assign first, second, and third place, but the top-ranked proposal may be considerably better than the ones ranked second and third, whereas the ones ranked fourth, fifth, and sixth may be similar to each other in quality. These differences among intervals are not reflected in the numerical assignment. Other examples would be ratings on a Likert scale such as "Strongly agree," "Agree," "Neutral," "Disagree," "Strongly disagree," or classifications for client ability such as "Dependent," "Needs partial assistance," "Independent." An ordinal data scale indicates a greater or lesser degree of something or reflects a "precedes" or "superior" concept.

### Interval Data

**Interval data** are also ordered in a logical sequence. However, the intervals between the numbers are considered equal and represent actual amounts. These are continuous data. Examples are intelligence scores, degrees of temperature, and magnitude rating scales. Items are ordered on a continuum; however, there is no zero starting point. For example, temperatures can fall below zero, or participants can be asked to rate the magnitude of a particular stimulus on a 1 to 10 scale, where the intervals are assumed to be equal.

### Ratio Data

**Ratio data** are also continuous numbers with equal intervals between them, but unlike interval data, they have a meaningful zero point. In other words, the zero point indicates a total absence of the ability or property being measured. For instance, there can legitimately be zero range of motion or visual acuity. Other examples of ratio data include time, weight, and income. Ratio data can be multiplied and divided to reveal proportions. For example, if a goniometer is used to measure elbow extension in a child with cerebral palsy, and the right elbow is measured at 160 degrees of extension and the left elbow is measured at 80 degrees of extension, one could report that the right elbow extends twice as far as the left.

As you can see, each data type builds on the previously described characteristics. Nominal data are separated into categories; with ordinal data, these categories can be rank-ordered; with interval data, the values between categories are equal, but there is no zero starting point; and finally, with ratio data, a real zero point exists. In healthcare research, ratio data are the most common type.

### Parametric and Nonparametric Data

Interval and ratio data are **parametric data**, whereas nominal and ordinal data are **nonparametric data**. This distinction is important because different statistics are appropriate for parametric and nonparametric data. Although most descriptive statistics can be used with both parametric and nonparametric data (the exception being that the mean and standard deviation cannot be used on nominal data), different inferential statistics must be used with the two data types. This is due to the properties of the data, such as the data being ordered or the intervals between numbers being equal. Some tests are not powerful enough to cope with unordered, unequal data, whereas others are. Table 5-2 summarizes the categories of data with their corresponding parametric and nonparametric classifications and types of appropriate statistical tests.

**Parametric tests** are appropriate when:

1. The sample is randomly selected, thereby helping to ensure the sample is representative of the population of interest and that the variables being measured fall within the normal distribution for that population.
2. Variables are measured in a manner that generates interval or ratio data.
3. Random assignment or matching of inquiry groups is completed to ensure similarity between the two groups.

Conversely, **nonparametric tests** should be used when:

1. Random selection has not occurred, so the sample is not considered representative of the population of interest, and variables are probably not normally distributed.
2. Variables have been measured in a manner that generates nominal or ordinal data.
3. The number of participants in the sample is small.

Because nonparametric tests have less statistical power, substantial differences must be found between sets of scores before those differences are considered meaningful. Nonparametric statistics are frequently used in healthcare research because pathological human conditions are being studied. The variables of illness or pathology are often not distributed normally in the target population. Also, locating many participants with the requisite pathology is often difficult, so samples tend to be smaller.

**TABLE 5-2 ■ Categories of Data With Corresponding Classifications and Statistical Tests**

| Category of Data | Classification | Appropriate Descriptive Statistics | Appropriate Inferential Statistics |
|---|---|---|---|
| **Nominal**<br>(named categories; unordered) | Nonparametric | ■ Frequencies<br>■ Percentages<br>■ Mode | ■ Pearson's chi-square<br>■ Fisher's exact<br>■ Goodman and Kruskal's tau b |
| **Ordinal**<br>(ordered categories; unequal intervals) | Nonparametric | ■ Frequencies<br>■ Percentages<br>■ Mode<br>■ Median | ■ Pearson's chi-square<br>■ Spearman rho<br>■ Wilcoxon rank sum<br>■ Mann-Whitney<br>■ Kruskal-Wallis<br>■ Kendall's tau |
| **Interval**<br>(ordered data; equal intervals; no zero starting point) | Parametric | ■ Frequencies<br>■ Percentages<br>■ Mean<br>■ Median<br>■ Mode<br>■ Range<br>■ Standard deviation | ■ *t* test<br>■ Analysis of variance (ANOVA)<br>■ Analysis of covariance (ANCOVA) |
| **Ratio**<br>(equal intervals with zero point) | Parametric | ■ Frequencies<br>■ Percentages<br>■ Mean<br>■ Median<br>■ Mode<br>■ Range<br>■ Standard deviation | ■ *t* test<br>■ Analysis of variance (ANOVA)<br>■ Pearson product-moment correlation |

### TIPS & INSPIRATION

- If your topic of interest can be explored quantitatively, consider the type of data generated (nominal, ordinal, interval, or ratio). After identifying the type of data, use Table 5-2 to determine appropriate descriptive and inferential statistics.

## Descriptive Statistics

Descriptive statistics involves analysis of numerical data to summarize or describe the inquiry sample and outcomes. Data from quasi-experimental and nonexperimental inquiries are often analyzed, at least in part, with descriptive statistics. Since these designs may lack manipulation, randomization, or control, it is difficult or inappropriate to make inferences from a sample to a population of interest (the purpose of inferential statistics) if these criteria are not met. Descriptive statistics can include frequencies and percentages, measures of central tendency, and measures of variation, which are discussed next.

### Frequencies and Percentages

Frequencies and percentages can describe a sample or their responses. **Frequency** is the number of times a specific variable or response occurs in a data set. For example, in a sample of 46 participants, the frequency or count of participants who reported feeling stressed at work was 35. The **percentage** is calculated by dividing the frequency (35 participants who reported stress) by the total scores or sample (46 participants) multiplied by 100 (76% of the sample reported stressful feelings). Percentages are often preferred because they account for the total number of scores and reflect the magnitude of the frequency. For example, if 35/46 participants were

### BOX 5-2 ■ Calculation of Percent Change

**Calculation:**

[(After score - Before score) / Before score] × 100 = Percent change

**Example:**

[(19 - 28) / 28] × 100 = -32.14%

stressed (76%), that is quite different than if 35/157 participants were stressed (22%). In both cases, 35 participants reported feeling stressed, but the former example is a much larger portion of the total. In some cases, it may also be helpful to report the **percent change** or the percentage of increase or decrease from one score to another. Using the prior example, if a participant's stress levels were assessed before and after an 8-week stress reduction program, you could report the percent change between their before score (28/40) and their after score (19/40). This calculation is illustrated in Box 5-2. Negative numbers indicate decreases in scores, and positive numbers indicate increases. In this example, the participant's reported stress score decreased by 32.41%.

### Measures of Central Tendency

**Central tendency** is a single average value that describes a set of data. The three measures of central tendency are the mean, median, and mode. The **mean**, commonly referred to as the average, is computed by adding all the scores and dividing by the total number in the group. The **median** is the midpoint among all the scores. Each score must be listed from the highest to the lowest, or vice versa, to locate the score that falls in the center. For example, a ranked order of IQ scores might be as follows: 150, 100, 98, 75, and 50. The median would be 98 because that score falls in the middle. For lists with an even number of scores, the protocol is to average the two middle-most scores. Finally, the **mode** is the most commonly occurring score or answer. For instance, in an inquiry on employment status and quality of life, participants could be asked if they are employed full time, part time, or are unemployed. If most respondents indicated they are employed full time, this category would be the mode. It is also possible for there to be more than one mode (bimodal)—say, if equal numbers of participants were employed full time and part time. Each measure of central tendency has advantages, and use is typically dictated by the type of data being analyzed. Salkind (2017) provides some additional guidelines:

- Use the mode when you have nominal data, namely, data arranged in mutually exclusive categories.
- Use the median when your set of scores includes several outliers that will skew the mean.
- Use the mean when you have interval or ratio data that does not include outliers. (pp. 74–75)

### Measures of Variation

**Measures of variation**, which describe the spread or variability of scores, include the range and standard deviation. The **range** is the simplest and is calculated by subtracting the lowest score in the set from the highest score. In essence, a range explains the continuum in which the participants scored, perhaps IQ scores from 90 to 120, resulting in a range of 30. The range could have practical implications as in the following scenario: You are asked to conduct a therapeutic intervention on Monday for a class of 7-year-olds with a mean IQ of 100 whose scores ranged from 90 to 110; on Tuesday, you are scheduled to conduct the same intervention with a group of 7-year-olds with a mean IQ of 100 whose scores ranged from 60 to 120. In the second group, you might need more assistance or have to structure the session differently to meet the needs of children with a wider array of cognitive abilities. The **standard deviation** indicates how the scores are grouped around the mean. A small standard deviation indicates scores clustered close to the mean, whereas a larger standard deviation denotes a wider spread in scores. The standard deviation can also determine consistency of a particular variable; a standard deviation of zero signifies no variability.

## Inferential Statistics

**Inferential statistics** are used to draw conclusions or make inferences about the population of interest from a smaller chosen sample, or to determine the probability of phenomena observed in a sample occurring in the larger population from which the sample was drawn. Inferential statistics can be divided into three groups:

1. Tests of statistical significance
2. Tests of correlation
3. Tests of comparison

### Tests of Statistical Significance

**Statistical significance** refers to outcomes attributed to a specific cause or intervention rather than chance alone. For example, in a classic experimental design where one group (experimental) receives an experimental treatment and another group (control) does not, tests of statistical significance would allow you to decide whether changes in the posttest scores between the groups are statistically significant—meaning changes can be attributed to the treatment rather than to chance.

Significance testing is based on the laws of probability. It answers the questions: What is the probability that this change occurred because of events in the inquiry, and what is the probability that this change would have occurred anyway, by chance? Tests of statistical significance result in a **confidence level**, which represents the probability you have that the scores or responses are not a chance occurrence.

Typically, in the social sciences, 5 out of 100 occurrences of a phenomenon being caused by chance is a reasonable number to accept, and any result better than that is statistically significant. This result would imply that you are 95% certain that the treatment caused the improvement in posttest scores of the experimental group. The confidence level (or probability level) is expressed as $p \leq 0.05$. Some scientific endeavors require more stringent proof, and a standard of $p \leq 0.01$, or a 1 in 100 chance that the phenomenon occurred by chance, is set for those inquiries, otherwise known as a 99% success rate. Ultimately, it is up to the researchers to determine the acceptable significance level for their inquiry. See Box 5-3 for an example of statistical significance in an experimental design.

The four most common tests of statistical significance—the Pearson's chi-square test, the *t* test, the Wilcoxon rank test, and the Mann-Whitney test—are reviewed next.

**BOX 5-3 ■ Example of Statistical Significance in an Experimental Design**

Researchers were interested in the effects of Swedish massage on pain in patients with rheumatoid arthritis. In their randomized controlled trial, 60 patients were randomized into two groups: one that received Swedish massage for 8 weeks and one that received routine care for the same duration.

Chi-square tests were completed initially and revealed no significant differences between the groups at baseline. Analysis of covariance (ANCOVA) was used to compare the two groups postintervention. Results indicate that the Swedish massage group demonstrated significantly less severity of pain than the control group ($p = 0.01$), leading to the conclusion that Swedish massage is effective for pain reduction in this population (Sahraei et al., 2022).

#### *Pearson's Chi-Square Test*

**Pearson's chi-square test** ($X^2$), used with nominal and ordinal categorical data, is appropriate to determine if differences between observed and expected results of an inquiry are statistically significant, or if two groups (experimental and control) have similar characteristics. The chi-square can compare groups on a single variable or on multiple variables, one at a time, for characteristics such as gender, age, or diagnosis. The calculated value for the chi-square is evaluated using standardized tables that list critical values. When the chi-square exceeds the table value, the hypothesis is supported. In the case of Sahraei et al.'s (2022) study (Box 5-3) on the impact of Swedish massage on pain, chi-square tests were used to compare the study groups on the characteristics of gender, educational level, marital status, and occupational status. No significant differences were noted among the groups at baseline.

#### *t Test*

The paired or unpaired *t* tests, used with interval or ratio data, are appropriate to compare the mean scores of two groups to determine if there is a statistically significant difference. The **paired samples**

## BOX 5-4 ■ Example of *t* Tests

Bellinger et al. (2021) used paired *t* tests to determine whether physical, occupational, and speech therapy provided in the inpatient rehab setting to individuals recovering from COVID-19 resulted in improvements in self-care, mobility, orientation, and cognition. Statistically significant improvements ($p < 0.05$) were noted in all areas, which suggest these services may be vital to recovery from the disease (p. 1).

## BOX 5-5 ■ Example of a Wilcoxon Rank Test

A group of physical therapists investigated if the *Vestibular/Ocular-Motor Screen* (VOMS), a screen used to assess signs of concussion, could adequately detect changes after vestibular therapy for adolescents with concussions. Participants with symptoms such as balance deficits, dizziness, headaches, and light sensitivity were provided with vestibular physical therapy and administered the VOMS before and after the intervention. A Wilcoxon rank test was used in data analysis because the VOMS provided ordinal, nonparametric data. This statistical test revealed that posttest scores were significantly ($p < 0.001$) improved compared to pretest scores. The study suggests that the VOMS may be an effective tool to measure changes in vestibular and ocular motor function, but further testing may be necessary (Alsalaheen et al., 2020).

**(correlated) *t* test** is used when participants are compared with themselves (i.e., they serve as their own control) or when groups of individuals are compared after being matched on a particular characteristic. In this case, the pretest and posttest scores are compared for the first group, and the two scores from the matched pairs are compared for the second group. In the **independent samples (unpaired) *t* test**, which is the most common *t* test, the pretest and posttest means are compared for the experimental and control groups, and the two posttest scores are compared. If you have a directional hypothesis (meaning you expect the results to go a certain way), a one-tailed *t* test is used to determine the significance of results; if you have a nondirectional hypothesis (meaning you do *not* expect the results to go in a specific direction), a two-tailed *t* test should be employed to determine the direction of the significance, if any. The *t* test is quite powerful and can be used on groups of participants smaller than 30. Box 5-4 contains an example of a study employing *t* tests.

### *Wilcoxon Rank Test*

Wilcoxon rank tests, used with ordinal data, can compare the degree and direction of differences between two groups and are particularly useful for small sample sizes, usually fewer than 30 participants (Salkind, 2017). The **Wilcoxon signed rank test** (equivalent to the paired samples *t* test but for nonparametric data) is performed on paired scores and can determine the significance of the difference between either pretest and posttest scores for individuals or scores on matched pairs of participants. In the **Wilcoxon rank sum test** (equivalent to the independent samples *t* test but for nonparametric data), ranks are assigned to scores for all participants in the inquiry, and the ranks for all participants in each group are summed. The test determines the degree of difference between group total scores. An example of a study utilizing a Wilcoxon rank test is included in Box 5-5.

### *Mann-Whitney Test*

The **Mann-Whitney test** is another alternative to the *t* test for use with ordinal, nonparametric data. It compares the means of two independent groups and is equivalent to the independent samples *t* test. See Box 5-6 for an example.

## Tests of Correlation

**Correlational tests** determine the relationship or association between two or more variables or sets of scores. The two sets of scores can be from one group or two different groups. The objective is to find out how closely the scores covary—that is, whether they change together in a particular pattern, positively or negatively. If both scores increase, they are positively correlated; for example, height and weight scores for a group of participants would likely increase together. Conversely, if scores for ages over 60 years and scores for muscle strength were compared, age scores

### BOX 5-6 ■ Example of a Mann-Whitney Test

In studying the effects of nonimmersive virtual reality on functional independence in children with cerebral palsy, Goyal et al. (2022) employed a Mann-Whitney *U* ($p = 0.042$) test to investigate differences in self-care between the experimental (virtual reality) and control (traditional therapy) groups. The children's self-care skills were assessed before and after the interventions with the *WeeFIM*. This measure provides ordinal data (numerical scales used to rate self-care performance); therefore, a Mann-Whitney test was appropriate, and the results revealed significant improvements in the experimental group.

might increase, whereas strength scores would likely decrease. These scores are said to be negatively correlated. The two sets of scores can be illustrated on a scatter diagram, a graph with one score plotted on the vertical axis and the other plotted on the horizontal axis to illustrate how scores are distributed.

Tests for correlation yield a statistic called a **correlation coefficient**, expressed as *r*. The *r* may range from -1 (indicating a perfect negative relationship) to +1 (indicating a perfect positive relationship). A zero indicates that there is no relationship between the two variables. Decimal factors indicate *r* scores (e.g., 0.87 or -0.66). As with the previous tests, a significance level can be computed for an *r* score. It is important to remember that a relationship between variables does not indicate cause and effect; you can claim only that a positive or negative relationship between the variables has been found and no more. The most common correlational tests, including the Pearson product-moment correlation, Spearman rho, and regression analysis, are reviewed here.

### Pearson Product-Moment Correlation

The **Pearson product-moment correlation**, often called the **Pearson *r***, is used on ratio parametric data and is the most common correlational test. This test, which can be used on group or individual scores, indicates only systematic disagreements between scores and does not show the odd or occasional disagreement. It is often used to estimate reliability between tests, as in a test-retest situation, or between two raters to indicate interrater reliability. Box 5-7 describes a study that used Pearson correlations to determine the relationship between variables.

### BOX 5-7 ■ Example of Pearson Product-Moment Correlations

A correlational study explored the relationship between the physical activity level of individuals with spinal cord injury and their levels of pain, fatigue, and depression (Tawashy et al., 2009). Activity level (heavy, moderate, or mild) was measured using the *Physical Activity Recall Assessment* for individuals with spinal cord injury (PARA-SCI). Pearson correlations revealed that heavy intensity physical activity was strongly correlated with less fatigue ($r = -0.767$) and pain ($r = -0.612$) and increased self-efficacy ($r = 0.656$). For negative *r* values, the two attributes are inversely proportional; whereas for positive *r* values, the two attributes are directly proportional. To clarify, it is likely that as physical activity increases, fatigue and pain decrease, and self-efficacy increases. The researchers also found that mild physical activity was correlated with fewer symptoms of depression ($r = -0.565$; p. 304). Although it might be easy to assume a cause-and-effect relationship, one must remember that correlations only define relationships and cannot prove causation.

### Spearman Rho

The **Spearman rho** (denoted as ρ or $r_s$), also called Spearman's rank correlation coefficient, is equivalent to the Pearson *r*, but is used with ordinal, nonparametric data. It is used in descriptive research resulting in nonparametric data, when items have been ranked, to compare two sets of rankings to see if there is any relationship between them. See Box 5-8 for an example of a study using the Spearman rho.

### Simple Regression Analysis

**Simple regression analysis** is a technique that can be used after the correlation coefficient has been established. When a relationship is found between two variables, you can attempt to predict future scores for

## BOX 5-8 ■ Example of Spearman Rho

Researchers studying the impact of emotional intelligence on perceived stress surveyed 51 entry-level occupational therapy doctorate (OTD) students who were in their first, second, or third year of the program. They used a Spearman rho correlation to determine that a statistical association exists ($r_s = -0.391$), namely a negative correlation between emotional intelligence and perceived stress (Carpenter et al., 2023, p. 1). In other words, higher emotional intelligence may be associated with lower levels of perceived stress. This information could support curricular innovations to improve students' emotional intelligence and their ability to manage stress.

the dependent variable based on the scores on which the correlation coefficient was found. There are multiple types of regression analysis (other types are discussed later in this chapter), but simple regression involves only one independent (predictor) variable.

### Tests of Comparison

The tests described previously cannot cope with more than two variables, but **tests of comparison**, can compare *three or more* variables or sets of scores at a time. The most common tests of comparison are the analysis of variance, analysis of covariance, Kruskal-Wallis test, and multiple regression analysis, which are reviewed next.

#### *Analysis of Variance*

**Analysis of variance** (ANOVA), used with interval or ratio (parametric) data, is a statistical technique that can compare the mean scores of three or more groups in one study. If a study intends to answer multiple questions or is multifactorial, using the ANOVA may be most appropriate. The ANOVA yields an *F* ratio, which is evaluated using a standardized table to determine whether a significant difference exists between the largest and smallest of the study group means. If you wish to see if there are significant differences between any of the other means, you must use another test known as a **post hoc comparison**. Some of the most common post hoc tests are Tukey's honestly significant difference test, Student-Newman-Keuls comparison, and Scheffé's method (Portney, 2020). Box 5-9 provides an example of a study that utilized an ANOVA and a post hoc comparison.

## BOX 5-9 ■ Example of ANOVA

Researchers explored the effect of coordination training on tennis skills via randomization of participants to an experimental group (who received traditional tennis skills practice plus tailored coordination programming) and a control group (who received traditional practice only). Backhand and forehand techniques were assessed before the training, after 8 weeks of training, and again as a follow-up 1 week after training ended. A one-way ANOVA was used to compare both groups at baseline, with no significant differences noted. A two-way repeated measure ANOVA (2 study groups × 3 measures) showed significant interaction between the study groups and backhand or forehand assessments at three points in time. Thus, overall differences existed between the means of all the groups, but using ANOVA alone will not reveal where the differences lie. A post hoc comparison (Bonferroni's) indicated that the experimental group performed better after the intervention than the control group, thereby supporting the hypothesis that coordination training can improve tennis skills (Zetou et al., 2012).

#### *Analysis of Covariance*

The **analysis of covariance** (ANCOVA), also used with parametric data, controls for initial differences between groups. If pretest scores reveal that the dependent variable is substantially different for the groups because of extraneous variables such as age or sex, an ANCOVA can account for these extraneous variables by treating them as covariates and extracting their effect from the data. If the groups are made more equitable to begin with, the final results can be compared and judged more fairly. See Box 5-3 for an example of a study that used an ANCOVA.

#### *Kruskal-Wallis Test*

The **Kruskal-Wallis test** is equivalent to the one-way ANOVA, except it is used on nonparametric ordinal

### BOX 5-10 ■ Example of Kruskal-Wallis Test

Chiarello et al. (2010) examined family priorities for activity and participation for children with cerebral palsy. In addition to identifying family priorities (dependent variable) in three primary categories (daily activity, productivity, and leisure), they were interested in knowing whether the priorities differed based on age and gross motor skills (independent variables). The Kruskal-Wallis test and post hoc comparisons were used to analyze differences in the number of priorities for each age group and gross motor level. Some significant differences were noted in the results.

data. Like other nonparametric tests, this test is based on rankings of scores on the dependent measure in which all participants are put into one group during the ranking procedure and then put back into their original treatment groups for the remaining analysis. For example, if you were interested in the impact of stress level (independent variable) on healthcare students' academic performance (dependent variable), students could be grouped into low, moderate, and high stress groups, and academic performance could be measured on a 0–100 scale. The Kruskal-Wallis test could help determine if the independent variable (stress level) groups have statistically different academic performance (dependent variable). Similar to the ANOVA, the Kruskal-Wallis test alone cannot identify which specific independent variable groups are different; therefore, a post hoc comparison would be needed. Box 5-10 provides an example of a study that used the Kruskal-Wallis test.

### *Multiple Regression Analysis*

**Multiple regression analysis** is a statistical technique used for making predictions about the study (dependent) variable by understanding the effects of two or more independent (predictor) variables. Sometimes, this procedure can be used to imply causal relationships; in other instances, it may be used to simply explore relationships. It is possible to take the procedure a step further by untangling the relative contributions of each independent variable;

### BOX 5-11 ■ Example of Regression Analysis

Trabelsi et al. (2021) explored whether sleep quality and physical activity (independent variables) are predictors of mental well-being (dependent variable) in older adults during the COVID-19 lockdown. Multiple linear regression revealed a predictive relationship, with changes in sleep quality and physical activity foretelling changes in well-being. Specifically, reductions in sleep quality and physical activity were associated with decreased mental well-being.

**stepwise regression** is employed to examine the independent variables in various combinations to see which combination is most useful in predicting the occurrence of the dependent variable. See Box 5-11 for an example of a study in which regression analysis was used.

### TIPS & INSPIRATION

- The calculations for many statistics are complicated and often completed with statistical software. Some common software examples are Stata, SAS/STAT, or SPSS; Microsoft Excel can also be used. Only those students and healthcare professionals pursuing a research doctorate or dedicated statistical coursework might be able to perform these calculations without the help of a statistician or faculty member. It is okay to ask for help!
- If you have reviewed this chapter and can articulate the differences between descriptive and inferential statistics and some of the most common statistics used in healthcare inquiries, you are right where you need to be. The next chapter provides additional details to help you understand the statistical information in existing literature as well as how other quantitative design features can drive decisions about statistical analysis.
- Choices about the sampling method, data collection tools, and data analysis of quantitative inquiries may be based on convenience, logistics, inquiry purpose, and the topic of interest. Considering all aspects well before an inquiry and collaborating with others can be keys to success.

## CHAPTER SUMMARY

1. Describe the most common sampling methods used in quantitative research.
   - The population of interest is the broader group of people to which you hope to generalize your results. Sampling involves selecting a smaller subset of the population of interest to participate in the inquiry.
   - One of two sampling methods, nonprobability sampling or probability sampling, is used once the participant inclusion and exclusion criteria and the recruitment methods are identified.
   - Nonprobability sampling involves selecting participants based on other phenomena, such as location or convenience access, instead of being selected randomly. The most common type of nonprobability sampling is convenience sampling. Other variations include quota sampling, purposive sampling, and snowball sampling.
   - Probability sampling is a method that ensures that all members of the population of interest have an equal chance of being selected for the study sample. Simple random sampling is the most popular type of probability sampling. Other options include stratified random sampling, systematic random sampling, cluster sampling, or multistage cluster sampling.
2. Recall factors used to determine sample size in quantitative research.
   - Ideally, a sample should accurately represent the population of interest from which it was drawn in order to allow generalization of the results found in the sample to the population.
   - The purpose and logistics of the inquiry and statistical analysis may be used to justify the sample size.
   - Two important statistical concepts related to sample size are the confidence interval (or margin of error) and the confidence level (which represents the degree of certainty that the scores or responses of the population would fall within this range).
3. Explain the most common data collection tools used in quantitative research.
   - Data collection tools for quantitative inquiry include observation, surveys and interviews, record review, equipment, and assessments.
4. Differentiate between descriptive and inferential statistics used in quantitative data analysis.
   - Descriptive statistics describe, organize, and summarize numerical data. Descriptive statistics are best suited for small samples without random selection.
   - Inferential statistics are used to test a hypothesis or make inferences about a population from the sample findings; therefore, they require sufficient samples that are randomly selected.
5. Identify the four types of data analyzed in quantitative data analysis.
   - Nominal data are the numbers applied to nonnumerical categories, in no particular order (e.g., 1 = women; 2 = men).
   - Ordinal data are the numbers applied to categories, but in a rank order with unequal intervals (e.g., Maximum assist: 4; Moderate assist: 3; Minimal assist: 2; No assist: 1).
   - Interval data are ordered data with equal intervals and no zero starting point (e.g., degrees of temperature).
   - Ratio data are ordered data with equal intervals *with* a zero starting point (e.g., weight).
6. Recognize the most common descriptive and inferential statistics.
   - Common descriptive statistics include frequencies, percentages, measures of central tendency (mean, median, mode), and measures of variation (range, standard deviation).
   - Inferential statistics can include tests of statistical significance, tests of correlation, and tests of comparison.
     - Tests of statistical significance, including Pearson's chi-square, *t* test, Wilcoxon rank test, and Mann-Whitney test, can determine the probability that an outcome can be attributed to a specific cause or intervention rather than chance alone.
     - Tests of correlation, including Pearson product-moment correlation, Spearman rho, and simple regression analysis, can determine the relationship or association between two or more variables or sets of scores.
     - Tests of comparison, including ANOVA, ANCOVA, Kruskal-Wallis test, and multiple regression analysis, can compare *three or more* variables or sets of scores at a time.

## TEST YOUR KNOWLEDGE

1. Which of the following is a type of nonprobability sampling?
   a. Simple random sampling
   b. Cluster sampling
   c. Purposive sampling
   d. Systematic random sampling
2. Why is convenience sampling frequently used in healthcare research?
   a. Because it is the easiest and least expensive of all sampling methods
   b. Because it is the most rigorous
   c. Because it ensures the sample is representative of the population of interest
   d. Because there are ethical concerns with other sampling methods
3. A larger sample size usually transfers to more accurate results. True or false?
4. Which data collection tool is MOST APPROPRIATE to measure hand strength?
   a. Observation of a client grasping objects
   b. Use of equipment such as a dynamometer
   c. An interview to ask the client about their hand strength
   d. A review of the client's medical record
5. Which of the following BEST describes surveys used in quantitative research?
   a. They are unstructured, leading to a greater understanding of the topic.
   b. They can include abbreviations to keep the survey short.
   c. They can gather detailed responses to open-ended questions from larger samples.
   d. They are a cost-effective method for gathering numerical data from a sample.
6. Identify the type of data (nominal, ordinal, interval, ratio) for each item.
   a. Types of arthritis
   b. Temperatures
   c. Likert scale ratings
   d. Knee range of motion
7. What is the primary purpose of descriptive statistics?
   a. To identify relationships among inquiry variables
   b. To generalize findings to a larger population
   c. To summarize the main features of a dataset
   d. To determine the statistical significance of results
8. Identify the type of statistic (descriptive or inferential) for each item.
   a. Mean
   b. *t* test
   c. ANOVA
   d. Standard deviation

Answer key appears at the end of this text.

## NEXT STEPS

1. Locate a quantitative inquiry on a topic of interest. Identify the purpose of the inquiry and the sampling method used. Was the sampling method appropriate for the intended purpose? Why or why not? Did the authors justify how they arrived at the final sample? What are the advantages and disadvantages of the sampling method used?
2. Find three quantitative inquiries on your topic and outcome of interest. For each inquiry, identify the data collection tool(s) used to assess the outcomes. Did the inquiries employ the same or differing data collection tools? If the tools were similar, how could this information be helpful in designing your inquiry? If the tools differed, what are the advantages and disadvantages of each tool?
3. Examine the data collection, data analysis, and results sections of an existing quantitative inquiry. Identify the type of data generated by the data collection tools. Does the type of data align with the statistical methods used? (*Hint:* See Table 5-2.) Share how the data collection tools, data analysis, and results align with the inquiry's purpose.

## REFERENCES

Alsalaheen, B., Carender, W., Grzesiak, M., Munday, C., Almeida, A., Lorincz, M., & Marchetti, G. (2020). Changes in vestibular/ocular-motor screen scores in adolescents treated with vestibular therapy after concussion. *Pediatric Physical Therapy, 32*(4), 331–337. https://doi.org/10.1097/PEP.0000000000000729

American Physical Therapy Association. (2022). *Tests and measures.* American Physical Therapy Association website. https://www.apta.org/patient-care/evidence-based-practice-resources/test-measures

American Statistical Association. (2013). *When you consult a statistician . . . What to expect.* ASA Statistical Consulting Section. https://higherlogicdownload.s3.amazonaws.com/AMSTAT/f6e8f6fd-6343-44e2-aa52-8b4e405c5457/UploadedImages/SCSBrochure%202013.pdf

Asher, I. E. (2014). *Occupational therapy assessment tools: An annotated index* (4th ed.). AOTA Press.

Bellinger, L., Ouellette, N. H., & Robertson, J. L. (2021). The effectiveness of physical, occupational, and speech therapy in the treatment of patients with COVID-19 in the inpatient rehabilitation setting. *Perspectives of the ASHA Special Interest Groups, 6*(5), 1291–1298. https://doi.org/10.1044/2021_PERSP-21-00024

Boateng, G. O., Neilands, T. B., Frongillo, E. A., Melgar-Quiñonez, H. R., & Young, S. L. (2018). Best practices for developing and validating scales for health, social, and behavioral research: A primer. *Frontiers in Public Health, 6,* Article 149. https://doi.org/10.3389/fpubh.2018.00149

Burlingame, J., & Blaschko, T. M. (2009). *Assessment tools for recreational therapy and related fields* (4th ed.). Idyll Arbor.

Carpenter, A. (2023). *How to increase survey response rates.* Qualtrics. https://www.qualtrics.com/experience-management/research/tools-increase-response-rate

Carpenter, H. A., Edwards, C., & Richardson, S. (2023). How traits of emotional intelligence affect perceived stress in entry-level doctor of occupational therapy students. *The Internet Journal of Allied Health Sciences and Practice, 22*(1), Article 11. https://nsuworks.nova.edu/ijahsp/vol22/iss1/11

Chiarello, L. A., Palisano, R. J., Maggs, J. M., Orlin, M. N., Almasri, N., Kang, L., & Chang, H. (2010). Family priorities for activity and participation of children and youth with cerebral palsy. *Physical Therapy, 90*(9), 1254–1264. https://doi.org/10.2522/ptj.20090388

Chudoba, B. (2023). *How much time are respondents willing to spend on your survey?* SurveyMonkey.com. https://www.surveymonkey.com/curiosity/survey_completion_times

Fischer, J., Corcoran, K., & Springer, D. W. (2020). *Measures for clinical practice and research* (6th ed., Vols. 1 and 2). Oxford University Press.

Fowler, F. J., Jr. (2014). *Survey research methods* (5th ed.). SAGE Publications.

Goyal, C., Vardhan, V., & Naqvi, W. (2022). Non-immersive virtual reality as an intervention for improving hand function and functional independence in children with unilateral cerebral palsy: A feasibility study. *Cureus, 14*(6), e26085. https://doi.org/10.7759/cureus.26085

Hayati, M., Bagherzadeh, R., Mahmudpour, M., Heidari, F., & Vahedparast, H. (2023). Effect of teaching health-promoting behaviors on the care burden of family caregivers of hemodialysis patients: A four-group clinical trial. *BMC Nursing, 22*(1), 1–12. https://doi.org/10.1186/s12912-023-01604-2

Holtom, B., Baruch, Y., Aguinis, H., & Ballinger, G. A. (2022). Survey response rates: Trends and a validity assessment framework. *Human Relations, 75*(8), 1560–1584. https://doi.org/10.1177/00187267211070769

Morton, S. M. B., Bandara, D. K., Robinson, E. M., & Atatoa Carr, P. E. (2012). In the 21st century, what is an acceptable response rate? *Australian and New Zealand Journal of Public Health, 36*(2), 106–108. https://doi.org/10.1111/j.1753-6405.2012.00854.x

Portney, L. G. (2020). *Foundations of clinical research: Applications to evidence-based practice* (4th ed.). F.A. Davis.

Revilla, M., & Ochoa, C. (2017). Ideal and maximum length for a web survey. *International Journal of Market Research, 59*(5), 557–565. https://doi.org/10.2501/IJMR-2017-039

Sahraei, F., Rahemi, Z., Sadat, Z., Zamani, B., Ajorpaz, N. M., Afshar, M., & Mianehsaz, E. (2022). The effect of Swedish massage on pain in rheumatoid arthritis patients: A randomized controlled trial. *Complementary Therapies in Clinical Practice, 46,* 101524. https://doi.org/10.1016/j.ctcp.2021.101524

Salkind, N. J. (2017). *Statistics for people who (think they) hate statistics: Using Microsoft Excel 2016* (4th ed.). SAGE Publications.

SurveyMonkey. (2023). *Survey sample size.* SurveyMonkey.com. https://www.surveymonkey.com/mp/sample-size

Tawashy, A., Eng, J., Lin, K., Tang, P., & Hung, C. (2009). Physical activity is related to lower levels of pain, fatigue and depression in individuals with spinal-cord injury: A correlational study. *Spinal Cord, 47*(4), 301–306. https://doi.org/10.1038/sc.2008.120

Trabelsi, K., Ammar, A., Masmoudi, L., Boukhris, O., Chtourou, H., Bouaziz, B., Brach, M., Bentlage, E., How, D., Ahmed, M., Mueller, P., Mueller, N., Hsouna, H., Elghoul, Y., Romdhani, M., Hammouda, O., Paineiras-Domingos, L. L., Braakman-Jansen, A., Wrede, C., ... Hoekelmann, A. (2021). Sleep quality and physical activity as predictors of mental wellbeing variance in older adults during COVID-19 lockdown: ECLB COVID-19 international online survey. *International Journal of Environmental Research and Public Health, 18*(8), 4329. https://doi.org/https://www.mdpi.com/1660-4601/18/8/4329

Walonick, D. S. (2010). *Survival statistics.* StatPac.

Zetou, E., Vernadakis, N., Tsetseli, M., Kampas, A., & Michalopoulou, M. (2012). The effect of coordination training program on learning tennis skills. *Sport Journal, 15*(1), 1.

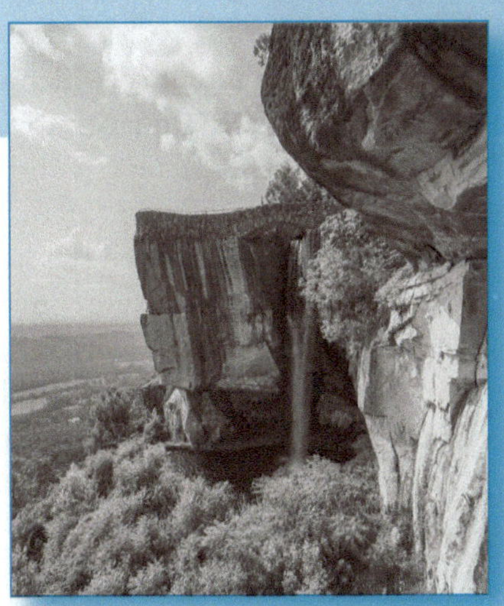

Chapter 6

# Critical Appraisal of Quantitative Research

LEARNING OUTCOMES

*The information provided in this chapter will assist you to:*

6.1 State the importance of critical appraisal.
6.2 Describe reliability and validity in quantitative research.
6.3 Identify threats to internal and external validity in quantitative research.
6.4 Identify threats to reliability in quantitative research.
6.5 Critically appraise the components of a quantitative research study.
6.6 Recall additional resources for critical appraisal of research.

## Importance of Critical Appraisal

In Chapters 4 and 5, you reviewed the prominent features of quantitative inquiry, the most common quantitative designs, and the quantitative technical elements of sampling, data collection, and data analysis. Now that you understand these components, it is time to shift your focus to the *quality* of the quantitative research you located. Not all research is created equal, and just because a study is published or available from a reputable source does not make it high quality or applicable to your purpose. This process of assessing the quality of an individual study is called **critical appraisal**. This chapter provides detailed guidance on critically appraising quantitative studies.

Critical appraisal is important regardless of whether you plan to conduct an evidence-based practice project or a research study. In evidence-based practice, critical appraisal is necessary for making informed decisions when applying the existing research to current practice. Consider that all research is flawed to some degree, but critical appraisal helps you determine if you can live with the existing flaws or biases. In other words, is the study you are reviewing of high enough quality that you feel reasonably comfortable applying it to practice? For example, you might choose not to apply information from a study with methodological shortcomings, vague conclusions, and many biases. Likewise, if you are planning to conduct a research study, scrutinizing the existing research on your topic can allow you to understand the challenges you might face, address prior methodological issues in your design, and ensure adequate justification for your study.

## Validity and Reliability in Quantitative Research

To begin the critical appraisal process, you must first understand the concepts of validity and reliability related to quantitative research.

High Falls, Lookout Mountain, Georgia.

## Validity

**Validity** is "the extent to which a concept is accurately measured in a quantitative study" (Heale & Twycross, 2015, p. 66). Validity involves two components–internal and external validity. **Internal validity** relates to how well the study methods, data collection, and analysis were conducted to limit bias. In contrast, **external validity** is the degree to which the outcomes can be applied to other similar groups or situations. Various threats to internal and external validity exist and are discussed here, along with the potential biases that may occur.

### *Threats to Internal Validity*

1. **Intervention methods.** When something unplanned happens to the participants or the environment during a study, such as a subject having an injury or inadvertently receiving another intervention, outcomes can be impacted. This is a type of **intervention bias**, which can be limited with careful sampling and controlling participants' activities during the study. Intervention bias can include **co-intervention** (when participants receive another intervention during the study that may impact results) and **contamination** (when participants in a control group receive the study intervention accidentally).
2. **Maturation.** Maturation refers to the participants' growth, development, or changes that occur naturally over time and may influence pretest and posttest measurements. For example, it might be difficult to determine if a year-long remedial writing program has improved a child's handwriting, or if that improvement would have occurred anyway with the passage of time. This is referred to as **timing bias**.
3. **Data collection methods.** If the same test is used several times throughout the study, participants may experience a practice effect and score higher simply because they have practiced the test. Additionally, if the test involves performing an activity to demonstrate strength or endurance, repeatedly performing the test could also increase the participants' skills. If equipment is used to collect data and the equipment is not accurately calibrated or is in poor condition, it may give inaccurate readings. Surveys or interviews could include cultural, racial, intelligence, or language biases that would influence the results. These scenarios represent **measurement bias**.
4. **Participant selection methods.** Participants who volunteer for a study are likely different from those selected to participate, but there is an element of volunteerism for all participants because of the consent process which may result in **sampling bias**. This can be controlled by using more than one study group and by randomly assigning participants to the groups.
5. **Participant attrition or mortality.** However well a study is designed, it is difficult to prevent participant attrition because of illness, a geographic move, or death. An inadequate sample could result in the inability to draw meaningful conclusions; therefore, extra participants should be recruited to account for these losses. This is particularly important in a case study.

### *Threats to External Validity*

The concepts of internal and external validity must be balanced, as many of the controls that increase internal validity (rigorous methodology, highly controlled study environments, strict testing procedures, and randomization of participants) can compromise the relevancy and application of research findings to real-life scenarios. Threats to external validity include the following:

1. **Hawthorne effect.** If participants perform better on a study task simply because they are being observed, and not necessarily because of the treatment they receive, they are said to exhibit the Hawthorne effect. This situation is named after a series of experiments completed with factory workers at the Hawthorne Works, an electric company in Illinois, in the early 1900s. In these experiments, worker productivity increased regardless of manipulation of environmental and psychological variables; this increase was attributed to the extra attention the workers received from the researchers (Franke & Kaul, 1978). This represents **attentional bias**.
2. **Description of methods.** When researchers report on their studies, they must describe their

methods sufficiently so others can replicate them. Without adequate methodological details, replication is unlikely, and results cannot be confidently generalized, thereby threatening external validity.

3. **Sample.** Is the sample being studied truly representative of those in the larger population? If not, generalizability, or the extent to which the sample's results are also found in the larger population, may be limited. This is another example of **sampling bias**. Randomly selecting the sample from the population of interest is a sound way to increase the likelihood that the study results can be applied to the larger population.
4. **Multiple treatments.** In a study in which participants are given more than one treatment as the independent variable, the results cannot be generalized to other settings where only one of those treatments is used. Effects of more than one treatment must be viewed as cumulative and intermingled. Studies that use a single treatment as the independent variable and a single measure for the dependent variable have greater external validity.
5. **Researcher interaction.** Sometimes participants react to a study in a certain way because of their relationship with the researcher, whether positive or negative. Similarly, the researchers may unintentionally alter their interactions with participants based on their own perceptions or feelings. These are particularly important considerations if the dependent variable involves interpersonal relationships or emotion-laden topics. This is known as **researcher bias**. While not always feasible, blinding, consistent training, and involving multiple researchers who are unknown to the participants are effective ways to combat this concern.

## Reliability

**Reliability** is the extent to which study outcomes are consistent or can be replicated in repeated experiments. Reliability also refers to the degree to which a data collection tool produces consistent results over time (test-retest), across test items (split-half), within an individual rater (intrarater), and among different raters (interrater). Each of these types of reliability will be discussed in the next section. If there is consistency among several measures of the same phenomenon, and across outcomes from similar studies, you can have more confidence in the study's results. Threats to the reliability of a quantitative study include study design features as well as the data collection methods.

### *Threats to Reliability*

1. **Participant fatigue.** If participants are expected to perform physical or mental tasks repeatedly, they may become tired and not perform to the best of their abilities, and results could be affected. Physiological abilities can change in response to diurnal or circadian rhythms, which may result in different results for the same person at different times. Scheduling testing and other performance tasks with adequate breaks can decrease subject fatigue.
2. **Participant motivation.** Participants are not always interested in the study and may not perform at their best because of decreased motivation or mood. They may even dislike participating in the study, which would certainly influence the effort they put forth in testing procedures. In this case, test results can vary and may not reliably indicate participants' abilities. Recruiting participants with a vested interest in the study's purpose and results can combat this issue.
3. **Participant learning.** If there are repeated tests using the same instrument within the study, participants are likely to achieve some learning. They may perform better on later tests simply because they have learned the material on the test rather than because of an experimental intervention. This is called **recall bias**, and using various data collection methods can decrease the impact of subject learning.
4. **Participant ability.** Participants' ability to respond to certain questions or tasks may vary according to their skill level or knowledge of the topic. Responses may vary for the same participant. For example, a participant may create a response to appease the examiner or to make

themselves look more favorable. This might be especially true if a relationship already exists between the participant and researcher or if a sensitive or embarrassing topic is being investigated. Self-report data collection methods are especially prone to these concerns. Preserving a distinct researcher-participant relationship and handling sensitive topics appropriately can minimize this concern.

5. **Quality of data collection tools.** A tool is reliable if the same results occur during repeated administrations over time. **Test-retest reliability** is concerned with the consistency of scores over time. Specifically, if participants are measured regarding some characteristic now and then remeasured on the same characteristic later in time, the scores should be similar, assuming that the conditions and the characteristic being measured are stable. **Split-half reliability** concerns the extent to which different parts of an instrument measure the same thing. For instance, are two different items on a test for self-esteem both actually measuring components of self-esteem? If not, the whole test may be suspect, and the compiled score may not truly represent the subject's self-esteem score. To assess this type of reliability, the test is divided into two parts, and participants' scores on the two groups of items are compared. A high correlation between sets of items indicates a higher degree of reliability (Heale & Twycross, 2015).
6. **Rater abilities.** The consistency with which a data collection tool is administered to participants can impact study outcomes. **Intrarater reliability** is the degree to which each rater or observer is consistent in their ratings. Multiple repetitions of the same test by one rater should yield consistently similar results, thus ensuring consistent administration and testing procedures by that rater. **Interrater reliability** is the extent to which different raters or observers perceive the same person or characteristic similarly. Specifically, if two different raters administer an assessment on the same subject, the scores should be relatively similar. Both intrarater and interrater reliability can be increased by clearly operationalizing all study variables and conducting formalized training in administering interventions and assessments.
7. **Test environment.** Changes in the environment from test to test can influence a subject's responses. Distractions such as noise or interruptions are particularly intrusive on test results. Controlling the study environment so that participants are tested under the same conditions each time can minimize environmental influences.

### TIPS & INSPIRATION

- Realize all research has flaws and potential sources of bias, but what is most important is that the results and conclusions are viewed while *considering* the flaws or biases. In some cases, the flaws may be too great to accept the conclusions, but in others, valuable information can still be gained from a study. Do not become so focused on the flaws that you miss the good stuff!
- If you plan to conduct your own inquiry, compare your proposed inquiry design to the threats to validity and reliability. This process can help you identify potential issues that you may be able to control for in the design phase. You will not be able to control all threats (and that is okay!), but you should be aware of them when interpreting your results.

## Components of Quantitative Research Critical Appraisal

As discussed in Chapter 4, there are many quantitative study designs, each with strengths and challenges. To learn how to appraise a quantitative study, it is best to break the article down by study components.

Table 6-1 provides a comprehensive template for appraising a quantitative study, and each component is discussed separately so that you understand what to look for. The template provided in Table 6-1 includes three columns for completion:

1. **Study Details:** where you will summarize information about the quantitative study being reviewed

**TABLE 6-1 ■ Critical Appraisal of Quantitative Study Template**

***Study Reference:*** (insert reference for the study being appraised here)

| Study Components | Study Details | Appraisal* | Potential Biases/ Limitations |
|---|---|---|---|
| **Purpose** | **Study's purpose:** | **Purpose was clearly stated:**<br>☐ Yes—If yes, indicate where:<br>____________________<br>☐ No | |
| **Literature review** | **Main points of the literature review:**<br>**Need for the study:** | **Sufficient literature on the topic was reviewed:**<br>☐ Yes ☐ No<br>**Need for the study is clear:**<br>☐ Yes ☐ No | |
| **Setting** | **Setting type** (e.g., inpatient rehab unit, skilled nursing facility, public school system, drug and alcohol clinic, community senior housing complex):<br>**Geographic location** where study took place (e.g., United States, Australia, rural/urban): | **The setting is sufficiently described:**<br>☐ Yes ☐ No<br>**Setting applies to your purpose:**<br>☐ Yes ☐ No | |
| **Sampling and recruitment** | **Sampling method:**<br>Nonprobability (convenience, quota, purposive, snowball):<br>Probability (simple random, stratified random sampling, systematic random sampling, cluster):<br>**Recruitment method:**<br>**Description of subjects/ participants** (include pertinent demographics such as age, diagnoses): | **Sample size:** __________<br>**Sample size was justified:**<br>☐ Yes ☐ No<br>**Sampling method is appropriate for study purpose:**<br>☐ Yes ☐ No<br>**Recruitment method is appropriate for study purpose:**<br>☐ Yes ☐ No<br>**Sample is appropriate for study purpose:**<br>☐ Yes ☐ No<br>**Sample applies to your purpose:**<br>☐ Yes ☐ No | |
| **Design and level of evidence** | Describe the **study design** (e.g., RCT, two group pretest-posttest, one group pretest-posttest, time series, repeated measures, cohort design, case study, correlational): | **Quantitative level of evidence:**<br>☐ I ☐ II ☐ III ☐ IV ☐ V<br>**Design is appropriate for study purpose:**<br>☐ Yes ☐ No<br>**Institutional Review Board approval/ exemption:**<br>☐ Yes ☐ No ☐ Unsure | |

*Continued*

**TABLE 6-1 ■ Critical Appraisal of Quantitative Study Template—cont'd**

***Study Reference:*** (insert reference for the study being appraised here)

| Study Components | Study Details | | | Appraisal* | Potential Biases/ Limitations |
|---|---|---|---|---|---|
| **Procedures** | Briefly summarize the methodology, or what the researchers did in the study. Be sure to include any interventions as well as who carried them out. | | | **Procedures are sufficiently described to allow replication:**<br>☐ Yes ☐ No<br>**Those carrying out the procedures have sufficient training or experience in the subject area:**<br>☐ Yes ☐ No ☐ Unsure<br>**Procedures avoided contamination:**<br>☐ Yes ☐ No ☐ Unsure<br>☐ N/A<br>**Procedures avoided co-intervention:**<br>☐ Yes ☐ No ☐ Unsure<br>☐ N/A | |
| **Data collection tools** | ***Tool*** | ***Constructs measured*** | ***When administered*** | **Tools included:**<br>☐ Standardized tools<br>☐ Non-standardized tools<br>**Standardized tools are valid:**<br>☐ Yes ☐ No ☐ Unsure<br>☐ N/A<br>**Standardized tools are reliable:**<br>☐ Yes ☐ No ☐ Unsure<br>☐ N/A<br>**Efforts were made to promote reliability and validity of nonstandardized tools:**<br>☐ Yes ☐ No ☐ Unsure<br>☐ N/A | |
| **Data analysis** | What **type of data** did the study produce (nominal, ordinal, interval, ratio)?<br>What **statistical methods** were used? | | | **Data analysis methods are appropriate for the resulting data:**<br>☐ Yes ☐ No | |
| **Results** | State the **study results** in layperson's terms: | | | **Results are statistically significant:**<br>☐ Yes ☐ No ☐ N/A<br>**Results are clinically significant/ meaningful:**<br>☐ Yes ☐ No ☐ N/A | |

*Continued*

**TABLE 6-1 ■ Critical Appraisal of Quantitative Study Template—cont'd**

***Study Reference:*** (insert reference for the study being appraised here)

| Study Components | Study Details | Appraisal* | Potential Biases/ Limitations |
|---|---|---|---|
| **Conclusions** | Concisely summarize the **study conclusions**: | **Conclusions are appropriate given the study information provided:** ☐ Yes ☐ No | |
| **Applicability (Check all that apply)** | ☐ Background information (justifies a need, defines key terms, establishes theoretical background)<br>☐ Shows the effectiveness or support for a proposed intervention<br>☐ Supports methodology (may include procedures, data collection methods or tools, data analysis).<br>☐ Other: | | |

*For each "No" response, indicate the potential biases/concerns (for example, researcher bias, sampling bias, inadequate description, missing information) in the corresponding far-right column. Exercise caution in applying research with 50% or greater "No" responses.

2. **Appraisal:** where you will appraise the study components (i.e., Is the information provided in the study sufficient, appropriate, and of good quality?)
3. **Potential Biases/Limitations:** where you will clearly outline your concerns related to each "No" response in the Appraisal column

## Study Purpose

The purpose should be a clear and concise statement conveying the aim of the inquiry. The purpose is frequently stated in the article's *Abstract* or embedded in the *Introduction*. In some cases, you will find it explicitly stated (The purpose of this study is to ...); some journals use headings in their abstracts to highlight important features, and often one of the headings is *Purpose* or *Aim*. In other instances, it may take some digging to uncover the purpose amid other study details. Some authors may provide a PIO or PICO question that they hope to address in the inquiry in lieu of a separate purpose statement. Ultimately, a clearly stated purpose is important because it is the guiding principle for all other decisions made in the study design. In the Purpose section of Table 6-1, you should briefly summarize the study's purpose under Study Details, and then indicate whether the purpose was clearly stated. If the purpose was stated clearly, justify your response by sharing where you located this information. If the purpose was not stated or was unclear, describe your concerns in the Potential Biases/ Limitations column.

## Literature Review

The literature review, discussed in detail in Chapter 3, should proceed logically, connecting one idea to the next to effectively summarize the existing literature on a topic and identify the gaps or need for the present study. The literature review should define all key terms and reasonably address the scope of literature on a topic. For topics where research is relatively sparse, the literature review may be shorter; for well-researched topics, more articles might be included to justify the inquiry. In the Literature Review section of Table 6-1, briefly summarize the main points of the literature review and the need for the study, and then indicate if the information is sufficient to understand the topic and establish the need. This is definitely a judgment call, but if you feel the literature review is inadequate or the need is not supported, be sure to indicate what other literature might have been helpful to discuss or what you found to be missing in the far right column of the table.

## Setting

The setting comprises the type of facility (for example, inpatient rehab unit, public school system, community senior housing complex) and the geographic location (for example, United States, India, or urban or rural communities) where the study occurred. The setting is an important consideration in determining if the study's outcomes can be reasonably generalized to your facility or location. For example, outcomes of a study on children's handwriting legibility in rural India may not apply to children in an urban school in the United States because the educational systems and resources available vary. Study settings may also include virtual ones, such as interventions offered via video conferencing, but the locations of participants still bear mentioning. In the Setting section of Table 6-1, identify the type of setting and geographic location of the study and indicate whether the setting is sufficiently described. A sufficient description includes all relevant details to place the study within context. While you might wish you had more detail in some instances, keep in mind that most journals restrict the length of articles, so authors must prioritize what information to include. It is helpful to ask, "If I knew more about X, would that significantly alter my appraisal of this article?" A quality setting description, which you might find integrated into an article's *Methods, Procedures,* or *Subjects* (or *Participants*) sections, is concise and avoids extraneous details. If relevant details are missing, be sure to note those under the Potential Biases/Limitations column.

### Sampling and Recruitment

The sampling and recruitment methods for a study are often found within the *Procedures* or *Methods* section of an article or within a dedicated *Sample* section. Here are some key points to consider when appraising sampling and recruitment methods:

- **What type of nonprobability or probability sampling did they use?** Recall that each sampling method varies in purpose, strengths, and challenges, which are important to consider when appraising quantitative research. (See Chapter 5 for a review of sampling methods.) For example, convenience sampling is common in healthcare research as it is a practical way to gain participants, but the results may not be generalizable beyond the setting or to the larger population. Random assignment or matching of participants in different study groups can decrease potential biases. Summarize the sampling method used by the researchers and consider how it aligns with the study's purpose, and then share potential biases/limitations in the last column.
- **What was the sample size?** Clarify how *many* participants were included in the study and if the sample size was justified. To justify a sample, the researchers should explain how they arrived at the final sample, including acknowledging any participants lost to attrition. A sample can also be justified via statistical methods (how many participants are needed to reveal statistically significant results if they exist), but in many studies, this will not be the case.
- **Were the participants recruited via direct contact, mail/email, flyers, online/social media, or other methods?** Where were they recruited from (for example, a support group, a unit of a hospital, or a senior center), and who did the recruiting (Was it a member of the research team? Someone unassociated with the research? Or did they use a passive form of recruitment, such as a flyer posted on a publicly visible bulletin board?) should be explained by the authors. Consider if there are potential biases in the recruitment methods and if the methods align with the study's purpose.
- **Was a relevant description of the participants provided?** A quality description should include the relevant characteristics of the participants to allow you to understand who they were so that you can decide if they are similar to your population of interest. Relevant details will be based on the study's purpose and may include gender, age, years of experience, diagnoses, living situations, or other study-specific components.

#### TIPS & INSPIRATION

- No sampling method is inherently bad or good. In making your appraisal, you must consider the study's purpose and scope and your intended application of the research to decide if the method was reasonable and if the study's conclusions are appropriate and meaningful for you.

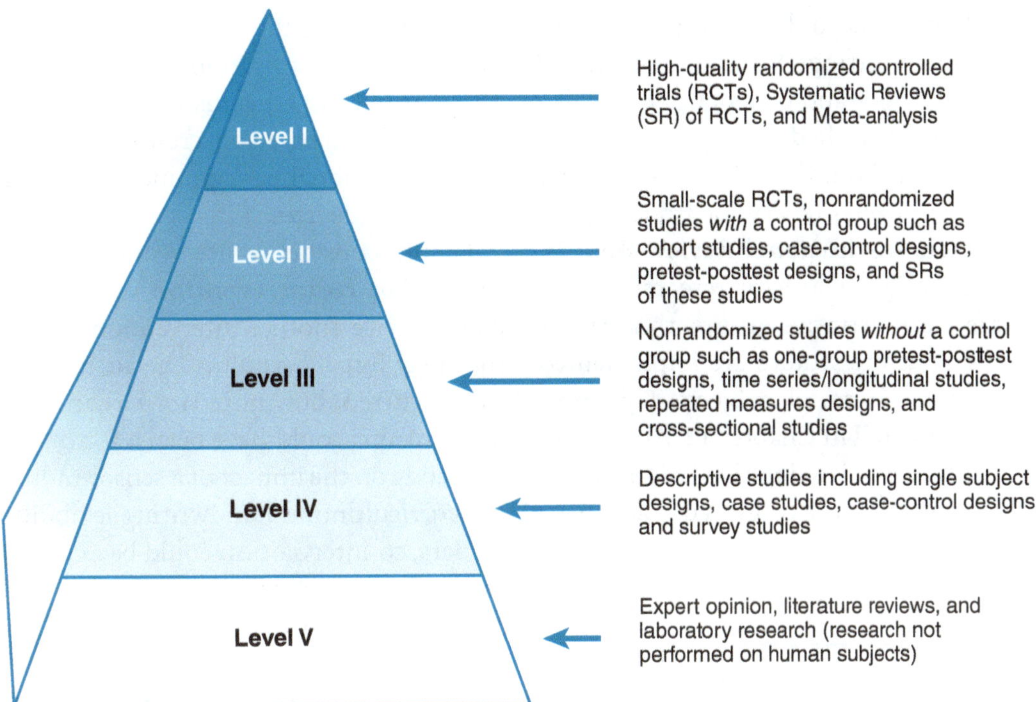


Figure 6-1 Quantitative levels of evidence.

## Design and Level of Evidence

Quantitative research designs (described in Chapter 4) vary in rigor and can be classified into levels of evidence based on the relative strength of the design. Several scales exist for categorizing quantitative research into levels of evidence, and one of the most used hierarchies is from the Oxford Centre for Evidence-Based Medicine (Howick et al., 2011; OCEBM Levels of Evidence Working Group, 2011). For our purposes, a simplified classification system, adapted from several scales, is included in Figure 6-1 (Howick et al., 2011; Joanna Briggs Institute, 2013; National Collaborating Centre for Methods and Tools, 2023; OCEBM Levels of Evidence Working Group, 2011; Polit & Beck, 2021).

On this scale, a level I study has the greatest strength or rigor, and a level V study has the least. Level I studies include high-quality randomized controlled trials, systematic reviews, and meta-analyses. **Systematic reviews** and **meta-analyses**, discussed in greater detail in Chapter 10, are study designs that synthesize results from multiple individual studies. Levels of evidence are primarily based on methodological rigor (for example, whether the study groups were randomized or if a control group was used) and aspects of internal validity. However, the levels fail to account for real-world scenarios and challenges to external validity (Polit & Beck, 2021). Therefore, the level of evidence cannot "provide you with a definitive judgment about the quality of evidence" (Howick et al., 2011, p. 2), and it is just one aspect of your comprehensive critical appraisal.

At this point in your appraisal, you should identify the design and corresponding level of evidence of the study being appraised. Sometimes the design type is explicitly named in the article's *Abstract*, *Design*, or *Methods* section. However, in other instances, you might need to determine the design based on the procedures—namely, whether the features of randomization, control, and manipulation were used. Ultimately, you must decide if the design is appropriate for the study's purpose. Recall that certain topics lend themselves more easily to rigorous study, whereas others cannot be studied under such strict conditions. For example, if you are researching a rare neurological disorder, you will likely find case studies or accounts from experts who have treated clients with this condition. However, if you are interested in more commonly occurring diagnoses or treatments, you might find larger-scale and more rigorous studies conducted in many settings. So, although a level I study boasts greater rigor and confidence in results, some topics cannot be studied appropriately under these conditions. You should also indicate whether the study was Institutional Review Board (IRB) approved or exempted. **Institutional Review Boards**, also called ethics review boards or research review committees, are administrative groups that review research proposals before studies are implemented to ensure protection of research subjects. This topic is covered in greater detail in Chapter 12. Any potential biases or limitations related to the design should be noted in the corresponding column of Table 6-1.

### TIPS & INSPIRATION

- Although level I quantitative studies are the most rigorous, know that they are sometimes difficult to translate to practice because the procedures are very strict.
- Do not be discouraged if you do not find level I or II studies on your topic. Many topics cannot be effectively studied under such rigorous conditions, and using a control group could present ethical issues. A good level III or IV study for many topics is acceptable.

### Procedures

A study's **procedures** include any interventions provided, who provided the intervention, what materials were used, and any other pertinent action steps. This information is typically found in an article's *Procedures* or *Methods* section. In your appraisal of the study procedures, you should briefly summarize the steps taken and consider if they are sufficiently described to allow someone else to replicate them. If relevant details are missing and impact your overall understanding of the study methods and outcomes, this should be clarified in the Potential Biases/Limitations section. Next, consider if those carrying out the procedures have sufficient training or experience in the subject area. At times, this could be explicitly stated within an article. For example, in a study exploring the management of chronic lymphedema, the authors may specify that those conducting the intervention held the Complete Lymphedema Certification from the Academy of Lymphatic Studies. In other instances, training or expertise may be inferred based on a researcher's prior scholarly work, educational background, clinical background, or academic degrees.

Finally, consider if intervention bias is a concern. Recall that **co-intervention** occurs when participants receive another intervention during the study that may impact results. The authors may share if this occurred, but more times than not, you must decide if this could have been a factor. For example, in a study on the impact of a sensorimotor handwriting curriculum on handwriting legibility of second graders, co-intervention could be a factor if children received typical classroom instruction or other therapeutic interventions during the study time frame. Ethically, it would be improper to withhold these other activities, so any positive study outcomes might be attributed to several interventions. If no intervention was offered in a study (for example, in the case of a descriptive survey design), this item would be marked N/A. **Contamination** occurs when participants in a control group accidentally receive the study intervention. Contamination is less likely when participants in experimental and control groups are in separate locations, participate in the study at separate times, or interact with different research team members. This item would also be marked N/A if the study did not involve a control group.

### Data Collection Tools

Recall from Chapter 5 that observations, surveys or interviews, record review, equipment, and assessments may be used to gather or measure study outcomes in quantitative research. In many research articles, the data collection tools are discussed in a dedicated section, but in others, this information might be embedded in the *Methods* or *Procedures* section. In the appraisal template (Table 6-1), you should identify each tool used, the constructs it measured, and when the tool was administered. For example, in a study of the impact of an online stress management program for healthy adults, the Perceived Stress Scale (tool) was used to measure psychological stress (construct measured) at baseline and at the study's conclusion (when administered; Stächele et al., 2020).

**BOX 6-1 ■ Example of Tool Validity and Reliability Information**

"The PSS demonstrated good reliability (Cronbach alpha = .84–.86) (45, 46) and has been used as a sensitive measure to track perceived stress in longitudinal studies [e.g., (34, 47, 48)]. The validation of the German translation (N = 2,463) of the PSS-10 has shown, in line with previous research, strong positive correlations with depression, anxiety, fatigue, and negative correlations with life satisfaction (46)" (Stächele et al., 2020, pp. 4–5).

Next, it is vital to consider the reliability and validity of each data collection tool. Data from low-quality measures or inconsistent procedures may lead to inaccurate study conclusions. **Reliability** is the degree to which a data collection tool produces consistent results over time (test-retest), across test items (split-half), within an individual rater (intrarater), and among different raters (interrater). **Construct validity** is how well the tool measures the construct it intends to measure. Standardized tools, processes, and equipment have undergone testing to establish the degree of reliability and validity, and authors typically cite this information in their articles. Box 6-1 provides an example of how validity and reliability might be reported in an article. Occasionally, the authors may not include this information for a standardized tool, and it will be up to you to search *beyond* the article you are appraising to confirm whether the tool is valid and reliable.

Many studies employ non-standardized tools, including those developed by the researchers (often said to be author-generated), when no standardized tools or methods exist to gather the exact information they are interested in. While this may seem like a poor choice, it is often the only option for gathering data about unique practice scenarios, diagnoses, and new interventions or constructs. All research must start somewhere, and many of the widely accepted data collection tools in existence today resulted from this type of foundational research. When using non-standardized measures, it is prudent to discuss how and why the tools were developed, including item creation, review by experts, pilot testing, and any other efforts taken to increase the content validity of the tool prior to its use. **Content validity** refers to how well the items or questions on a tool represent all aspects of the construct being explored. Details about the data collection process can also help you make a judgment about the reliability of these non-standardized tools. To complete your appraisal in this section of Table 6-1, indicate the type of tools used (standardized versus non-standardized) and their validity and reliability. Be sure to note any potential biases/limitations with the data collection tools and methods in the last column of the template.

**TIPS & INSPIRATION**

- As you appraise a study, do not hesitate to contact the authors if you have questions. The authors' contact information is often included in the article or is readily available through an online search. Most authors are more than willing to assist others interested in their area of study.

### Data Analysis

The simplest way to identify a quantitative study is to review the data analysis methods. If the study yielded numbers as data and the researchers analyzed that data with descriptive or inferential statistics, you can conclude that the design is quantitative. Most quantitative research articles have a dedicated section describing the data analysis methods. In some cases, you might find this information integrated into the *Procedures* section or the beginning of the *Results* section. In your appraisal, you must assess if the data analysis methods were appropriate for the resulting data. First, consider the type of data that was generated in the study—nominal, ordinal, interval, or ratio. See Chapter 5 for a review of these data scales. Next, identify the type of statistics the researchers used in the study. Finally, compare the data type and statistics used to Table 5-2 to determine appropriateness. For example, in a study exploring the use of mindfulness on weight loss, participants are weighed at baseline and after participating in structured education on mindful eating and applying these practices over 8 weeks. Weight represents ratio data since this scale has equal intervals from one pound to the next, with a zero starting point. The researchers use a paired samples *t* test to compare the participants' baseline and final weights to determine whether statistically significant changes occurred. Using Table 5-2, ratio data is a type of parametric data for which a *t* test is appropriate.

You can take this a step further by also considering the purpose of the study and the number of outcomes. Recall that descriptive statistics are used to describe or summarize outcomes, whereas inferential statistics are used to compare interventions or samples to test for statistical significance or to examine correlations between variables. Also, some inferential statistics can only be used to compare two different scores (for example, a *t* test to compare the baseline and final weights of participants in the prior example). However, advanced statistical tests are required to cope with more than two variables or scores. For example, an ANOVA can compare three or more groups or variables within one study. The purpose of the statistical tests used should align with the study's purpose to increase your confidence in the outcomes noted. Any concerns with the data analysis methods should be indicated in the Potential Biases/Limitations column of the provided template (Table 6-1).

## Results

Quantitative research articles usually include a *Results* or *Outcomes* section, where the study results are shared in narrative form. Tables or figures may also be included to illustrate the outcomes. Results can be reported in terms of statistical or clinical significance, or both. **Statistical significance** refers to outcomes attributed to a specific cause or intervention rather than chance alone. **Clinical significance**, also called practical significance, represents clinically meaningful outcomes (Carpenter et al., 2021). Many outcomes with a small **effect size**, or magnitude of change, could still be deemed clinically important. For example, an intervention that results in a small reduction in the number of falls for geriatric clients at risk for falls would be valuable.

**TABLE 6-2 ■ Common Effect Sizes (Chen et al., 2010; Cohen, 1988; Cohen, 1992; Funder & Ozer, 2019)**

| Effect Sizes | Small | Medium | Large |
|---|---|---|---|
| Cohen's *d* | 0.2 to <0.5 | 0.5 to <0.8 | ≥0.8 |
| Pearson *r* | <0.2 | 0.2 to <0.4 | ≥0.4 |
| Eta- squared ($\eta^2$) | 0.01 to <0.06 | 0.06 to <0.14 | ≥0.14 |
| Spearman rho ($\rho$ or $r_s$) | 0.1 | 0.3 | ≥0.5 |
| Odds ratio | ~1.5 | ~2.5 | ≥4 |

Recall that tests of statistical significance result in a **confidence level**, which represents the probability that the outcomes are not a chance occurrence. The confidence level is commonly set at $p \leq 0.05$, meaning you are 95% certain the outcomes are not due to chance. If the confidence level is set at $p \leq 0.01$, you can be 99% confident that the outcomes are not due to chance. The sample size influences statistical significance, and increasing the sample size can increase the likelihood of statistically significant results. For this reason, an effect size may be calculated and reported to highlight whether the magnitude of change is small, medium, or large (Sullivan & Feinn, 2012). Table 6-2 includes the most common effect sizes and accepted values for comparison to those reported in the articles you are appraising.

An accurate appraisal of the results hinges on your ability to understand the study's results and summarize them in layperson's terms. Reviewing the

### TIPS & INSPIRATION

- In appraising the articles, do not let the statistics intimidate you. Consulting a basic statistical text such as Salkind and Frey's (2020) *Statistics for People Who (Think They) Hate Statistics* or seeking assistance from a faculty mentor or statistician can help you make sense of the numbers.

*Discussion* section of the article can also be helpful in processing what the results mean and understanding limitations that may have impacted them. Note your concerns and any limitations in the last column of Table 6-1.

### Conclusions

The study's conclusions represent the "take-home message," and the researchers frequently offer practical implications of the research or recommendations for future inquiries. After you summarize the study's conclusions, now is the time to consider your appraisal of all other study components. Are the conclusions appropriate given these other details? Some key aspects to consider include the following:

- **Does the study design align with the study outcomes?** Be wary of studies claiming to prove the effectiveness of interventions or treatments. Recall that only experimental designs can determine cause-and-effect relationships. If a quasi-experimental design was used, the researchers might appropriately conclude that the results *support* the use of the intervention or treatment, rather than confirm effectiveness.
- **Are the clinical implications appropriate given the study procedures?** If the authors suggest applying the information to a larger population, be cautious if the sample is small, there are concerns with the quality of the outcome measures used, or the procedures introduce significant opportunities for bias.
- **Did the authors acknowledge limitations in the study?** Remember that all research is flawed, and the authors' recognition of the limitations/potential biases signifies ethical research practices. A study with no reported limitations or biases should be considered circumspect. It is also entirely possible that you might consider limitations beyond those explicitly stated by the authors.

### Applicability

Finally, you must consider how this appraised study specifically applies to your purpose, population, or practice setting. Whether you are conducting an evidence-based practice project or a research study, now is the time to determine if and how the study information will be useful to you. In the last section of Table 6-1, check all items that apply. For example, the study may provide useful background information, including establishing the theoretical background or need for your inquiry or defining key terms. This information could be useful in drafting your literature review if you plan to conduct a formal inquiry. The study may confirm the effectiveness of or suggest positive outcomes related to a planned practice intervention. If you plan to complete an evidence-based practice project, locating multiple good-quality studies that support a planned intervention is recommended. The study may also provide insight into appropriate study procedures, data collection methods and tools, and data analysis methods. This information could be helpful in designing your own inquiry procedures, including making decisions about the timing, duration, and other inquiry logistics. If you derive other useful information from a study not encompassed by these categories, an additional section is included for you to provide clarification.

Novak (2012) proposed the metaphor of a traffic light as a framework for applying research to clinical practice. High-quality evidence showing a treatment intervention to be ineffective or to cause harm is given a red light—meaning the recommendation is to abstain from using the treatment in question. Application with caution (yellow light) is recommended for treatments with low-quality evidence or inconclusive evidence, or if the studied population differs from your clients. In these cases, clinical judgment should be exercised with consideration given to the clinical situation, your skills, and any similarities that can be drawn between the study sample and your clients or inquiry participants. Treatments substantiated with strong clinical evidence and studies conducted with similar populations and in similar situations to the current practice scenario would be given a green light—meaning the treatment is recommended. Finally, as you review your article appraisal, a good rule is to exercise caution in applying studies if concerns related to 50% or more of the study components were noted.

## TIPS & INSPIRATION

- When considering the conclusions and application of a study, always reflect on whether the topic and intervention fall within your scope of practice.
- Be aware of your preconceived ideas as you complete your appraisal. Looking for only studies that support your ideas may result in a flawed rationale, a poorly designed inquiry, or worse yet, the use of inappropriate clinical interventions. Be fully open to discovering the best evidence on your topic.
- The more studies you appraise, the more skilled you will become in knowing what to look for. Allowing a little extra time for your first few appraisals is a good idea.

## CAPs and CATs

Appraising research can be time-consuming since there are many components to consider. So, it bears mentioning here that sometimes you can access appraisals completed by others, thereby saving you valuable time. These appraisals come in the form of **critically appraised papers** (CAPs), which are short analyses of individual studies, and **critically appraised topics** (CATs), which are summary appraisals of multiple studies on a single topic or intervention. First, CAPs are completed on individual studies, and then they are compiled to complete a CAT. CATs result in a clinical bottom line or summary of recommendations, and in many cases, these recommendations are formally published as **clinical practice guidelines**. Conditions for publication typically include collaboration by multiple individuals to critically appraise the literature and set forth practice recommendations. Expert consensus may also be used when the involved parties have extensive experience or advanced training in the subject area. The popularity of clinical practice guidelines has grown due to their proven ability to enhance clinical practice, contain costs, and improve client outcomes. Previously completed CAPs and CATs are often available through professional organizations and institutional repositories. If you locate a CAT on a topic of interest, be sure to check the completion or revision date. CATs completed some time ago may not incorporate more recent studies and should be considered cautiously. Various templates exist for completing CAPs and CATs, and two such templates are provided in Appendices C and D if you need them.

## CHAPTER SUMMARY

1. State the importance of critical appraisal.
   - Critical appraisal is the process of assessing the quality of an individual study.
   - Critical appraisal can help you make informed decisions about applying existing research to current practice, justify the need for an inquiry, and understand and avoid methodological issues in your own research.
2. Describe reliability and validity in quantitative research.
   - Validity refers to how well a study/tool measures the concepts it intends to measure.
   - Internal validity relates to how well the study methods, data collection, and analysis were conducted to limit bias, whereas external validity is the degree to which the outcomes can be applied to similar groups or situations.
   - Reliability is the extent to which study outcomes are consistent or can be replicated in repeated inquiries.
   - Reliability also refers to the degree to which a data collection tool produces consistent results over time (test-retest), across test items (split-half), within an individual rater (intrarater), and among different raters (interrater).
3. Identify threats to internal and external validity in quantitative research.
   - Threats to internal validity include intervention bias (contamination or co-intervention), maturation of participants (timing bias), measurement bias, sampling bias, and subject attrition or mortality.
   - Threats to external validity include the Hawthorne effect (attentional bias), limited description of the study methods, sampling bias, multiple treatments, and researcher bias.

4. Identify threats to reliability in quantitative research.
   - Threats to reliability include subject fatigue, motivation, learning, and ability, as well as the quality of the data collection tools, the raters' abilities, and the test environment.
5. Critically appraise the components of a quantitative research study.
   - Table 6-1 provides a comprehensive template for appraisal of a quantitative research study by component.
   - A quality appraisal includes a summary of relevant study details (column 1), the appraisal or determination if the study components are sufficient, appropriate, and of good quality (column 2), and the identification of potential biases or limitations (column 3).
   - The chapter details each component of a quantitative research study to guide you through an appraisal.
   - Quantitative research can be classified into levels of evidence (I–V, with I being the most rigorous and V the least) based on a study's methodological strength or rigor. Levels of evidence cannot be used definitively to assess the quality of a study; aspects of external validity must also be considered.
   - Statistical significance refers to outcomes attributed to a specific intervention rather than chance alone. Clinical significance refers to meaningful clinical outcomes.
   - After an appraisal is complete, you must consider if and how the study applies to your purpose, population, and setting. Exercise caution in applying studies where concerns were noted related to 50% or more of the study components.
6. Recall additional resources for critical appraisal of research.
   - A critically appraised paper (CAP) is an appraisal of an individual study.
   - A critically appraised topic (CAT) is a summary appraisal of multiple studies on a single topic or intervention that results in a clinical bottom line or recommendations.
   - CATs and CAPs completed by others are available through various professional organizations or institutional repositories and are sometimes formally published as clinical practice guidelines.

## TEST YOUR KNOWLEDGE

1. Which of the following BEST describes critical appraisal?
   a. Evaluation of existing research for application to practice or future research
   b. Assessment of a study's rigor to determine publication potential
   c. Detailed review of existing research to avoid duplication in future research
   d. Confirmation of effective interventions for evidence-based practice
2. What term describes when participants receive another intervention during the study that may impact results?
   a. Sampling bias
   b. Contamination
   c. Timing bias
   d. Co-intervention
3. The Hawthorne effect is also known as what type of bias?
   a. Timing bias
   b. Sampling bias
   c. Measurement bias
   d. Attentional bias
4. What type of reliability involves the consistency of scores over time?
   a. Test-retest reliability
   b. Intrarater reliability
   c. Split-half reliability
   d. Interrater reliability
5. In the quantitative level of evidence hierarchy in Figure 6-1, which of the following would be classified as a level III study?
   a. A survey of South African healthcare professionals on the use of homeopathic medicine
   b. An article published in a professional journal by a nurse on medication adherence
   c. A study comparing participants' quality of life before, immediately after, and 6 months after a mindfulness program.
   d. An experimental study with randomization of children to intervention and control groups
6. If outcomes of a study indicate a large effect size, what does this mean?
   a. The confidence level was set at $p \leq 0.05$ and should be adjusted.
   b. The study has significant limitations and biases present.

c. A substantial or meaningful difference is present in the results.
d. There is greater confidence that the results are due to chance.

7. Which of the following studies would be MOST APPROPRIATE to apply to your setting?
   a. A study with quality design features and relevance to your setting and population
   b. A study that is level I or II quantitative evidence
   c. A study in which the outcomes align with your personal beliefs
   d. A study that shows effectiveness of the intervention you are interested in
8. What is a CAT?
   a. Comprehensive appraisal template
   b. Comparison analysis topic
   c. Critically appraised topic
   d. Critical analysis task

Answer key appears at the end of this text.

## NEXT STEPS

1. Locate a quantitative inquiry on a topic of interest. Identify any threats to validity and reliability. Based on what you find, would you apply this research? Why or why not?
2. Try to locate five quantitative inquiries on a topic of interest with one inquiry for each level of evidence (I–V). If you are successful, compare the design features and purpose of each study. How do they differ, and what unique information results from each one? If you cannot locate one inquiry for each level of evidence, consider why this might be. Can you find multiple inquiries clustered within only certain levels of evidence for this topic? Why might this be?
3. Locate a quantitative inquiry on a topic of interest and use Table 6-1 to complete a full appraisal. Use the text to guide you through this process.

## REFERENCES

Carpenter, R., Waldrop, J., & Carter-Templeton, H. (2021). Statistical, practical and clinical significance and Doctor of Nursing Practice projects. *Nurse Author & Editor, 31*(3-4), 50–53. https://doi.org/10.1111/nae2.27

Chen, H., Cohen, P., & Chen, S. (2010). How big is a big odds ratio? Interpreting the magnitudes of odds ratios in epidemiological studies. *Communications in Statistics—Simulation and Computation, 39*(4), 860–864. https://doi.org/10.1080/03610911003650383

Cohen, J. (1988). *Statistical power analysis for the behavioral sciences* (2nd ed.). Routledge.

Cohen, J. (1992). A power primer. *Psychological Bulletin, 112*(1), 155–159. https://doi.org/10.1037/0033-2909.112.1.155

Franke, R. H., & Kaul, J. D. (1978). The Hawthorne experiments: First statistical interpretation. *American Sociological Review, 43*(5), 623–643. https://doi.org/10.2307/2094540

Funder, D. C., & Ozer, D. J. (2019). Evaluating effect size in psychological research: Sense and nonsense. *Advances in Methods and Practices in Psychological Science, 2*(2), 156–158. https://doi.org/10.1177/2515245919847202

Heale, R., & Twycross, A. (2015). Validity and reliability in quantitative studies. *Evidence-Based Nursing, 18*(3), 66–67. https://doi.org/10.1136/eb-2015-102129

Howick, J., Chalmers, I., Glasziou, P., Greenhalgh, T. Heneghan, C., Liberati, A., Moschetti, I., Phillips, B., & Thornton, H. (2011). *The 2011 Oxford CEBM levels of evidence* (Introductory Document). Oxford Centre for Evidence-Based Medicine. https://www.cebm.ox.ac.uk/resources/levels-of-evidence/ocebm-levels-of-evidence

Joanna Briggs Institute. (2013). *JBI levels of evidence.* https://jbi.global/sites/default/files/2019-05/JBI-Levels-of-evidence_2014_0.pdf

National Collaborating Centre for Methods and Tools. (2023). *6S Search Pyramid Tool: Searching for research evidence.* McMaster University. https://www.nccmt.ca/tools/6s-search-pyramid

Novak, I. (2012). Evidence to practice commentary: The Evidence Alert Traffic Light Grading System. *Physical & Occupational Therapy in Pediatrics, 32*(3), 256–259. https://doi.org/10.3109/01942638.2012.698148

OCEBM Levels of Evidence Working Group. (2011). *The Oxford 2011 levels of evidence.* Oxford Centre for Evidence-Based Medicine. https://www.cebm.ox.ac.uk/files/levels-of-evidence/cebm-levels-of-evidence-2-1.pdf

Polit, D. F., & Beck, C. T. (2021). *Nursing research: Generating and assessing evidence for nursing practice* (11th ed.). Wolters Kluwer.

Salkind, H. J., & Frey, B. B. (2020). *Statistics for people who (think they) hate statistics* (7th ed.). SAGE Publications.

Stächele, T., Domes, G., Wekenborg, M., Penz, M., Kirschbaum, C., & Heinrichs, M. (2020). Effects of a 6-week internet-based stress management program on perceived stress, subjective coping skills, and sleep quality. *Frontiers in Psychiatry, 11,* Article 463. https://doi.org/10.3389/fpsyt.2020.00463

Sullivan, G. M., & Feinn, R. (2012). Using effect size—Or why the *P* value is not enough. *Journal of Graduate Medical Education, 4*(3), 279–282. https://doi.org/10.4300/JGME-D-12-00156.1

Chapter 7

# Qualitative Research Design and Methods

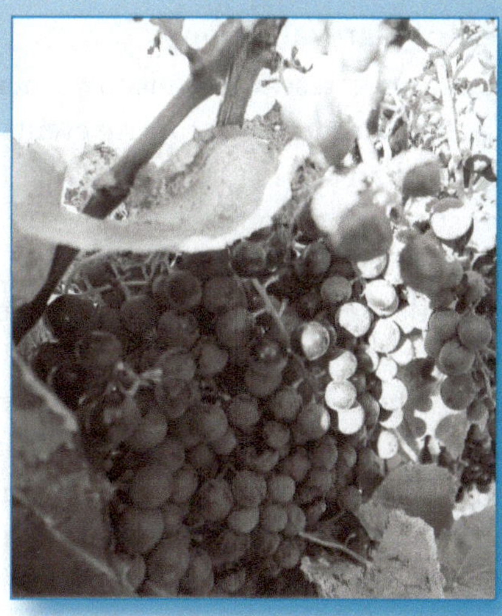

LEARNING OUTCOMES

*The information provided in this chapter will assist you to:*

7.1 Define qualitative research.

7.2 Describe the prominent features of qualitative research, including use of natural settings; focus on perspectives, meaning, and values of participants; and flexible procedures.

7.3 Compare quantitative and qualitative research.

7.4 Describe six common qualitative designs.

## What Is Qualitative Research?

**Qualitative research** is the study of people, events, and social phenomena within natural contexts, or real-world settings. Instead of numerical data, qualitative research generates "thick description" or narrative data that must be processed to draw conclusions (Geertz, 1973). While quantitative research aims to statistically describe or determine relationships among variables, qualitative research aims to uncover how or why something happens. For example, quantitative methods could be used to explore the impact of student-centered programming on the academic success of first-generation college students. Researchers could compare students' grades before and after the programming to determine any effect. Using qualitative methods, researchers could explore students' perceptions of supports and barriers to academic success. In this case, researchers could use qualitative methods to understand the lived experience of a first-generation college student. The information gained could help design future programming and target resources to best support this student group.

Historically, qualitative research was employed in the fields of anthropology, history, and political science. However, the approach has now been widely adopted in psychology, sociology, education, and healthcare due to the benefits of exploring the experiences of clients and professionals in their natural contexts. This chapter describes the major qualitative research designs and their advantages and disadvantages. Of course, there are many more designs than those presented here, but these should get you started. Let us begin with the prominent features of qualitative research.

## Features of Qualitative Research

Three key features characterize qualitative research:

1. Use of natural settings
2. Focus on participants' perspectives, meaning, and values
3. Flexible procedures

Vineyards, Keuka Lake, New York.

### Use of Natural Settings

Qualitative research typically relies on natural settings and naturally occurring events and phenomena rather than constructed experiments carried out under strict conditions. Qualitative researchers immerse themselves in the field (at the study site), observing and talking to subjects (typically referred to as participants or informants in qualitative research), and gathering and analyzing data. They must establish rapport with the participants to foster the sharing of information, and for this reason, qualitative research may require extended periods of time. Rather than acquiring a snapshot view (such as that gained from a one-time survey), researchers get an intensely holistic view of the lived experiences of the individual, group, or community being studied.

Because naturalistic data emphasize these lived experiences, researchers can identify the meanings people place on the events, processes, and structures of their lives. As a qualitative study proceeds, participants' perceptions, assumptions, and judgments become clear and can be placed in the context of the social world around them. In healthcare, placing this information in context can be particularly helpful in understanding how patients view their illness and how they cope with it.

### Focus on Participants' Perspectives, Meaning, and Values

In qualitative research, the researcher attempts to capture the participants' perspectives, meanings, and values through deep attentiveness, empathetic understanding, and suspended preconceptions about the topics of focus. The researcher adopts a learner's role to gain a holistic view of the participants and their surroundings. The power of stories and narratives collected directly from participants or by embedding oneself in the daily lives of the individual, group, or community can lead to rich and powerful insights. For example, understanding the perspectives of individuals who use wheelchairs could shape public health policy and advocacy efforts related to accessibility.

### Flexible Procedures

Unlike quantitative research, in which strict procedures are employed, qualitative research involves relatively flexible procedures. In qualitative research, standardized or formal data collection tools are seldom used; the researchers serve as the data collection tool by observing participants and asking flexible probing questions to gain insight into the phenomena of interest. Questioning co-occurs with collecting information and making sense of it. One process drives the other, resulting in refining the problem and forming additional questions, which are then pursued in the field. In other words, as you learn more about the participants and the topic of interest, you can modify the questions you might ask on the spot. The processes of gathering and analyzing data are intermixed and can influence each other.

Table 7-1 further outlines the differences between quantitative and qualitative methods. Quantitative designs and their features are discussed in greater detail in Chapters 4 and 5.

### TIPS & INSPIRATION

- Review a research article's *Data Analysis* and *Results* sections to quickly identify if the study is a quantitative or qualitative design. The study is a quantitative design if you find statistical analysis, and the results are presented as numbers. The study is a qualitative design if you see narrative descriptions and identification of common words, behaviors, or themes. You may find studies that employed both methods simultaneously.

## Qualitative Designs

Most quantitative research begins with a theory that you want to test—for example, you might theorize that an educational intervention will positively impact fall risk in community-dwelling seniors. However, in qualitative research, the reverse is often the norm—meaning that you gather data to learn as much as you can about a group or community, and you then generate a theory from the data, which could be further tested in later quantitative experimentation. For example, as part of a qualitative inquiry, you could regularly observe and engage with seniors at a local community center to understand

**TABLE 7-1 ■ Comparison of Quantitative and Qualitative Research Methods**

| Features | Quantitative | Qualitative |
|---|---|---|
| **Purpose** | To describe variables, examine relationships among variables, or determine cause and effect | To understand how or why something happens |
| **Sampling** | ■ Probability or nonprobability sampling<br>■ May involve randomization | ■ Nonprobability sampling |
| **Procedures** | ■ Systematic, rigid<br>■ May involve manipulation and control | ■ Flexible<br>■ Naturally occurring situations and events |
| **Data Collection Methods** | ■ Observation<br>■ Surveys/interviews<br>■ Record review<br>■ Equipment<br>■ Assessments | ■ Fieldwork (observation)<br>■ Interviews/focus groups<br>■ Examination of photographs, written documents, and artifacts |
| **Resulting Data** | Numerical data | Narrative data or "thick" description |
| **Data Analysis** | Descriptive or inferential statistics | Grouping of common words or behaviors (nonstatistical) |
| **Data Presentation** | Tables, figures, graphs | Narrative descriptions, subject quotes |

factors that influence their attendance at the center, chosen social activities, and motivators to leave their homes. These factors may influence fall risk behaviors and could later be incorporated into a quantitative study to determine the relationship between these factors and fall risk. It also bears mentioning that sometimes researchers incorporate both quantitative and qualitative methods in one study to gain a more holistic understanding of the phenomenon under study. Quantitative methods can determine relationships among variables, but qualitative methods can take this a step further to understand why. These studies are called **mixed methods designs**, explored in further detail in Chapter 10. See Box 7-1 for an example of a qualitative study.

Qualitative research begins with broad questions about a topic or phenomenon to understand diverse experiences, cultures, social phenomena, and complexities of human behavior. The value of qualitative research in healthcare cannot be overstated. For example, a quantitative randomized controlled trial

**BOX 7-1 ■ Example of Qualitative Study**

A qualitative study explored the perceptions of clients with cancer in relation to their participation in a 12-week exercise program. They were previously diagnosed with cancer and had participated in a structured exercise program, representing naturally occurring circumstances. Borsati et al. (2023) used semi-structured interviews with a purposive sample of 21 clients to better understand the benefits, barriers, and other influences on their participation. The semi-structured interviews align with the flexible nature of qualitative research; the researchers used guiding questions to initiate the conversations, but likely exercised flexibility as necessary to keep the participants engaged and sharing throughout the interviews. The resulting data included thick descriptions focused on several emerging themes. The article includes direct participant quotes to support each theme.

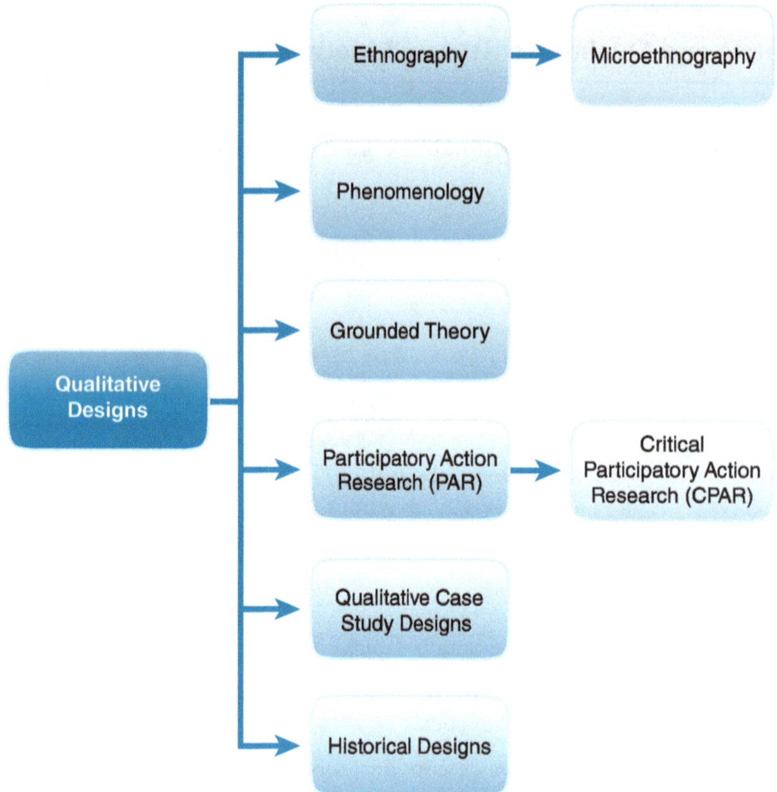


Figure 7-1 Common qualitative designs.

could prove the effectiveness of a therapeutic intervention, yet you might find that few clients are compliant with this intervention. Qualitative methods can be used to explore why the clients are unreceptive to the intervention—perhaps it is cost-prohibitive, too time-consuming, or conflicts with important familial traditions or cultural values. This information cannot be expressed with the numerical data garnered from quantitative methods. Also, while qualitative methods can provide clues about cause and effect, they cannot definitively determine causality. Qualitative designs do not produce numerical data and usually lack manipulation and control—all elements necessary for determining causality. The most common types of qualitative designs, highlighted in Figure 7-1, are reviewed here.

### TIPS & INSPIRATION

- As you review the features of qualitative research, you may think it is less rigorous than quantitative research, but do not be fooled. There is valuable information to be gained from qualitative research and steps can be taken to improve the validity and reliability of the findings. These are discussed further in Chapter 8.

## Ethnography

**Ethnography** is a qualitative design used to describe a collective culture or aspects of culture, which may include "shared patterns of behaviors, language, and actions of an intact cultural group in a natural setting" (Creswell & Creswell, 2023, p. 15). Ethnography originated in anthropology, intending to describe ethnic groups, but has been borrowed by the health sciences to describe the culture of healthcare systems, specialized schools, living facilities, or communities where services are rendered. Groups such as refugees or those experiencing homelessness or a specific medical condition can also be studied to understand better the group's behaviors, habits, beliefs, and cultural norms.

One of the primary methods of gathering data in ethnography is through observation, often called

**fieldwork.** During fieldwork, the researcher observes the environment, events, and participants in their natural context to explore and learn as much as possible. For example, researchers might be interested in studying the culture of a rehabilitation department that regularly introduces and uses complex, innovative treatment programming. In the initial fieldwork, the researchers would focus on learning about the basic structure and function of the culture (the department, facility, and policies); how many people are involved and their demographics; the relationships between those involved in the program; the language used by clients, staff, and administrators; and some historical data about the department and previous treatments. Ethnographers have biases and preconceived ideas about the group under study, just as other researchers do. Therefore, it is crucial to acknowledge these biases in an attempt to achieve an open mind before going into the field. A good first step is to make a list of assumptions and preconceived ideas before starting the inquiry and then revisit this list during the data analysis phase. Additional strategies to improve validity and reliability in qualitative research are discussed in Chapter 9.

The time spent in fieldwork can vary from several weeks to several years. The latter is typical of anthropological studies of foreign cultures in distant lands, whereas the former is more common in recent ethnographic studies, sometimes called **micro-ethnographies**, undertaken in healthcare. Most ethnographic studies probably fall on a timeline somewhere between the two. In addition to fieldwork, data may be gathered via interviews and examination of photographs, written documents, and artifacts. It has been said that an ethnography is strong if it teaches the reader how to behave according to the cultural norms of the setting or group (Bogdan & Biklen, 1998). See Box 7-2 for an example of an ethnography.

### BOX 7-2 ■ Example of an Ethnography

Lavalley (2023) wanted to better understand the role of occupational therapy in a community senior center and *how* occupation may include or exclude Latinx older adults. The researcher observed older adults and staff at the center, engaged in activities alongside them, reviewed documents, conducted interviews, and used field notes to gain a holistic view of the setting. Results indicate that inclusivity can be promoted by proactively offering activities of relevance and value to different cultures and in different languages consistently. This information may provide insight into how to structure occupational therapy activities in the future.

## Phenomenology

**Phenomenology** is a qualitative design focused on describing the "lived experiences of individuals about a phenomenon" from their perspective (Creswell & Creswell, 2023, p. 14). In healthcare, the phenomenon might include a condition, emotion, or diagnosis (for example, anxiety, grief, low vision, or multiple sclerosis), or participation in a specific treatment or group (for example, participation in preoperative education or attending a support group for cancer survivors). The aim is to understand and describe this experience for others who have not experienced it. Interviewing is the primary data collection method in phenomenological designs, though observation may also be used. Table 7-2 differentiates ethnography and phenomenology, as novice researchers sometimes confuse these designs. Box 7-3 provides an example of phenomenology.

### TIPS & INSPIRATION

- As you consider various qualitative research designs, search the literature for similarly designed studies in your discipline or practice area. Reviewing actual research studies that employed the designs discussed in this chapter can help you understand each design's purpose and overall process.

## Grounded Theory

**Grounded theory** originated in the 1960s and is an inductive qualitative research method used to construct theories (Glaser & Strauss, 1967). In most research methods, a theoretical base is chosen before

**TABLE 7-2 ■ Comparison of Ethnography and Phenomenology**

| Features | Ethnography | Phenomenology |
|---|---|---|
| **Central Question** | What is the culture of the site, community, or people? | What is the meaning, structure, and essence of one's lived experience? |
| **Purpose** | To understand the behaviors, habits, beliefs, and cultural norms of the group | To understand the lived experience of individuals experiencing a particular phenomenon |
| **Data Collection Methods** | ▪ Fieldwork (observation)<br>▪ Interviews<br>▪ Examination of photographs, written documents, and artifacts | ▪ Primarily interview<br>▪ Observations |
| **Duration** | Several weeks to several years | Typically shorter duration than an ethnography |

**BOX 7-3 ■ Example of Phenomenology**

Halsen et al. (2023) were interested in understanding the experience of preoperative education and exercise for community-dwelling older adults prior to hip replacement surgery. Using a phenomenological design, they purposively sampled four participants who previously participated in a preoperative program. Participants were interviewed to gain an in-depth understanding of challenges, benefits, and overall experience in the preoperative programming. The results provide support for individualized preoperative programming for this population to promote increased function postsurgery.

**BOX 7-4 ■ Example of Grounded Theory**

Literature supports the use of self-management strategies for those with diabetic foot ulcers, but little attention has been given to explaining the process by which these individuals engage (or do not engage) in self-management. The authors used a grounded theory approach with the aim of developing a theoretical model to explain engagement in self-management strategies from the perspective of individuals with diabetic foot ulcers. Through intensive interviews, a model highlighting five phases of engagement emerged, which may be used to better understand perceptions of individuals with diabetic foot ulcers and how to create programming to support them (Costa et al., 2021).

the study begins. This theoretical base helps you understand the existing problem and guides the development of the study's procedures. In contrast, with grounded theory, data are gathered and processed or coded. These codes represent concepts or ideas that emerge from the data, which may eventually be organized into a new theory. The name originates from the theory being grounded in the data. Grounded theory designs are typically time-intensive, with multiple cycles of data collection, data processing, and refinement of concepts to construct a theory (Corbin & Strauss, 2015). Box 7-4 provides an example of a grounded theory design.

### Participatory Action Research

**Participatory action research (PAR)** is a qualitative research method that involves participation and action by the individuals or groups being researched to promote change or action that will positively impact those being studied (Luborsky & Lysack, 2017). In other words, individuals who represent the participants may also serve as co-investigators. Researchers work collaboratively with the participants to understand and reflect on the participants' perspectives, strengths, and challenges; participants are equal partners in determining the research topic, study methods, and the eventual action taken to address the void or identified need (Baum et al., 2006). This type of research has grown in popularity and is frequently used to address public health disparities and social determinants of health (Jacobs, 2018). Social determinants of health are nonmedical factors that contribute to your state of health. These could include your living environment, social support, socioeconomic status, and access to education and healthcare. Another version of this design is **critical participatory action research** (CPAR), which "focuses intentionally on questions of power and injustice, intersectionality and action" (Fine & Torre, 2021, para. 8). In other words, CPAR centers on the inequity of resources, privileges, or opportunities of a specific group of people (for example, individuals experiencing homelessness, women working in a primarily male-dominated field, or racial or ethnic minority groups) with the aim of understanding those inequities and taking action to change them. A primary benefit of participatory action research is collaboration *with* those being studied (rather than research *on* them), which promotes their learning through action and empowerment for change. In some cases, the researcher may also be a member of the group being studied. This is illustrated in the example in Box 7-5.

### BOX 7-5 ■ Example of Participatory Action Research

Shaffer et al. (2020) used a participatory action approach to investigate using an online mindfulness-based course to reduce stress in parents affiliated with the U.S. Foreign Service who had children with special needs. Shaffer is an occupational therapist, mother of two children with autism, and a Foreign Service family member. She was intimately aware of the challenges of this unique population, including limited support due to frequent moves, cultural barriers, and varying regulations from country to country. This information was critical in developing accessible programming and allowed participants to reflect and share throughout the sessions so that future sessions could be modified to meet their needs best.

### TIPS & INSPIRATION

- Whether you plan to conduct your own inquiry or gather existing literature on a topic, consider the question you want to answer. If your question concerns how or why something happens, you will likely gather qualitative research, or at the very least, mixed-methods research.

## Qualitative Case Study Designs

**Qualitative case study designs** involve an in-depth longitudinal analysis of an individual, group, unit, community, institution, or event and the purpose is to answer *how* or *why* questions. Unlike quantitative case study designs, qualitative case studies explore naturally occurring contexts, circumstances, or cases, and they are typically bound by time and place (or setting) in order to keep the research sufficiently focused (Baxter & Jack, 2008; Stake, 1995; Yin, 2018). Researchers and evidence-based practitioners create a complete picture of the phenomenon they are exploring using multiple data sources over a sustained period (Yin, 2018). For example, healthcare practitioners might be interested in gaining a greater understanding of a particular client's circumstances regarding their disability, and how they managed or overcame it, to inform treatment practices in similar circumstances. Observations, interviews, videos of treatment sessions or the client's achievements, or review of artifacts such as assistive technology and the client's medical records could be useful to create a picture of the phenomenon over time and explain how or why a client may be more proactive or resilient in managing their condition than others. See Box 7-6 for an example of a qualitative case study.

## Historical Designs

**Historical designs** (or historiographies) use data from past events and circumstances to better understand current events or make predictions about the future. In healthcare, these designs can be beneficial

**BOX 7-6 ■ Example of a Qualitative Case Study**

Researchers used a qualitative case study to investigate *how* noncompliance with hand hygiene protocols impacts hospital-acquired infections and *why* healthcare workers were noncompliant. They chose this design because they were exploring how/why questions within a single hospital, and the phenomena in question were naturally occurring, complex, and multifaceted. Observation, review of records, and a questionnaire were used to garner data explaining barriers to compliance and to suggest potential actions to drive change within the setting in the future (Augustine et al., 2019).

for understanding social issues, healthcare policy, regulatory issues, ethical concerns, professional identities and roles, and the evolution of exemplary or deficient healthcare practices (Lewenson & McAllister, 2015). Historical data can include both primary and secondary sources. A **primary source** is an original account of an event, such as an eyewitness account, a journal written by someone who experienced an event, or photographs. A **secondary source** is information at least one step removed from the original source, such as a newspaper account (if the reporter did not actually observe the event), a book by another historian, or a clinical consult by a consultant who has not seen the client. A basic rule of historiography is that data sources should be predominantly primary sources, though an occasional secondary source may be used for support. Bias may creep in as the facts are altered in the telling from one person to the next; the greater the distance from the original source, the more distorted the story. Libraries, archival collections, museums, government offices, and private papers are additional places to look for data.

An historical study involves much more than making a chronology of an event. To understand an event and apply the information to present practice means knowing the context of the event, the assumptions behind it, and perhaps the event's impact on an institution or participants, both then and now. For example, consider how an historical analysis of the COVID-19 pandemic might impact future global healthcare crises, including treatment protocols, government actions, and civil liberties. One historian based their historical analysis of the COVID-19 pandemic within the context of epidemic history and prior work on the AIDS crisis (Forbes, 2021). What distinguishes an historical researcher from a collector of historical facts is generalization, or the ability to discern patterns or themes in the data and to infer information from them (Schwartz & Colman, 1988).

Healthcare students and professionals are well positioned to examine the development of their professions through historiography, with several examples available. Gutman (1978) described the influence of the U.S. military and occupational therapy reconstruction aides in World War I on the development of occupational therapy. One therapist proposed that the use of graded activity in occupational therapy originated in facilities where patients with tuberculosis were treated in the late 1800s (Creighton, 1993). Another researcher suggested that 19th-century practices of moral treatment and phrenology contributed to a loss of caring attitudes and actions in treating mental illness (Peloquin, 1993). In physical therapy, Moffat (1994) proposed that therapists look to the evolution of their profession to decide whether they can achieve their professional dreams. More recently, historical developments of trends in online education both within and outside healthcare disciplines have emerged (Belarmino & Bahle-Lampe, 2019; Betts et al., 2021).

**TIPS & INSPIRATION**

- Continue to review the literature on your topic with a critical eye. Did you find studies on your topic that employed various qualitative research designs? If so, those studies may provide insight into possible designs you could use to build on these prior inquiries. Consulting the *Conclusions* or *Future Research* sections of these studies can also spark ideas.
- If you plan to conduct an inquiry, do not feel you must choose between a quantitative and a qualitative inquiry. Mixed-methods designs incorporate both

quantitative and qualitative methods in one study to gain a more holistic understanding of the phenomenon of interest. These designs are discussed further in Chapter 10.

- Consider that qualitative designs often require fewer participants than quantitative designs; however, the data analysis is sometimes more cumbersome and time-consuming. The choice may ultimately come down to the question that you want to answer.

## CHAPTER SUMMARY

1. Define qualitative research.
   - Qualitative research is the study of people, events, and social phenomena within natural contexts, or real-world settings. Qualitative research results in narrative or "thick" descriptive data.
2. Describe the prominent features of qualitative research, including use of natural settings; focus on perspectives, meaning, and values of participants; and flexible procedures.
   - Qualitative research involves using natural settings and naturally occurring events or phenomena to gain a holistic view of the lived experiences of individuals, groups, or communities being studied.
   - Stories and narratives are gathered from participants to capture their perspectives, meanings, and values.
   - Qualitative research involves flexible procedures, including simultaneous data collection and processing, refining the problem, and forming additional questions as the study proceeds.
3. Compare quantitative and qualitative research.
   - Table 7-1 highlights the differences between quantitative and qualitative research.
   - Quantitative research is a systematic process used to describe variables, examine relationships among variables, or determine cause and effect. Quantitative research results in numerical data that is analyzed with statistics and presented in tables, figures, and graphs.
   - Qualitative research is a flexible process used to understand how or why something happens in naturally occurring settings. Qualitative research results in narrative or "thick" descriptive data that is analyzed by grouping common words or behaviors and presented in narrative descriptions or subject quotes.
4. Describe six common qualitative designs.
   - Ethnography answers, "What is the culture of the site, community, or people?" The purpose is to understand the group's behaviors, habits, beliefs, and cultural norms.
   - Phenomenology answers, "What is the meaning, structure, and essence of one's lived experience?" The purpose is to understand the lived experience of individuals experiencing a particular phenomenon.
   - Grounded theory is an inductive qualitative research method used to construct theories.
   - Participatory action research (PAR) is a qualitative research method that involves participation and action by individuals or groups being researched to promote change or action that will positively impact those being studied. Another version of the same design, critical participatory action research (CPAR), focuses on the inequity of resources, privileges, or opportunities of a specific group of people and taking action to change them.
   - Qualitative case study designs involve in-depth longitudinal analysis of an individual, group, or other units under naturally occurring circumstances to determine how or why something occurs.
   - Historical designs, or historiographies, use data from past events and circumstances to better understand current events or make predictions about the future.

## TEST YOUR KNOWLEDGE

1. Which of the following is TRUE of qualitative research?
   a. Qualitative research is less rigorous than quantitative research.
   b. Qualitative research produces numerical data.
   c. Qualitative research explores the lived experiences of participants.
   d. Qualitative research can determine cause and effect.
2. Which of the following BEST describes the features of qualitative research?
   a. Manipulation and control
   b. Subjectivity and in-depth understanding
   c. Precise procedures and statistical analyses
   d. Natural settings and causation

3. Historiographies may include both primary and secondary sources. Which of the following would be considered a PRIMARY source for a study on World War II?
   a. A book by an historian
   b. A photograph taken at that time period
   c. An interview with a current member of the U.S. military
   d. A news article by a reporter who did not observe the events
4. Which qualitative design involves those being studied as co-investigators?
   a. Participatory action research
   b. Primary participant research
   c. Participant-led research
   d. Subject-led action research
5. Which qualitative design is BEST to study the culture of a senior living community?
   a. Grounded theory
   b. Phenomenology
   c. Historiography
   d. Ethnography

Answer key appears at the end of this text.

## NEXT STEPS

1. Locate a qualitative research study on a topic of interest. Identify the how or why research question(s) being explored. Explain how this study's procedures align with the key features of qualitative research outlined in this chapter (use of natural settings; focus on perspectives, meaning, and values of participants; and flexible procedures).
2. Identify a topic of interest that could be studied via a qualitative research design. Recall that qualitative research designs generate narrative or "thick" descriptive data to answer how or why questions. What specific study design best aligns with your topic of interest and why? Consider advantages and disadvantages of each design in your justification.
3. Find a qualitative research article on a topic of interest; then locate a quantitative research article on the same topic. Use Table 7-1 to compare the design features between the two studies. What are the strengths and challenges of each design? Which one is more applicable to your purposes and why?

## REFERENCES


Augustine, L., McCollum, W., Brown, R., & Mourning-Star, P. (2019). A qualitative case study exploring hand-hygiene standards in an intensive care unit. *International Journal of Applied Management and Technology, 18*(1), 126–141. https://doi.org/10.5590/IJAMT.2019.18.1.09

Baum, F., MacDougall, C., & Smith, D. (2006). Participatory action research. *Journal of Epidemiology & Community Health, 60*(10), 854–857. https://doi.org/10.1136/jech.2004.028662

Baxter, P., & Jack, S. (2008). Qualitative case study methodology: Study design and implementation for novice researchers. *The Qualitative Report, 13*(4), 544–559. https://doi.org/10.46743/2160-3715/2008.1573

Belarmino, J. A., & Bahle-Lampe, A. (2019). A preliminary report on embracing online education in occupational therapy. *Open Journal of Occupational Therapy, 7*(3), 1–10. https://doi.org/10.15453/2168-6408.1554

Betts, K., Delaney, B., Galoyan, T., & Lynch, W. (2021). Historical review of distance and online education from the 1700s to 2021 in the United States: Instructional design and pivotal pedagogy in higher education. *Journal of Online Learning Research and Practice, 8*(1), 3–55.

Bogdan, R., & Biklen, S. (1998). *Qualitative research for education: An introduction to theory and methods.* Allyn & Bacon.

Borsati, A., Marotta, A., Ducoli, V., Dodi, A., Belluomini, L., Schena, F., Milella, M., Pilotto, S., Lanza, M., & Avancini, A. (2023). A qualitative study exploring the experiences and perspectives of patients with cancer attending a 12-week exercise program. *Sport Sciences for Health, 19*(3), 993–1001. https://doi.org/10.1007/s11332-023-01055-x

Corbin, J. M., & Strauss, A. (2015). *Basics of qualitative research: Techniques and procedures for developing grounded theory* (4th ed.). SAGE Publications.

Costa, I. G., Tregunno, D., & Camargo-Plazas, P. (2021). Patients' journey toward engagement in self-management of diabetic foot ulcer in adults with Types I and 2 diabetes: A constructivist grounded theory study. *Canadian Journal of Diabetes, 45*(2), 108–113.e2. https://doi.org/10.1016/j.jcjd.2020.05.017

Creighton, C. (1993). Graded activity: Legacy of the sanatorium. *American Journal of Occupational Therapy, 47*(8), 745–748. https://doi.org/10.5014/ajot.47.8.745

Creswell, J. W., & Creswell, J. D. (2023). *Research design: Qualitative, quantitative, and mixed methods approaches* (6th ed.). SAGE Publications.

Fine, M., & Torre, M. E. (2021). Critical participatory action research: Conceptual foundations. In *Essentials of critical participatory action research* (pp. 3–20). American Psychological Association.

Forbes, A. W. (2021). Covid-19 in historical context: Creating a practical past. *HEC Forum, 33*(1-2), 7–18. https://doi.org/10.1007/s10730-021-09443-x

Geertz, C. (1973). *Thick description: Toward an interpretative theory of culture.* Basic Books.

Glaser, B., & Strauss, A. (1967). *The discovery of grounded theory: Strategies for qualitative research.* Aldine.

Gutman, S. A. (1978). Influence of the U.S. military and occupational therapy reconstruction aides in World War I on the development of occupational therapy. *American Journal of Occupational Therapy, 49*(3), 256–262. https://doi.org/10.5014/ajot.49.3.256

Halsen, K., Svinøy, O. E., Hilde, G., & Langhammer, B. (2023). Better before—Better after: A qualitative phenomenology study of older adults' experiences with prehabilitation before total hip replacement. *Orthopaedic Nursing, 42*(6), 384–395. https://doi.org/10.1097/NOR.0000000000000988

Jacobs, S. D. (2018). A history and analysis of the evolution of action and participatory action research. *Canadian Journal of Action Research, 19*(3), 34–52. https://doi.org/10.33524/cjar.v19i3.412

Lavalley, R. (2023). Occupation's role in inclusion of Spanish-speaking older adults in a senior center. *OTJR: Occupation, Participation and Health, 43*(1), 74–80. https://doi.org/10.1177/15394492221093311

Lewenson, S. B., & McAllister, A. (2015). Learning the historical method: Step by step. In M. de Chesnay (Ed.), *Nursing research using historical methods: Qualitative designs and methods in nursing* (pp. 1–22). Springer

Luborsky, M. R., & Lysack, C. (2017). Design considerations in qualitative research. In R. R. Taylor, *Kielhofner's research in occupational therapy: Methods of inquiry for enhancing practice* (2nd ed., pp. 180–195). F.A. Davis.

Moffat, M. (1994). Will the legacy of our past provide us with a legacy for the future? *Physical Therapy, 74*(11), 1063–1066. https://doi.org/10.1093/ptj/74.11.1063

Peloquin, S. M. (1993). Moral treatment: How caring practice lost its rationale. *American Journal of Occupational Therapy, 48*(2), 167–173. https://doi.org/10.5014/ajot.48.2.167

Schwartz, K. B., & Colman, W. (1988). Historical research methods in occupational therapy. *American Journal of Occupational Therapy, 42*(4), 239–244. https://doi.org/10.5014/ajot.42.4.239

Shaffer, E. J., Lape, J. E., & Salls, J. (2020). Decreasing stress for parents of special needs children through a web-based mindfulness program: A pilot study. *Internet Journal of Allied Health Sciences and Practice, 18*(4), Article 16. https://doi.org/10.46743/1540-580X/2020.1887

Stake, R. E. (1995). *The art of case study research*. SAGE Publications.

Yin, R. K. (2018). *Case study research and applications: Design and methods* (6th ed.). SAGE Publications.

Chapter 8

# Qualitative Research: Technical Aspects and Data Analysis

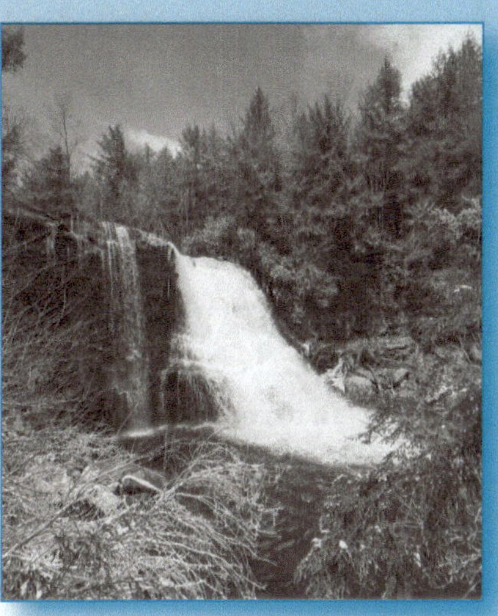

LEARNING OUTCOMES

*The information provided in this chapter will assist you to:*

8.1 Describe the most common sampling methods used in qualitative research.

8.2 Recall factors used to determine sample size in qualitative research.

8.3 Explain the most common data collection tools used in qualitative research.

8.4 Recognize the most common qualitative data analysis methods.

## Technical Aspects of Qualitative Research

Whether you aim to design and conduct your own qualitative inquiry or to review and understand an existing qualitative research study, you should be familiar with several important technical design elements. These include sampling methods, data collection tools, and data analysis. This chapter covers each of these topics in greater depth.

### Sampling Methods

In qualitative research, subjects are often referred to as **participants** or **informants**. Like quantitative research, the participant inclusion and exclusion criteria are specified at the outset of a qualitative inquiry. **Participant inclusion criteria** consist of characteristics or traits that participants must have to qualify for involvement in the inquiry (for example, male residents of a retirement community who are single or widowed), whereas **participant exclusion criteria** consider undesirable features for participants (for example, residing outside the inquiry site, or having impaired cognitive abilities that might impact involvement in inquiry procedures). While people (participants) are most commonly sampled in qualitative research, other items, including locations, events, records or documents, artifacts, or periods of time, can also be sampled. In these cases, parameters are clearly established to outline the focus of the inquiry and the criteria for the other items sampled. For example, if researchers were interested in exploring adverse events in one rehabilitation hospital, they might consider an historical review of medical records during the years of interest. The criteria may also define adverse events (medication errors, falls, etc.) and specify records that will provide the most insight (incident reports, therapy documentation, nursing notes, etc.).

Qualitative research with a narrow focus may target one site, geographic region, or event, which increases the likelihood that everyone in the **population of**

Swallow Falls, Oakland, Maryland.

**interest** (or all documents or observations of the event) can be included in the research sample. In cases in which this is impractical, **nonprobability sampling** is used to select a subset of participants in qualitative research.

TIPS & INSPIRATION

- If you plan to conduct a qualitative inquiry, look to prior research to determine if your proposed topic has been explored with another population. There may be value in exploring this topic with your population if you believe their perspectives may differ. Reviewing similar studies on your topic may provide insight into your inclusion and exclusion criteria.

### Nonprobability Sampling

Recall that in nonprobability sampling, the participants are selected based on some other phenomena, such as location, culture, a shared experience, or convenience access, instead of being selected randomly. Since qualitative research aims to capture the participants' perspectives, meanings, and values to explore how or why questions, purposive sampling is the most common method used. **Purposive sampling** involves selecting participants based on specific attributes, such as their diagnoses, clinical or personal experiences, culture, geographic location, or group membership. The purpose of the research dictates the specific selection criteria, hence the technique's name. In qualitative research, distinct information-rich cases are sought to explore the phenomena of interest. Potential reasons for the selection of cases are provided in Table 8-1.

**Quota sampling** is like purposive sampling in that the aim is still to identify participants based on specific criteria. However, with quota sampling, the proportion of certain attributes represented within the sample is specified. For example, if you were interested in exploring factors that motivated allied health practitioners to return to school for an advanced degree, gender may be an attribute of interest since perspectives may vary among genders. To be sure that all gender identities are represented, you could draw adequate samples from each gender group to represent the proportion of each gender occurring naturally in the population of interest.

Finally, **snowball sampling**, also known as referral sampling or chain sampling, involves selecting a small number of participants who meet the study criteria; these participants then refer others who also meet the same criteria. The process continues until a sufficient sample is achieved. This technique is useful for identifying participants who might otherwise be inaccessible or hesitant to participate. Existing participants may be able to encourage others to become involved by sharing their own commitment to the inquiry, including why they feel comfortable participating or what they see as motivators for participation. Snowball sampling can be particularly useful for inquiries on rare conditions, sensitive matters, or topics with perceived social stigma.

In many cases, participants in qualitative research are obtained through **convenience sampling**, which involves using participants simply because they are available. This cost-effective sampling technique focuses on recruiting participants from places the researchers readily have access to. Examples may include a hospital where they work, a community where they reside, or an organization they belong to. Using volunteers is also a common convenience sampling technique. However, consideration should be given to the fact that the perspectives of those who volunteer may differ significantly from those who do not. Multiple sampling methods may be employed depending on the inquiry's purpose and desired sample. See Box 8-1 for an example of sampling in a qualitative study.

**Recruitment**, discussed in further detail in Chapter 11, is the process of soliciting participants who meet the inclusion criteria. As in quantitative research, participants may be recruited via flyers, online postings, mailings, or word of mouth, and recruitment decisions can be made only after consideration of the goals, geographic location, funding, and other logistics of the inquiry. When the sample consists of items rather than people, public libraries, archival collections, museums, government offices, and newspapers can be additional sources.

**TABLE 8-1 ■ Types of Cases in Purposive Sampling**

| Type of Case(s) Selected | Explanation | Example |
|---|---|---|
| **Typical** | Cases are chosen because they are considered to be like the majority (i.e., typical). | A therapist might want to see how a typical person with hemiplegia proceeds through a specific rehabilitation program. |
| **Extreme or deviant** | After the norm for typical cases is established, the researcher might want to explore extreme cases to make a comparison. | A person with hemiplegia who does not complete the rehabilitation program or a person who completes the program in an extremely short time |
| **Comprehensive** | All the cases in a sample are examined. | All individuals with hemiplegia who completed a rehabilitation program within a particular site |
| **Unique case** | Case selection is based on unique or rare attributes. | A person with double lower extremity amputations who becomes an athlete |
| **Reputational case** | Case selection is based on the recommendation of experienced experts, based on its reputation. | A highly successful caregiver support program for persons caring for a spouse with dementia—an expert in caregiver support programs recommends the program because of its excellent reputation. |
| **Comparable case** | Selecting cases on the same relevant characteristics over time to compare results | Selection of one person with hemiplegia who completes a rehabilitation program for each month over a 6-month period |
| **Critical case** | Selection of one or more cases that makes the point dramatically | A program succeeding in a challenging location, or with especially low overhead costs, or a rehabilitation program showing an extremely high success rate with medically complex clients |

**BOX 8-1 ■ Example of Sampling in Qualitative Research**

In a study exploring the perceptions of family caregivers of older adults with dementia near the end of life, participants were recruited through *convenience sampling* from clinics associated with a university hospital in one city in Brazil. The researchers were affiliated with the university hospital where participants were initially recruited. Additional participants were identified from nearby private clinics (to which the researchers did not have convenient access) via *snowball sampling* (Pires de Andrade Lage Cabral et al., 2023).

**TIPS & INSPIRATION**

- To better understand sampling methods in qualitative inquiry, search the literature for qualitative studies in your discipline or practice area. What types of sampling were used, and how might those methods have impacted the results? Reviewing actual studies that employed various methods of nonprobability sampling discussed in this chapter can help you understand the process and need for each.

## Sample Size

Compared to quantitative studies, qualitative studies typically have much smaller sample sizes. However, methods for determining and justifying an adequate sample in qualitative research vary and are somewhat inconsistent and challenging (Creswell & Creswell, 2023; Malterud et al., 2016; Vasileiou et al., 2018). Some recommended sample sizes are provided in the literature by design type, including ethnography (multiple data sources on one cultural group), phenomenology (3–10), grounded theory (20–30), and qualitative case study designs (1–5; Creswell & Creswell, 2023, p. 198; Vasileiou et al., 2018, p. 4). However, these are not firm requirements. Also, because data collection and analysis often occur simultaneously in qualitative research, it may be difficult to predetermine an appropriate sample size (Johnson et al., 2020).

When determining the sample size in qualitative research, consideration must be given to the inquiry purpose, design, theoretical background, depth of data collection, and analysis methods. A larger sample may be needed if the study's purpose is very broad, the participant group is highly diverse, the theoretical background for the study is limited, or challenges exist with data collection and analysis (Malterud et al., 2016). These challenges may include varying interviewer or observer skills and duration and quality of interactions between the participants and the interviewer/observer that can impact the quality of data extracted. Conversely, smaller samples may be appropriate if the study's purpose is sufficiently narrow, the participant group is well defined, the study has a strong theoretical foundation, and procedural rigor is high (Malterud et al., 2016). **Procedural rigor** refers to the quality of a study's design and the thoroughness of data collection and analysis methods (Johnson et al., 2020).

**Theoretical saturation**, also termed **data saturation** or sampling until redundancy is reached, is another method used to justify a resulting sample in qualitative research (Creswell & Creswell, 2023; Johnson et al., 2020). The point of data saturation occurs in the data collection process when "new information is no longer emerging from data collection, new coding is not feasible, and/or no new themes are emerging" (Johnson et al., 2020, p. 141). In essence, this is the point at which you continue to uncover the same information from additional interviews or observations that you have already garnered from prior ones, or in your analysis, no new themes are discovered even though you are incorporating new data. This concept may be difficult to operationalize in a study because there is no strict procedure for determining saturation. Ultimately, it is a judgment call of the researchers that should be made after ensuring a sufficient quantity and quality of data have been collected to address the study's aims.

Finally, in some cases, the sample size may be justified by the available participants who meet the inquiry criteria. If the focus of the inquiry is exceptionally narrow or targets unique populations or phenomena, you may be able to include all participants in the setting, review all the documents, or observe all the critical events. When this is not possible, it is important to sample a range of people and materials so that you have diverse perspectives on the setting that align with the inquiry's purpose and design. Regardless, qualitative researchers should explain how they arrived at their final sample so that the results can be considered within this context.

### TIPS & INSPIRATION

- Know that samples of greater than 50 participants are the minority in qualitative research, and most are much smaller. Larger samples in qualitative research may result in more cumbersome data analysis and may not lead to contributions beyond those achieved with a smaller sample. If you are new to qualitative inquiry, consider a meaningful yet sufficiently narrow topic or a case study to keep the sample size manageable.

## Data Collection Tools

**Data collection** is the process of gathering data or measuring inquiry outcomes, and various tools can be used depending on the inquiry's purpose and design. Some of the previously described quantitative data collection tools (in Chapter 5) can also be used for qualitative data collection, with some differences noted. One important distinction with qualitative data collection is that it typically co-occurs with data analysis such that the analysis may prompt additional questioning or changes to the data collection process. Qualitative data collection tools can include the following:

1. Observation
2. Interviews and surveys
3. Focus groups
4. Record or artifact review

## Observation

**Observation**, as the name implies, involves watching participants or video recordings of participants. In qualitative inquiry, the method for documenting observations is often less formal than in quantitative research, though skilled observers are still needed to limit bias and accurately portray the results. With proper permission, qualitative researchers may audio or video record observations so that other researchers can check the veracity of the conclusions. However, if participants know they are being recorded, this could influence their actions. Observations may be used with any qualitative designs and are frequently used in conjunction with other data collection tools.

Observations, the primary data collection method in fieldwork, can occur within or from outside the context being studied, with the degree of researcher participation ranging from a complete observer to an active participant observer. The complete observer does not participate in any activities and looks at the scene as though through a one-way mirror. The active participant observer is deeply involved in the site activities, with little discernible difference between the observer and the participants. Most observers settle on a role somewhere between these two extremes. If you observe a classroom or a treatment setting, taking part in the teaching or treatment may be inappropriate, particularly if you do not possess the required credentials for the role or site. On the other hand, it may be reasonable for you to act as an assistant, which can help build rapport with the participants and allow you to gain a more holistic view of the setting and its culture. In either case, keeping a detailed record of your behavior is important to assess its possible influence on participants and the ensuing data collection. These detailed notes about your behavior and your observations are commonly referred to as **field notes**.

Field notes can be taken during or immediately after the observations occur, though a combination of both is typical. Field notes can serve multiple purposes, including constructing "thick" descriptions of study contexts, identifying biases, reflecting on study processes, and increasing rigor in data analysis (Phillippi & Lauderdale, 2018). Field notes can also supplement data from interviews and focus groups, which are discussed later in this chapter. Care should be taken to record, review, and clarify field notes during or as soon after the observations as possible; waiting too long increases the likelihood of overlooking salient details. The primary components of field notes are as follows:

1. **Description of observations:** Narrative script, dictations, or drawings recorded during observations (or immediately following them) to preserve contextual details for analysis. These details may include descriptions of the physical and social environment, the participants, observed actions and events, or potential researcher impact.
2. **Critical reflections of observations:** Researcher reflections recorded during and after observations to aid in data analysis and identify potential biases or additional data collection needed to fully address the study's aims (Phillippi & Lauderdale, 2018).

The timing of observations is another consideration. During initial observations, it is important to find out as much as possible about the roles and routines of the setting and participants. Selecting when to observe will depend on the purpose of the inquiry. For example, suppose the purpose is to gain a perspective on a community living facility's overall functioning and culture. In that case, you should observe at different times of the day, week, or year. Conversely, if the aim is to gain insight into the morning meeting process in a skilled nursing facility, you would likely observe during the morning meeting, perhaps several days per week, over multiple weeks. Finally, the duration of data collection varies greatly and often cannot be predicted at the start of the inquiry since it is impacted by the researcher's prior knowledge and the complexity and scope of the inquiry, site, or culture, several of which may be unknown until initial observations have begun.

### Interviews and Surveys

In contrast to interviews in quantitative research, which typically involve a set of well-developed questions, the format for an interview in qualitative research is often unstructured or semi-structured and includes primarily open-ended questions. An **unstructured interview** is an interview in which there is no set format, and the questions are not predetermined. The topic and aims of the study and interview are specified, and a skilled interviewer crafts the questions and directs the flow of the conversation as the interview progresses. This type of interview takes a great deal of skill and practice. Another option is a **semi-structured interview** in which the interviewer has a well-defined set of topics or guiding open-ended questions to address the inquiry goals. The guiding questions or topics need not be covered in the same order or with the exact same wording from interview to interview, as in a structured interview. Instead, the questions or topics may be interjected as they best fit in the flow of the conversation. In either case, the participant is encouraged to thoroughly discuss the topic at hand, give copious examples, and offer personal feelings and opinions. The length of each interview may vary from participant to participant. Some participants may be more willing to talk, have greater experience in the setting or insight into the topic, or even be interviewed multiple times if necessary.

Typically, interviews are audio- or video recorded and transcribed before data analysis begins. The advantage of video recording is that the participant's nonverbal reactions are preserved and can be revisited during data analysis. An interviewer may also keep field notes to record their thoughts, potential biases, topics they want to revisit, and the participant's reactions. Additional advantages and disadvantages of phone, in-person, or video interviews are discussed in Chapter 5. Interviews can be particularly effective for probing sensitive topics that are difficult to discuss or for topics that cannot be well addressed via more structured methods or observation. Some examples in healthcare include substance abuse, the stigma associated with mental illness, suicide, and sexuality.

Qualitative researchers may also use **surveys** to ask these open-ended questions. However, this written method tends to be less successful than an interview because the personal rapport is lost, participants are unlikely to write several pages of narrative describing personal experiences and feelings, and there is no opportunity for additional probing or clarifying questions to be asked. While a survey is more efficient and cost-effective than interviews, some open-ended questions on a survey are unlikely to yield the depth and breadth of data garnered from a quality interview. Recall that surveys are a particularly efficient way of gathering data from larger groups of people in quantitative research. With smaller samples in qualitative research, a survey may not be the best choice for capturing your participants' perspectives, feelings, and experiences. Additional considerations for survey distribution and design are included in Chapters 5 and 11.

### Focus Groups

A **focus group** is an interview or guided discussion on a specific topic with a small group of participants who share similar characteristics or experiences. For example, a focus group might be conducted with a group of clients who recently underwent heart valve replacement, a group of physical therapists who work in community-based practice settings, a group of females with postpartum depression, or a group of children who participate in adaptive sports programming. Although participants have some commonality tied to the topic being investigated, they may be quite diverse in other aspects. The inclusion criteria for a focus group should be thoughtfully considered to avoid power differentials or other differences that may cause discomfort with participation. In the previous example of females with postpartum depression, valuable information from a spouse or partner about their experiences could be incorporated. However, a mixed group may lead to the females' discomfort in sharing.

Typically, focus group participants have no prior relationships, which may reduce inhibitions that might be experienced when sharing with familiar individuals. Occasionally, focus groups are conducted with groups who already know each other, such as a group of employees from a rehabilitation department or a group of students from the psychology program at a university. When outlining your group's inclusion criteria, the inquiry's purpose, logistics, and participants' comfort and willingness to share are all important considerations.

A focus group discussion is guided by a researcher facilitator who shares thought-provoking questions, encourages participation among all focus group members, keeps the discussion going, and welcomes opposing views. A skilled facilitator asks additional probing questions as needed and takes care to avoid single members monopolizing the conversation. In addition to the facilitator, many focus groups incorporate a trained observer who studies nonverbal communication and group dynamics and takes notes.

A series of 8 to 12 carefully crafted questions in three categories is recommended for a successful focus group (Eliot & Associates, 2005). The facilitator also shares the ground rules for the discussion, such as respecting the opinions of others, sharing only what you feel comfortable with, staying on topic, and maintaining confidentiality. See Table 8-2 for the categories of focus group questions and examples. These questions are based on a potential study exploring physical and occupational therapy students' clinical rotation experiences. Research also supports integrating some activity-based questions to promote engagement; this might involve listing, ranking, sorting, selecting photos, or role-playing, to name a few (Colucci, 2007).

Focus groups can serve a variety of purposes in qualitative inquiry. Group interactions can prompt deeper discussions than may result from individual interviews (Katz-Buonincontro, 2022; Tausch & Menold, 2016). Participants may hone their own thoughts, generate new ones, or be more comfortable sharing after hearing the perspectives, ideas, beliefs, and opinions of others. Focus groups can be effective for program evaluation to solicit ideas for quality improvement. They are also commonly used in market research to gather opinions about products, services, or shared experiences. Finally, focus groups can serve as one element of a needs assessment. (For more information on needs assessments, see Chapters 2 and 13.) For example, focus groups could be used to gather data from members of a residential

**TABLE 8-2 ■ Focus Group Questions and Examples**

| Categories of Focus Group Questions | Explanation | Example |
|---|---|---|
| **Engagement** | ■ Questions used to open the discussion and prompt engagement<br>■ Start with simple questions that require little thinking<br>■ Avoid sensitive topics | ■ What was a favorite experience in your rotation?<br>■ What types of professionals did you interact with during your rotation? |
| **Exploration** | ■ Questions that are the primary focus of the discussion<br>■ Tied explicitly to the purpose of the inquiry<br>■ Most questions fall into this category | ■ What was the most challenging aspect of your rotation? Why?<br>■ What feedback did you receive on your rotation that was most helpful to you? Why do you think this feedback was helpful?<br>■ What would you do differently to prepare for your rotation?<br>■ How did the curriculum support you in your rotation?<br>■ What could have enhanced your experience in the rotation? |
| **Exit** | ■ Questions that give the participants a final opportunity to share anything else they feel is important to the topic that has not been previously shared | ■ What other information would you like to share about your experience? |

community about priorities for programming for children or from stakeholders within a healthcare system about a new rehabilitation unit. Regardless of the purpose, most focus groups involve 3 to 12 participants. Larger groups limit the ability to hear from everyone, and smaller groups may not generate sufficiently rich data (Eliot & Associates, 2005; Katz-Buonincontro, 2022). Multiple focus groups may sometimes be used to reach data saturation.

In addition to those advantages already mentioned, focus groups are efficient, convenient, and cost-effective because groups of individuals can be interviewed simultaneously. Also, geographically dispersed participants could be convened for an online focus group. However, there are several challenges with focus groups:

- **Potential biases:** Biases may result if leading questions are asked, select individuals dominate the conversation, or the facilitator is not skilled.
- **Confidentiality concerns:** Participants are typically asked to keep the identity of other participants and all information disclosed confidential, but this is not a guarantee.
- **Groupthink:** This phenomenon involves participants conforming to the thoughts of the group majority regardless of their own thoughts.
- **Limited communication:** Participants may falsely expect the focus group to proceed in a question-and-answer fashion rather than a dynamic conversation. Data collection may be impacted if the facilitator cannot quickly establish rapport with participants or if the participants feel uncomfortable participating for any reason (Tausch & Menold, 2016).
- **Lack of experimental control:** Even with a skilled facilitator, there is a risk of the conversation becoming derailed or leading.
- **Recruitment challenges:** Targeted groups may have limited time or willingness to participate or represent extremely rare conditions, increasing the burden on those meeting criteria. If patients or clients are the targeted participants, their physical or mental well-being could impact attendance and increase the likelihood of last-minute cancellations (Tausch & Menold, 2016).
- **Cumbersome data analysis:** The analysis involves a detailed examination of verbal and nonverbal responses in the context of group dynamics.

### Record or Artifact Review

Reviewing records or documents and examining artifacts can be appropriate data sources for qualitative research, especially historical designs. Recall from Chapter 5 that written documents may include patients' medical records, minutes of meetings and case conferences, letters, speeches, articles, books, diaries, graffiti, notes, membership lists, newsletters, newspapers, and illustrations. Records can be primary or secondary sources; **primary sources** are first-hand accounts about the topic or event, and **secondary sources** are accounts written by others not based on personal experiences. Artifacts may include physical materials such as adaptive equipment, adapted clothing, photographs, audio and video recordings, and films. Records and artifacts can be used as standalone data sources, or they can be used to supplement data acquired through observations, interviews, or focus groups. Box 8-2 provides an example of a qualitative study incorporating record and artifact review.

#### BOX 8-2 ■ Example of Qualitative Study With Record and Artifact Review

Peters (2011), an occupational therapist, wanted to explore the evolution of the occupational therapy profession, including how the beliefs and activities of the time and the influential scholars and leaders contributed to this evolution. This study was time-bound in the years 1950 to 1980. In compiling this extensive historical review, she examined and cited many professional documents, studies, meeting minutes, conference proceedings, audiotapes, and transcripts. She also incorporated her own journal entries and reflections, eyewitness accounts, presence at occupational therapy events and conferences, and interviews with others. Including many primary and secondary sources resulted in a detailed professional history.

There are various ways of obtaining and accessing documents and artifacts. Excellent sources include institutional libraries, professional organizations, national archives, museums, organizational records, and private collections. Snowball sampling can also be useful. For example, if you are fortunate enough to find one quality source or eyewitness, this could lead to others. With permission, you can copy, record, or video valuable information you locate for later review and reflection. For example, you could take photographs of objects, items on a bulletin board, writings from a journal entry, or images from a film.

### TIPS & INSPIRATION

- If you plan to conduct a qualitative inquiry, look at other studies on your topic and the outcome of interest. How was data gathered in the existing inquiries? Reviewing the data collection tools in existing inquiries can be extremely helpful in choosing an appropriate tool for your inquiry. More information about reliability and validity in qualitative research can be found in Chapter 9. Additional considerations in choosing a data collection tool are provided in Chapter 11.
- Many qualitative inquiries employ more than one data collection method to strengthen the credibility of the results. This can be an important consideration if you are designing your own qualitative inquiry or appraising an existing study.

## Qualitative Data Analysis

Recall that **data analysis** is the process of organizing and transforming data collected during an inquiry to make meaning of it. Qualitative data analysis involves coding and systematically processing narrative "thick" descriptive data, which is sometimes confused with the less rigorous practice of simply summarizing narrative data. **Coding** involves chunking data into smaller phrases or words that represent singular ideas, which can then be used to further process and interpret the data (Braun et al., 2019; Clarke & Braun, 2013; Portney et al., 2020). It also bears mentioning that while qualitative data analysis is discussed separately, this process frequently occurs in tandem with data collection, such that the analysis may prompt additional questioning or changes to the data collection process.

Qualitative analysis is primarily inductive, meaning the data leads to the identification of patterns, themes, a theory, or a comprehensive picture of the phenomena being studied. In contrast, the deductive approach, more common in quantitative research, begins with a theory or hypothesis, which is tested. Completing data analysis or even understanding the data analysis section of an existing published article can be intimidating. The rest of this chapter offers clear descriptions and examples of the most common qualitative data analysis methods with the dual aim of helping you understand existing research and determine what methods you might use to complete your own inquiry. Details about specific methods or how to use qualitative analytic software are beyond the scope of this text. You might consider soliciting help from a skilled qualitative researcher, faculty member, or mentor if you are engaging in your own inquiry.

### Thematic Analysis

**Thematic analysis** is a reflective inductive process of identifying and interpreting patterns or themes from qualitative data (Braun & Clarke, 2006; Clarke & Braun, 2013). This is one of the most common types of qualitative data analysis. While multiple methods exist, the most widely accepted is Braun and Clarke's (2006) six-step process:

1. **Become familiar with the data:** This step includes transcribing and then reading and rereading the data to grasp the scope of the content.
2. **Generate initial codes:** This step includes identifying interesting and meaningful parts of the data. **Codes** represent singular ideas extracted from small parts of the dataset (Braun et al., 2019). Many codes could be derived from one data set.
3. **Search for themes:** This step involves sorting and condensing codes into themes. **Themes** are recurrent ideas, concepts, or patterns within the dataset (Braun et al., 2019).

4. **Review themes:** This step comprises refining the themes. Themes are compared to the codes and may be combined, separated, or removed. There may be relationships among themes. For example, multiple themes may actually be subthemes of a primary theme. Additional comparison to the codes may be required.
5. **Name and define themes:** In this step, each distinct theme is concisely named and described.
6. **Presentation of analysis:** The final step incorporates the resultant themes and exemplars from the dataset (for example, passages from the data or participant direct quotes) into a report that addresses the study's purpose.

Braun et al. (2019) share additional guidelines for completing a thematic analysis. These guidelines are presented in Table 8-3.

The process of thematic analysis is reflective, fluid, and often overlapping. Reflection on the extracted codes and themes and repeated comparisons to the data are necessary to ensure the final report thoroughly represents the phenomena of interest. Maguire and Delahunt (2017) provide a step-by-step example of thematic analysis with data from a study that used a focus group. This example will be beneficial if you are new to this process.

### TIPS & INSPIRATION

- Qualitative data analysis is often more time-consuming than quantitative data analysis. Be patient, and do not rush the process. Taking your time as you repeatedly process and reflect on the data is important.

### Content Analysis

Like thematic analysis, **content analysis** is also a systematic process for identifying, describing, and interpreting qualitative data. Despite distinct differences,

**TABLE 8-3 ■ Guidance for Thematic Analysis**

| Question | Recommendations |
|---|---|
| **Is it necessary to have more than one person complete the thematic analysis?** | With reflective analysis, there is no right or wrong approach. However, having multiple coders, or someone to review your coding, may allow you to consider the data from a different perspective. This could strengthen your analysis. |
| **Should you quantify your themes?** | While you may be tempted to report frequencies or percentages when discussing themes, Braun et al. (2019) argue against this. The value of qualitative research lies in the rich description, and the numbers may detract from the truly meaningful information obtained. |
| **How do you know you have adequately analyzed the data?** | Your analysis should go beyond summarizing the data to explain what it means. Also, your resultant themes should not directly connect to your data collection questions (this is a sign you may be summarizing instead of analyzing). |
| **What should be avoided in the presentation of analysis?** | Avoid stating that the themes emerged from the data, which implies that the themes existed already. Through this reflective data analysis process, you develop the themes. |
| **What other questions can help refine your themes?** | ■ Is each theme sufficiently strong (based on data) and distinct (clearly discernible from other themes; focused on one concept)?<br>■ If themes overlap, does this represent separate themes or some other relationship (for example, subthemes)?<br>■ Do the themes answer the inquiry question(s)?<br>■ Are the connections between the themes and the data clear?<br>■ Have you used examples directly from the dataset to explain and support each theme? |

these processes are often confused or falsely considered synonymous (Braun & Clarke, 2006; Vaismoradi et al., 2013). The primary difference is the potential to *quantify* data in content analysis by recording the frequency of words, phrases, or themes (Elo & Kyngäs, 2008; Vaismoradi et al., 2013). For example, you could analyze interview transcripts from a study exploring stress among 25 doctoral students in allied health programs. By tabulating common words or phrases in the dataset, you might find that 20/25 or 80% of the students' responses include the word "grades," prompting you to theorize that grades may be a common source of stress among this population. This is an example of **manifest analysis**, or simply taking the data at face value. However, a word of caution here—more frequent responses may not always equate with greater importance or significance. For example, a term or phrase might be commonly used in a particular setting or culture or perceived as more socially acceptable than what participants really think or feel (Vaismoradi et al., 2013).

Upon closer inspection of the data in the prior example, you find that most phrases that incorporate grades also mention the cost of schooling. Taking your analysis a step further, you could explore why the concepts of grades and cost of schooling are frequently stated together. Patterns in the data might suggest that those with more financial support (for example, parents who pay for the schooling or a partner who works) are less likely to report feelings of stress in balancing the demanding coursework with a job. This interpretive analysis is also termed **latent analysis**, which involves considering the context of the data and what it might mean. Content analysis can involve manifest analysis, latent analysis, or both; thematic analysis involves both.

Content analysis is primarily a **deductive** process, meaning that it is based on some prior knowledge of the topic. Perhaps the current inquiry is based on the outcomes of prior studies or a well-established theoretical framework. In other words, you already have some strong ideas about the data and what you might find. In contrast, the **inductive** approach, used in thematic analysis, is more appropriate when you have little knowledge or preconceived ideas about the topic. Content analysis involves three primary steps, which incorporate similar processes to those used in thematic analysis:

1. **Preparation:** This step involves transcription, becoming familiar with the data through reading and rereading, and determining whether manifest or latent analysis (or both) will be used.
2. **Organizing:**
   a. **If inductive (i.e., you have no preconceived ideas about the data):** Coding occurs, and then codes are organized and condensed into categories (termed themes in thematic analysis). As the categories and subcategories are organized, they are named and defined.
   b. **If deductive (i.e., you have preconceived ideas about the data and how to organize it):** A categorization matrix is created based upon prior research and expectations about the data. Then, data are coded and organized within this matrix.
3. **Reporting:** This last step involves effectively presenting the outcomes, which may include a visual depiction, model, table, or narrative description of the categories. Reporting should also include a detailed description of the analysis since this process has much flexibility (Elo & Kyngäs, 2008).

Additionally, **intercoder reliability**, or the degree to which independent coders code data consistently similar, is a marked feature in content analysis used to improve confidence in the inquiry's outcomes. As noted in Table 8-3, this element is not necessarily a concern in thematic analysis since there are no definitive right or wrong answers in a reflective analysis. Instead of having others review your coding to see if it is "correct," you might consider having someone review your data to help you consider other perspectives you may have missed. In either analysis method, if multiple people code, review, or analyze the data, a description of this process in the written report can highlight the thoroughness of the analysis and lend credibility to the outcomes. To summarize, the themes derived from content analysis may be linked to quantifiable data and/or qualitative data, whereas themes identified via thematic analysis capture meaningful points in qualitative data alone

(Braun & Clarke, 2006; Elo & Kyngäs, 2008; Vaismoradi et al., 2013). Table 8-4 further compares thematic analysis and content analysis.

### TIPS & INSPIRATION

- Consider having multiple people analyze qualitative data and compare resultant observations and themes. This process can allow you to consider perspectives you may not have originally considered, adding credibility to your analysis process and results.

### Constant Comparative Analysis

**Constant comparative analysis**, the primary analysis method in grounded theory designs, is a process of coding, sorting, and organizing qualitative data to form a theory (Chun Tie et al., 2019; Glaser & Strauss, 1967). The process begins with separating data into manageable chunks (referred to as **incidents**) to identify similarities and differences. Incidents could include interviews with different people, observations of an activity or event, examination of multiple artifacts, or data from a case study over time.

The data from each incident is compared and transformed into codes; codes are compared and transformed into categories, and eventually, categories are compared and transformed into concepts. As the name implies, this type of analysis requires comparison at each step to generate "successively more abstract concepts and theories through an inductive process of comparing data with data, data with category, category with category, and category with concept. Comparisons then constitute each stage of analytic development" (Charmaz, 2006, p. 187). Grouping similar data, categories, or concepts signifies conceptual commonalities among these constructs.

Constant comparative analysis allows exploration of complex phenomena and theory generation through rigorous iterative methods that can limit bias. The continual comparisons promote an openness to new ideas and perspectives and a

**TABLE 8-4 ■ Thematic Analysis Versus Content Analysis**

| Thematic Analysis | Content Analysis |
|---|---|
| Purpose: To identify and interpret patterns or themes from qualitative data | Purpose: To *quantify*, describe, and interpret qualitative data |
| Primarily inductive (codes developed as the analysis proceeds) | Primarily deductive (codes predetermined); may also be inductive |
| Focused on interpretation | Focused on description, though attempts can be made to interpret |
| Incorporates manifest and latent analysis | May incorporate manifest *or* latent analysis (or both) |
| Involves analysis of primarily text | May involve analysis of text, audio, or images |
| Best used when:<br>■ You have limited knowledge of the topic<br>■ There are limited studies on the topic<br>■ You have *no* preconceived ideas about the outcomes or themes | Best used when:<br>■ You have existing knowledge of the topic<br>■ There are existing studies on the topic<br>■ You have preconceived ideas about the outcomes or themes |
| Presentation of analysis:<br>■ Detailed qualitative narrative summary of the phenomenon of interest, likely supplemented with excerpts from the data (i.e., participant responses, quotes, etc.) | Presentation of analysis:<br>■ May include a qualitative narrative summary of the phenomenon of interest, likely supplemented with excerpts from the data (i.e., participant responses, quotes, etc.).<br>■ May also include tables or figures if data is quantified |

**BOX 8-3 ■ Example of Study With Constant Comparative Analysis**

Researchers conducted semi-structured interviews with 13 new athletic trainers to explore what aspects of a mentoring relationship they found most beneficial during their transition to practice. They used constant comparative analysis to compare data within each interview transcript and then among interview transcripts. The data analysis section of their article describes how multiple phases of comparison were undertaken to identify, separate, combine, and define categories and eventually generate a theory to explain the perceived benefits of informal mentoring (Walker et al., 2021).

comprehensive understanding of the phenomena of interest. However, the method can be extremely time-consuming and challenging for a novice researcher. This method requires high-level interpretive skills and is frequently used with a team of researchers who collaborate. See Box 8-3 for an example of a study that used constant comparative analysis.

### Interpretive Phenomenological Analysis

**Interpretative phenomenological analysis (IPA)** is an idiographic qualitative analysis method used primarily with phenomenological study designs. An idiographic approach focuses on understanding personal lived experiences or phenomena rather than generalizing findings to larger groups. This method of analysis is participant-focused, meaning there should be great effort from the researcher to set their own biases aside to retain the depth and meaning of the experience from the perspective of those who experienced it. IPA is a very flexible approach, but it can be time-consuming and complicated for novice researchers (Charlick et al., 2016; Pietkiewicz & Smith, 2012). See Box 8-4 for an example of a study that used IPA. This method generally involves the following steps:

1. Reading and rereading interview transcripts multiple times while noting observations and reflections related to the content, language, and potential interpretations.
2. Transforming the researcher's notes into emerging themes or units of meaning.
3. Condensing, separating, and grouping themes to illustrate relationships.
4. Continuing to analyze each transcript or case by comparing it to prior themes but also being open to new ones.
5. Searching for patterns across transcripts or cases.
6. Finalizing and interpreting meanings among the patterns and thoroughly describing the lived experience in the final report.

(Charlick et al., 2016; Pietkiewicz & Smith, 2012; Priest, 2002)

**BOX 8-4 ■ Example of Study With Interpretive Phenomenological Analysis**

Researchers conducted two focus groups with five adults with rheumatic disease to explore their lived experiences of mindfulness training. The researchers used interpretive phenomenological analysis to process the data. Their article details the steps of repetitive reading of the transcripts, initial coding/theming, comparing themes across cases, and condensing and organizing the final themes. The resultant two themes were "responding to pain and improved psychological wellbeing" (Hawtin & Sullivan, 2011, p. 139). The narrative description of the themes further explains the meaning of these themes, the lived experience of the disease, and the incorporation of mindfulness as a treatment remedy.

**TIPS & INSPIRATION**

- Continually reflect on your perspectives, views, and prior knowledge as you process qualitative data to limit bias.

### A Priori Coding

Many of the previously discussed qualitative data analysis methods are examples of **emergent coding** (also called **a posteriori coding** or **in vivo coding**), meaning the codes (and categories or themes) are extracted from the data *after* it is collected. **A priori coding**, on the other hand, refers to coding in which categories or themes are named *before* data collection. The categories or themes are selected during the design of the inquiry, and they usually take the form of multiple research questions you hope to answer.

When using the a priori method, word or concept coding is used to determine if the components of interest from the research questions are present in the data. With word coding, the research questions are broken down into key words or phrases considered to represent the variables of interest in the inquiry, and the transcripts are reviewed to identify the occurrence and frequency of the identified words or phrases. In concept coding, the transcripts are assessed to ascertain if the participants mention key concepts. This process is more difficult than word coding because a concept can be elusive, and it takes skill to determine if groups of words indeed represent the concept. Once transcripts have been word or concept coded, you must decide if there is sufficient occurrence of each research question theme, either in weight or frequency, to be considered meaningful or relevant for further discussion and sharing. Many researchers new to qualitative methods find the a priori method more feasible and less intimidating than the previously discussed data analysis methods.

## TIPS & INSPIRATION

- Coding and analysis of qualitative data are complicated and often completed with software packages. Some common qualitative analysis software examples are NVivo or Atlas.TI. Microsoft Excel can also be used. Only those students and healthcare professionals pursuing a research doctorate or dedicated coursework on qualitative research methods might be able to perform qualitative analysis without the help of a skilled qualitative researcher or faculty. It is okay to ask for help!
- The steps for qualitative data analysis outlined in this chapter should provide a guide for you, but it is not essential to follow these steps rigidly. Remember that qualitative data analysis requires some degree of flexibility and much reflection as you fully consider the depth of data and what it might mean.
- Choices about the sampling method, data collection tools, and data analysis of qualitative inquiries may be based on convenience, logistics, inquiry purpose, and the topic of interest. Considering all aspects well before an inquiry and collaborating with others can be keys to success.

## CHAPTER SUMMARY

1. Describe the most common sampling methods used in qualitative research.
   - Subjects in qualitative research are often referred to as participants or informants.
   - Nonprobability sampling, which involves selecting participants based on other phenomena, such as location, culture, a shared experience, or convenience access, is used in qualitative research. The most common type of nonprobability sampling in qualitative research is purposive sampling. Other variations include quota sampling, snowball sampling, and convenience sampling.
   - Some qualitative inquiries may incorporate more than one sampling method.
2. Recall factors used to determine sample size in qualitative research.
   - Variability exists in determining and justifying an adequate sample in qualitative inquiries. In many cases, the sample size cannot be predetermined because data collection and analysis frequently co-occur.
   - Sample size may be justified by the purpose, design, and scope of a qualitative inquiry, the available participants (for cases in which the targeted population is very unique or limited), or theoretical saturation.
   - Theoretical saturation, also called data saturation, refers to the point in the data collection process at which no new information is emerging.
3. Explain the most common data collection tools used in qualitative research.
   - Data collection tools for qualitative research include observation, interviews or surveys, focus groups, and record or artifact review.
4. Recognize the most common qualitative data analysis methods.
   - Qualitative data analysis involves coding and systematically processing narrative "thick" descriptive data. Coding is chunking the data

into smaller words or phrases that represent singular ideas, which can then be further processed and interpreted.

- The most common qualitative analysis methods are thematic analysis, content analysis, constant comparative analysis, interpretive phenomenological analysis, and a priori coding.
  - Thematic analysis is a reflective inductive process of identifying and interpreting patterns or themes from qualitative data. Braun and Clarke's (2006) six-step process is the most commonly used and is most appropriate when you have no preconceived ideas about the data or potential outcomes.
  - Content analysis is a primarily deductive process for *quantifying*, describing, and interpreting qualitative data. This method is most appropriate when you have existing knowledge or preconceived ideas about the topic, data, or outcomes.
  - Constant comparative analysis is primarily used with grounded theory designs and involves coding, sorting, and organizing qualitative data to form a theory.
  - Interpretive phenomenological analysis (IPA) is used with phenomenological designs to understand personal lived experiences and involves a flexible yet complex process to transform the data into themes or units of meaning.
  - In a priori coding, categories or themes are named before data collection. This process, which involves word or concept coding to determine if there is sufficient occurrence of a theme within the data to be considered meaningful or relevant, is often more feasible and less intimidating than other methods of qualitative data analysis.

## TEST YOUR KNOWLEDGE

1. Which type of nonprobability sampling is MOST COMMON in qualitative inquiries?
   a. Quota sampling
   b. Snowball sampling
   c. Purposive sampling
   d. Convenience sampling
2. The sample size is usually determined before a qualitative inquiry begins. True or false?
3. Which of the following is commonly used to justify the sample size in qualitative inquiry?
   a. Randomization
   b. Power analysis
   c. Stratification
   d. Theoretical saturation
4. A larger sample size in qualitative research usually transfers to more accurate results. True or false?
5. Which data collection tool is MOST APPROPRIATE to explore the perspectives of individuals with substance abuse disorders?
   a. Review of medical records of individuals with substance abuse disorders
   b. Individual interviews with individuals with substance abuse disorders
   c. Observations of individuals with substance abuse disorders
   d. A focus group with individuals with substance abuse disorders
6. Which of the following is TRUE about focus groups?
   a. Questions are typically unstructured, leading to a greater understanding of the topic.
   b. Specialized skills are not necessary to facilitate a focus group.
   c. A minimum of 15 participants is best for an effective focus group.
   d. Groupthink is a distinct advantage of focus groups.
7. Which type of qualitative analysis is MOST APPROPRIATE for a grounded theory design?
   a. A priori coding
   b. Content analysis
   c. Constant comparative analysis
   d. Interpretive phenomenological analysis
8. Identify whether each item refers to thematic analysis OR content analysis.
   a. Primarily inductive
   b. Can be used to quantify qualitative data
   c. Useful if you have preconceived ideas about the themes
   d. Always incorporates manifest and latent analysis

Answer key appears at the end of this text.

## NEXT STEPS

1. Locate a qualitative inquiry on a topic of interest. Identify the purpose of the inquiry and the sampling method used. Was the sampling method appropriate for the intended purpose? Why or

why not? Did the authors justify how they arrived at the final sample? If so, explain how.

2. Find three qualitative inquiries on your topic and outcome of interest. For each inquiry, identify the data collection tool(s) used to assess the outcomes. Did the inquiries employ the same or differing data collection tools? Did any of the studies employ multiple data collection tools? How could this information be useful in designing an inquiry of your own?
3. Examine an existing qualitative inquiry's data collection, analysis, and results sections. Share how the data collection tools, data analysis, and results align with the purpose of the inquiry. Are the results reflective of the data? Why or why not?

## REFERENCES

Braun, V., & Clarke, V. (2006). Using thematic analysis in psychology. *Qualitative Research in Psychology, 3*(2), 77–101. http://dx.doi.org/10.1191/1478088706qp063oa

Braun, V., Clarke, V., Hayfield, N., & Terry, G. (2019). *Answers to frequently asked questions about thematic analysis.* https://cdn.auckland.ac.nz/assets/psych/about/our-research/documents/Answers%20to%20frequently%20asked%20questions%20about%20thematic%20analysis%20April%202019.pdf

Charlick, S., Pincombe, J., McKellar, L., & Fielder, A. (2016). Making sense of participant experiences: Interpretative phenomenological analysis in midwifery research. *International Journal of Doctoral Studies, 11,* 205–216. https://doi.org/10.28945/3486

Charmaz, K. (2006). *Constructing grounded theory: A practical guide through qualitative analysis.* SAGE Publications.

Chun Tie, Y., Birks, M., & Francis, K. (2019). Grounded theory research: A design framework for novice researchers. *SAGE Open Medicine, 7,* 1–8. https://doi.org/10.1177/2050312118822927

Clarke, V., & Braun, V. (2013). Teaching thematic analysis: Overcoming challenges and developing strategies for effective learning. *The Psychologist, 26*(2), 120–123.

Colucci, E. (2007). "Focus groups can be fun": The use of activity-oriented questions in focus group discussions. *Qualitative Health Research, 17*(10), 1422–1433. https://doi.org/10.1177/1049732307308129

Creswell, J. W., & Creswell, J. D. (2023). *Research design: Qualitative, quantitative, and mixed methods approaches* (6th ed.). SAGE Publications.

Eliot & Associates. (2005). *Guidelines for conducting a focus group.* https://datainnovationproject.org/wp-content/uploads/2017/04/4_How_to_Conduct_a_Focus_Group-2-1.pdf

Elo, S., & Kyngäs, H. (2008). The qualitative content analysis process. *Journal of Advanced Nursing, 62,* 107–115. https://doi.org/10.1111/j.1365-2648.2007.04569.x

Glaser, B., & Strauss, A. (1967). *The discovery of grounded theory: Strategies for qualitative research.* Aldine.

Hawtin, H., & Sullivan, C. (2011). Experiences of mindfulness training in living with rheumatic disease: An interpretive phenomenological analysis. *British Journal of Occupational Therapy, 74*(3), 137–142. https://doi.org/10.4276/030802211X12996065859283

Johnson, J. L., Adkins, D., & Chauvin, S. (2020). A review of the quality indicators of rigor in qualitative research. *American Journal of Pharmaceutical Education, 84*(1), 138–146. https://doi.org/10.5688/ajpe7120

Katz-Buonincontro, J. (2022). *How to interview and conduct focus groups.* American Psychological Association. https://doi.org/10.1037/0000299-000

Maguire, M., & Delahunt, B. (2017). Doing a thematic analysis: A practical, step-by-step guide for learning and teaching scholars. *The All Ireland Journal of Teaching and Learning in Higher Education, 9*(3), 3351–33514. http://ojs.aishe.org/index.php/aishe-j/article/view/335

Malterud, K., Siersma, V. D., & Guassora, A. D. (2016). Sample size in qualitative interview studies: Guided by information power. *Qualitative Health Research, 26*(13), 1753–1760. https://doi.org/10.1177/1049732315617444

Peters, C. O. (2011). Powerful occupational therapists: A community of professionals, 1950–1980. *Occupational Therapy in Mental Health, 27*(3–4), 199–410. https://doi.org/10.1080/0164212X.2011.597328

Phillippi, J., & Lauderdale, J. (2018). A guide to field notes for qualitative research: Context and conversation. *Qualitative Health Research, 28*(3), 381–388. https://doi.org/10.1177/1049732317697102

Pietkiewicz, I., & Smith, J. A. (2012). A practical guide to using interpretive phenomenological analysis in qualitative research psychology. *Psychological Journal, 18*(2), 361–369.

Pires de Andrade Lage Cabral, B., Martino Buttros, G., Leite Brito, E. M., Giacomin, K. C., & Guimarães Assis, M. (2023). End-of-life perspectives according to family caregivers of older adults with dementia: A qualitative study. *Dementia, 22*(2), 346–358. https://doi.org/10.1177/14713012221148524

Portney, L. G., Fritz, H., & Lysack, C. (2020). Qualitative research. In L. G. Portney, *Foundations of clinical research: Applications to evidence-based practice* (4th ed., pp. 297–316). F.A. Davis.

Priest, H. M. (2002). An approach to the phenomenological analysis of data. *Nurse Researcher, 10*(2), 50–63. https://doi.org/10.7748/nr2003.01.10.2.50.c5888

Tausch, A. P., & Menold, N. (2016). Methodological aspects of focus groups in health research. *Global Qualitative Nursing Research, 3,* 1–12. https://doi.org/10.1177/2333393616630466

Vaismoradi, M., Turunen, H., & Bondas, T. (2013). Content analysis and thematic analysis: Implications for conducting a qualitative descriptive study. *Nursing & Health Sciences, 15*(3), 263–405. https://doi.org/10.1111/nhs.12048

Vasileiou, K., Barnett, J., Thorpe, S., & Young, T. (2018). Characterising and justifying sample size sufficiency in interview-based studies: Systematic analysis of qualitative health research over a 15-year period. *BMC Medical Research Methodology, 18*(1), 1–18. https://doi.org/10.1186/s12874-018-0594-7

Walker, S. E., Singe, S. M., & Cavallario, J. M. (2021). The role mentoring plays in the transition to practice of newly credentialed athletic trainers. *Journal of Athletic Training, 56*(3), 227–233. https://doi.org/10.4085/1062-6050-0242.20

# Chapter 9

# Critical Appraisal of Qualitative Research

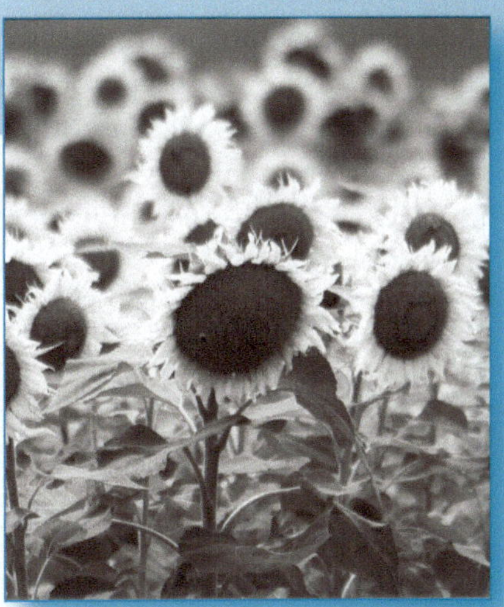

## LEARNING OUTCOMES

*The information provided in this chapter will assist you to:*

9.1 State the importance of critical appraisal.
9.2 Describe reliability and validity in qualitative research.
9.3 Identify the four components of trustworthiness and potential strategies to address each component.
9.4 Critically appraise the components of a qualitative research study.

## Importance of Critical Appraisal

In Chapters 7 and 8, you reviewed the prominent features of qualitative inquiry, the most common qualitative designs, and the qualitative technical elements of sampling, data collection, and data analysis. Now that you understand these basic components, it is time to shift your focus to the *quality* of the qualitative research you located. Not all research is created equal, and just because a study is published or available from a reputable source does not make it high quality or applicable to your purpose. This process of assessing the quality of an individual study is called **critical appraisal**. This chapter provides detailed guidance on critically appraising qualitative studies. As previously discussed, critical appraisal is important regardless of whether you plan to conduct an evidence-based practice project or a research study. Critical appraisal can help you make informed decisions about applying existing research to current practice, justify the need for an inquiry, and understand and avoid methodological issues in your own research. However, the process of appraising qualitative research differs significantly from appraising quantitative research, namely because the design features are different.

## Validity and Reliability in Qualitative Research

To begin the critical appraisal process, you must first understand the concepts of validity and reliability related to qualitative research. Qualitative research is often criticized because the methods are perceived as less rigorous, with more flexibility and reflexivity (Cypress, 2017; Golafshai, 2003; Noble & Smith, 2015). However, the concepts of validity and reliability can still be applied to qualitative research with a shift in understanding. In qualitative research, **validity** refers to the soundness of the data collection methods and the consistency between the data and

Sunflower Field, Asheville, North Carolina.

the results; **reliability** relates to the use of consistent and precise research procedures (Cypress, 2017; Noble & Smith, 2015). Care should be taken during the design of a qualitative study to adopt strategies to improve the study's validity and reliability, or overall rigor (Cypress, 2017).

Lincoln and Guba (1985) proposed four components of trustworthiness that can help you further assess the reliability and validity of a qualitative study. **Trustworthiness** is the degree of confidence in the study methods and findings. The four components, along with their definitions and useful strategies, are presented in Table 9-1.

Many concerns related to rigor in qualitative research can be adequately addressed in the design phase and through detailed note taking and reflection during the study. In addition, providing detailed descriptions of the study setting, participants, data collection and analysis methods, as well as the researcher's role, assumptions, beliefs, and their relationship and involvement with the participants represent best practice in qualitative research. As you move into critical appraisal of qualitative research, this depth of information will be used to make decisions about the quality or soundness of the research.

**TABLE 9-1 ■ Four Components of Trustworthiness**

| Component | Definition | Strategies to Address Component |
|---|---|---|
| **Credibility** | Confidence that the results are "true" or accurate | ■ Data collection over an extended period.<br>■ Data collection with a range of participants.<br>■ **Member checking**: involves asking participants to verify the data and your interpretations. This can be completed at various stages throughout the research.<br>■ **Triangulation**: using multiple data sources/perspectives to validate results. This could include using multiple methods of data collection (observation, interviews, focus group), multiple data sources (people from different sites, different points in time, different stakeholders), a team of researchers, or multiple theories to analyze and interpret the data. |
| **Transferability** | Confidence that the results can be applied to other similar contexts or situations | ■ Ensuring adequate "thick" description of the study participants and setting, so others can determine if your findings may apply to their setting and clients. |
| **Dependability** | Confidence that the data are consistent with the results | ■ Using an audit trail. An **audit trail** is a record that traces the research process (and your decision-making) from data collection through data analysis to results. The purpose is to illustrate your thought process and to show that your analysis is logical.<br>■ **Peer review**: involves having a researcher not involved with the study evaluate if the study data supports your results. |
| **Confirmability** | Confidence that steps were taken to limit bias | ■ Triangulation<br>■ Using an audit trail<br>■ Peer review<br>■ Using multiple researchers<br>■ Member checking<br>■ Having the researchers keep a reflective journal about their decisions and perspectives as the study progresses.<br>■ Clearly outline the researcher's perspectives, assumptions, and beliefs in the study manuscript so the results can be viewed considering this information. |

(Lincoln & Guba, 1985)

Concerns with trustworthiness can lead to bias in the research. The primary biases of concern in qualitative research are participant, sampling, and researcher bias. **Participant bias** involves the participants responding in a way that does not accurately represent their views. They might do this to conform to what they think the researchers perceive as socially acceptable or desirable. **Sampling bias** may be a concern when the sample is primarily composed of volunteers; the views of volunteers might differ significantly from those who choose not to volunteer. Finally, **researcher bias** may be introduced, particularly during the data collection and analysis phases, if strategies are not taken to minimize this potential. Interview questions could be leading, and the data could be interpreted to align with preconceived ideas. Many of the strategies in Table 9-1 can be used to minimize the risks of bias in qualitative research.

### TIPS & INSPIRATION

- Qualitative research is inherently flexible and reflective, which introduces the potential for bias. Ultimately, you must decide if the authors used sufficient strategies to limit bias so that you feel comfortable accepting and perhaps applying the conclusions. Reviewing a study for the strategies noted in Table 9-1 is an excellent first step.
- If you plan to conduct your own inquiry, compare your proposed inquiry design to the strategies in Table 9-1. Are there other strategies that you could use without significant increases in time and resources? It is unlikely that you will employ all these strategies, but making efforts in the design phase to use those that you can is essential if you want your results to be meaningful to others.

## Components of Qualitative Research Critical Appraisal

As discussed in Chapter 7, qualitative study designs vary in purpose and strengths. To appraise a qualitative study, breaking the article down by study components is effective. Table 9-2 provides a comprehensive template for appraising a qualitative study, and each component is discussed separately so that you understand what to look for. The template provided in Table 9-2 includes three columns for completion:

1. **Study Details:** where you will summarize information about the qualitative study being reviewed
2. **Appraisal:** where you will appraise the study components (i.e., Is the information provided in the study sufficient, appropriate, and of good quality?)
3. **Potential Biases/Limitations:** where you will clearly outline your concerns related to each "No" response under the Appraisal column

### Study Purpose

The purpose should be a clear and concise statement conveying the aim of the inquiry. The purpose is frequently stated in the article's *Abstract* or embedded in the *Introduction*. In some cases, you will find it explicitly stated (The purpose of this study is to ...); some journals use headings in their abstracts to highlight important features, and often one of the headings is *Purpose* or *Aim*. In other instances, it may take some digging to uncover the purpose amid other study details. Some authors may provide a PIO or PICO (population, intervention, comparison intervention [if applicable], and outcomes) question that they hope to address in the inquiry in lieu of a separate purpose statement. Some qualitative studies may have multiple aims, which may be less precise than those in quantitative research. For example, the aim of a qualitative inquiry may be to explore the views of a group of people or to describe an experience, culture, or process. Ultimately, a clearly stated purpose is important because it is the guiding principle for all other decisions made in the study design. In the Purpose section of Table 9-2, you should briefly summarize the study's purpose under Study Details, and then indicate whether the purpose was clearly stated. If the purpose was stated clearly, justify your response by sharing where you located this information. If the purpose was not stated or was unclear, describe your concerns in the Potential Biases/Limitations column.

### Literature Review

The literature review, discussed in detail in Chapter 3, should proceed logically, connecting one idea to the next to effectively summarize the existing literature

**TABLE 9-2 ■ Critical Appraisal of Qualitative Study Template**

***Study Reference:*** (insert reference for the study being appraised here)

| Study Components | Study Details | Appraisal* | Potential Biases/ Limitations |
|---|---|---|---|
| **Purpose** | **Study's purpose:** | **Purpose was clearly stated:**<br>☐ Yes—If yes, indicate where:<br>____________________<br>☐ No | |
| **Literature review** | **Main points of the literature review:** | **Sufficient literature on the topic was reviewed:**<br>☐ Yes ☐ No | |
| | **Need for the study:** | **Need for the study is clear:**<br>☐ Yes ☐ No | |
| | **Theoretical perspective:** | **A theoretical perspective was identified:**<br>☐ Yes ☐ No | |
| **Setting** | **Setting type** (e.g., inpatient rehab unit, rural community with limited healthcare access, drug and alcohol clinic, community senior housing complex, support group for those with breast cancer): | **The setting is sufficiently described:**<br>☐ Yes ☐ No | |
| | **Geographic location** where study took place (e.g., United States, Australia, rural/urban): | **Setting applies to your purpose:**<br>☐ Yes ☐ No | |
| **Sampling and recruitment** | **Nonprobability sampling method(s)** (convenience, quota, purposive, snowball): | **Sample size:** __________<br>**Sample size was justified:**<br>☐ Yes ☐ No<br>**Sampling method is appropriate for study purpose:**<br>☐ Yes ☐ No | |
| | **Recruitment method:** | **Recruitment method is appropriate for study purpose:**<br>☐ Yes ☐ No | |
| | **Description of participants** (include pertinent demographics such as age, diagnoses): | **Sample is sufficiently described:**<br>☐ Yes ☐ No<br>**Sample applies to your purpose:**<br>☐ Yes ☐ No | |

*Continued*

**TABLE 9-2 ■ Critical Appraisal of Qualitative Study Template—cont'd**

***Study Reference:*** (insert reference for the study being appraised here)

| Study Components | Study Details | Appraisal* | Potential Biases/ Limitations |
|---|---|---|---|
| **Design and level of evidence** | Describe the **study design** (e.g., ethnography, phenomenology, grounded theory, participatory action research, qualitative case study, historical design): | **Qualitative level of evidence:**<br>☐ I ☐ II ☐ III ☐ IV ☐ N/A<br>**Design is appropriate for study purpose and aligns with theoretical perspective:**<br>☐ Yes ☐ No<br>**Institutional Review Board approval/ exemption:**<br>☐ Yes ☐ No ☐ Unsure | |
| **Data collection methods** | Briefly summarize the **data collection methods** (e.g., observations, interviews, surveys, focus groups, or record/ artifact review) and include who collected the data: | **Data collection methods are sufficiently described:**<br>☐ Yes ☐ No<br>**Those carrying out the data collection have sufficient training or experience in the subject area:**<br>☐ Yes ☐ No ☐ Unsure<br>**The role of the researcher(s) and their relationship to the participants are adequately described:**<br>☐ Yes ☐ No ☐ Unsure<br>☐ N/A<br>**The theoretical perspective, assumptions, and potential biases of the researcher(s) are described:**<br>☐ Yes ☐ No ☐ Unsure | |
| **Data analysis** | Describe the **data analysis methods** (e.g., thematic analysis, content analysis, constant comparative analysis, interpretive phenomenological analysis, a priori coding): | **Data analysis methods are adequately described:**<br>☐ Yes ☐ No<br>**An audit trail is described:**<br>☐ Yes ☐ No | |
| **Trustworthiness** | Describe evidence of **credibility** (confidence results are "true" or accurate):<br><br>Describe evidence of **transferability** (confidence results can be applied to similar contexts or situations): | **Credibility present:**<br>☐ Yes ☐ No<br><br>**Transferability present:**<br>☐ Yes ☐ No | |

*Continued*

**TABLE 9-2 ■ Critical Appraisal of Qualitative Study Template—cont'd**

***Study Reference:*** (insert reference for the study being appraised here)

| Study Components | Study Details | Appraisal* | Potential Biases/ Limitations |
|---|---|---|---|
| | Describe evidence of **dependability** (confidence data are consistent with the results): | **Dependability present:** ☐ Yes ☐ No | |
| | Describe evidence of **confirmability** (confidence steps were taken to limit bias): | **Confirmability present:** ☐ Yes ☐ No | |
| **Resultant themes** | Explain the **resultant themes** in layperson's terms: | **Results are consistent with the data collected:** ☐ Yes ☐ No<br>**A meaningful picture of the phenomena studied resulted:** ☐ Yes ☐ No | |
| **Conclusions** | Concisely summarize the **study conclusions**: | **Conclusions are appropriate given the study information provided:** ☐ Yes ☐ No | |
| **Applicability (Check all that apply)** | ☐ Background information (justifies a need, defines key terms, establishes theoretical background)<br>☐ Shows support for a proposed intervention<br>☐ Supports methodology (may include procedures, data collection methods or tools, data analysis)<br>☐ Other: | | |

*For each "No" response, indicate the potential biases/concerns (for example, researcher bias, sampling bias, inadequate description, missing information) in the corresponding far-right column. Exercise caution in applying research with 50% or greater "No" responses.

on a topic and identify the gaps or need for the present study. The literature review should define all key terms and reasonably address the scope of literature on a topic. For topics with relatively sparse research, the literature review may be shorter; for well-researched topics, more articles might be included to justify the inquiry. The literature review for a qualitative study often includes the theoretical perspective of the researchers. The **theoretical** (or philosophical) **perspective** is a framework used to understand phenomena and human actions and interactions, which can be used to contextualize how we (or the researchers) view the topic. See Box 9-1 for an example of a theoretical perspective.

In the Literature Review section of Table 9-2, briefly summarize the literature review's main points, the need for the study, and any theoretical perspectives,

**BOX 9-1 ■ Example of a Theoretical Perspective in Qualitative Research**

Occupational therapy researchers used a qualitative study to describe the decision-making experiences of children, parents, and occupational therapy practitioners. The theoretical perspective, shared in the introduction of their article stems from the philosophical base of the profession of occupational therapy, which is rooted in client-centered care. The researchers differentiate between client (child)-centered care versus simply child-friendly care, and advocate for strengthening child-centered participation and decision-making (O'Conner et al., 2021).

and then indicate whether the information is sufficient to understand the topic and establish the need. This is definitely a judgment call, and if you feel the literature review is inadequate or the need is not supported, be sure to clearly indicate what other literature might have been helpful to discuss or what you found to be missing in the far right column of the table.

## Setting

The setting comprises the type of facility, group, or community (for example, a public school system, a support group for those with a recent amputation, a senior housing complex, or a community with limited healthcare access) and the geographic location (for example, United States, Australia, or urban or rural communities) where the study occurred. As noted previously, the setting is an important consideration in determining if the study's outcomes can be reasonably generalized to the facility and location you are interested in. It is also important to consider where the study occurred and how this may have supported or hindered the data gathering. For example, participants may feel more comfortable answering questions of a personal or sensitive nature one on one with the researcher in their home versus in a group or an unfamiliar institutional setting. In the Setting section of Table 9-2, identify the type of setting and geographic location of the study, and note whether the setting is sufficiently described. A sufficient description includes all relevant details to place the study within context. While you might wish you had more detail in some instances, keep in mind that most journals restrict the length of articles, so authors must prioritize what information to include. It is helpful to ask, "If I knew more about X, would that significantly alter my appraisal of this article?" A quality setting description, which you might find integrated into an article's *Methods*, *Procedures*, or *Participants* sections, is concise and avoids extraneous details. If relevant details are missing, be sure to note those under the Potential Biases/Limitations column.

## Sampling and Recruitment

The sampling and recruitment methods for a study are often found within the *Procedures* or *Methods* section of an article or within a dedicated *Sample* section. Here are some key points to consider when appraising sampling and recruitment methods of qualitative research:

- **What type of nonprobability sampling did they use?** Recall that qualitative studies may incorporate multiple sampling techniques to arrive at a purposive yet diverse sample. (See Chapter 8 for a review of qualitative sampling methods.) While the sampling methods in qualitative research may not lend themselves to generalization beyond the setting or to a larger population, this is often not the goal of the research to begin with. Summarize the sampling method used by the researchers and consider how it aligns with the study's purpose, and then share potential biases/limitations in the last column.
- **What was the sample size?** Clarify how *many* participants were included in the study and if the sample size was justified. For a qualitative sample to be justified, the researchers should explain how they arrived at the final sample; this may include using a sample size recommended in or based on prior literature, sampling until theoretical saturation is achieved, using all participants if the number is limited, or rationalizing the decision through consideration of study factors including the purpose, scope, duration, and other design features. In qualitative research, sampling may also occur at several levels, including initial sampling and then continued sampling, to explore new concepts as they are discovered in the data.
- **Were the participants recruited via direct contact, mail/email, flyers, online/social media, or other methods?** The authors should explain where participants were recruited and who did the recruiting. For example, were participants recruited from a support group, a hospital unit, or a community event? Did a research team member do the recruiting, or was it someone not associated with the research? Or did they use a passive recruitment method, such as a flyer posted on a publicly visible bulletin board? If the qualitative research involves observations of an event, site, community, or culture of people (of which the researchers are not already a part), this section may also include a description of how the researchers accessed the event, site, or community. Consider whether there

are potential biases in the recruitment methods and if the methods align with the study's purpose.

- **Was a relevant and sufficiently detailed description of the participants provided?** A quality description should include the relevant characteristics of the participants to allow you to understand who they were so that you can decide if they are similar to your population of interest. Relevant details will be based on the study's purpose and may include gender, age, years of experience, diagnoses, living situations, or other study-specific components.

### TIPS & INSPIRATION

- Qualitative research most often employs purposive sampling. Do not be concerned with the lack of blinding or randomization in qualitative research, as these strategies do not align with the aims of qualitative research.
- Sometimes the sample size is justified through a flow diagram indicating how the sampling process and data collection proceeded throughout the study. These diagrams can be handy when continuous sampling becomes necessary to solicit additional perspectives or further explore new concepts as they are extracted from the initial data collection and analysis.
- A small sample size in qualitative research is typically not considered a limitation if the sample is sufficiently justified. For example, if the authors state that sampling was continued until theoretical saturation was achieved, the sample would be considered adequately justified.

## Design and Level of Evidence

Chapter 7 reviews some of the most common qualitative research designs, but variations of these designs as well as additional qualitative designs exist. Regardless of the design, a primary benefit of qualitative research is the flexibility in the design, data collection, and data analysis to explore topics of interest. Additionally, the "thick" description generated in qualitative research is extremely valuable in understanding the perspectives and experiences of those being studied; this information is often missing when more rigid quantitative designs are employed. However, the regarded design flexibility and rich narrative data result in challenges when assessing rigor or assigning a level of evidence to a qualitative study. In fact, there is some debate as to the appropriateness of assigning levels of evidence to qualitative research since it may be challenging to consider all the design variations and details, as well as how one might accurately assess the author's narrative conclusions (Daly et al., 2007; Jackson et al., 2010; Lumsden, 2019). However, if you intend to use qualitative research to inform healthcare practice and policy decisions, some criteria for assessing the rigor of the design and application of the results are warranted.

Several researchers have proposed levels of qualitative evidence based on a study's relative strength of the theoretical perspective, sampling process, data collection and analysis methods, and soundness of the conclusions for application beyond the study participants (Daly et al., 2007; Jackson et al., 2010). For our purposes, a recommended classification system based on features impacting generalizability of the results is provided in Table 9-3 (Daly et al., 2007; Jackson et al., 2010); the higher the level of evidence, the greater the potential to generalize or apply the research beyond the study participants.

On this scale, a level I qualitative study has the greatest strength or rigor and is the most likely to be generalizable beyond the study participants. Marked features of level I qualitative research include aims of building on prior research, strong theoretical foundations, larger and more diverse samples, and meticulous data collection and analyses with evidence of theoretical saturation of all views noted. The conclusions clearly connect the results to the theoretical foundation and prior literature and provide recommendations on how the outcomes can be applied to similar groups or sites. In contrast, level IV qualitative research, which is restricted to very small samples or one or more unique cases, is significantly less likely to be generalized to those beyond the sample. These designs aim to explore new concepts or rare conditions and may result in recommendations for future research. Levels II and III fall within this continuum and are marked by increasingly sound research practices, diverse samples, and other design features. It is important to note that this classification system is only a guide in determining the relative strength of a qualitative study, and you must thoroughly consider

**TABLE 9-3 ■ Qualitative Levels of Evidence and Features**

| Features | Level I Generalizable Studies | Level II Conceptual Studies | Level III Descriptive Studies | Level IV Case Studies |
|---|---|---|---|---|
| | *Most generalizable* ← | | | → *Least generalizable* |
| **Theoretical perspective** | **Always** included | **Always** included | **Seldom** included | **May** be included |
| **Sample** | **Diverse** participants from **multiple** sites or groups supported by prior literature and theoretical perspective | Sample from **one or more** sites supported by the theoretical perspective; may not be diverse | Sample often restricted to **one** site/group, often limited diversity | Very **small** sample or single case(s) |
| **Data collection and analysis methods** | ■ Often involves **multiple** data sources<br>■ Extremely detailed analysis focused on identification of conceptual themes<br>■ Evidence of theoretical saturation and consideration of unique or isolated views (and continued sampling to explore these) | ■ Often involves **more than one** data source<br>■ Detailed analysis<br>■ Analysis focuses on identification of conceptual themes (moves beyond summarizing data) | ■ Involves **one or more** data sources<br>■ Analysis focuses on summarizing views or experiences | ■ Involves **one or more** data sources<br>■ Analysis restricted to thick description |
| **Conclusions** | ■ Builds on prior research<br>■ Ties the results to the theoretical perspective and comprehensive literature review<br>■ Addresses how the results can be applied to other sites or groups and cites additional literature to support these recommendations | ■ May build on prior research<br>■ Ties the results to the theoretical perspective and prior literature | ■ Describes views but not why they exist<br>■ Focuses on participant quotes that exemplify views | ■ Provides insight into new topic or case<br>■ Least likely to be applied directly to practice<br>■ Recommends future research |

(Daly et al., 2007; Jackson et al., 2010)

all design features and aspects of trustworthiness in your critical appraisal. For example, while most case studies are not generalizable (or intended to be, based upon their aims), it is entirely possible that a case study focused on multiple cases with a variety of data collection sources over time could move beyond the level IV rating (Jackson et al., 2010).

At this point in your appraisal, you should identify the design and the level of evidence of the study being appraised. Sometimes the design type is explicitly named in the article's *Abstract*, *Design*, or *Methods* section. However, because of the variety of qualitative designs and design variations, you might need to determine the design based on the aims and other study features. In assigning the level of evidence, know that qualitative studies focused on theory generation would not fall within this classification system (Daly et al., 2007). The theory generated would require further testing, so you should indicate N/A for the level of evidence if you encounter this scenario. Next, you must decide whether the design was appropriate for the study's purpose and aligns with the theoretical perspective. You should also indicate if the study was Institutional Review Board (IRB) approved or exempted. **Institutional Review Boards**, also called ethics review boards or research review committees, are administrative groups that review research proposals before studies are implemented to ensure protection of research participants. This topic is covered in greater detail in Chapter 12. Any potential biases or limitations related to the design should be noted in the corresponding column of Table 9-2.

### TIPS & INSPIRATION

- In some instances, a study's design may only be identified as "qualitative" in an article. In this case, be sure to examine the study's purpose and other design features to clearly identify the specific design type (from Chapter 7) in your appraisal. The concern is more about the design features than the specific terminology used to describe the design.
- Qualitative research is distinctly valuable in answering how or why questions and developing a deep understanding of the targeted sample's perspectives, behaviors, and beliefs. Do not make the mistake of comparing the levels of qualitative research to those of quantitative designs.
- Do not be discouraged if you do not find level I or II qualitative studies on your topic. If your topic is more novel or rare, a level III or IV study may provide recommendations for future research that you can build upon.
- The literature review and theoretical perspective are the foundation of a qualitative research study. All other aspects of the design should align with and flow from these details. Studies with limited literature reviews or a lack of a strong theoretical perspective fall at the weakest end of the qualitative research continuum (which is okay!). These studies still have an important purpose, but you must consider this information when determining how to use this research.

### Data Collection Methods

Recall from Chapter 8 that various methods (or tools) can be used to gather data in qualitative inquiries. These tools can include observations, interviews or surveys, focus groups, or record/artifact reviews. In many research articles, the data collection tools are discussed in a dedicated section, but in others, this information might be embedded in the *Methods, Procedures,* or *Data Collection* section. In the appraisal template (Table 9-2), you should clearly identify each tool used, how and when the tool was used, and by whom. It is important to consider the role of the researcher(s) and their relationships (if any) with the participants. Researchers using convenience samples from sites to which they already have access may have prior relationships with the participants, which could impact data collection positively or negatively; participants may feel more comfortable with the researcher and therefore be more open and honest when sharing information. Conversely, participants may be more inclined to provide information they perceive as acceptable or pleasing to the researcher, which may not represent honest or truthful responses.

Another consideration is the researcher's prior perspectives, assumptions, and potential biases. All researchers bring their unique experiences, values, beliefs, and assumptions to the research process, and despite the best attempts, bias may still creep in. Disclosure of a researcher's previously held assumptions and beliefs represents ethical research practice. You might find this information distributed throughout a journal article in the *Introduction, Literature Review, Methods,* or *Discussion* sections. The theoretical perspective, discussed earlier, can also provide important information about this topic.

Finally, you should consider the researcher's experience and training in the topic and data collection methods. Many qualitative data collection methods require advanced skills. For example, it takes great skill to facilitate a focus group discussion, including building rapport, making participants feel comfortable, steering the conversation appropriately, and giving participants the space to explore the topic. While a researcher's experience or training may not be explicitly stated in an article, citations of their prior work on the topic in the literature review, their affiliations and credentials, information contained in their biography as part of the article, or a quick online search could be used to confirm this information. To complete your appraisal in this section of Table 9-2, describe the data collection methods and answer each question in the appraisal column to the best of your ability based upon the information you have. The N/A option for the researcher's

**BOX 9-2 ■ Example of Data Collection Methods From a Qualitative Inquiry**

From a prior example in which the occupational therapy researchers sought to describe the decision-making experiences of children, parents, and occupational therapy practitioners, they explain how they conducted semistructured interviews within the homes of children and their parents and in clinical settings or via phone with occupational therapy practitioners. They provide additional details regarding the interview structure, language, and techniques employed with the children to establish rapport and elicit their participation. In this article, the information appears in a dedicated section titled *Data Generation* (O'Conner et al., 2021).

role and the relationship to participants should be utilized for studies in which there was no direct contact between the researchers and the sample, for example, in record review. Be sure to note any potential biases/limitations with the data collection tools and methods in the last column of the template. See Box 9-2 for an example of data collection methods from a qualitative inquiry.

### Data Analysis

The easiest way to identify a qualitative study is to review the data analysis methods. If the study yielded narrative data or "thick" description, and the authors describe a coding and analysis process, you can conclude that the design was qualitative. Most qualitative research articles have a dedicated section describing the data analysis methods. In some cases, you might find this information integrated into the *Procedures* section or the beginning of the *Results* section. In your appraisal, you must assess whether the data analysis methods were adequately described. This is a judgment call and often a difficult one to make. The authors might describe the analysis using one of the previously introduced processes: thematic analysis, content analysis, constant comparative analysis, interpretative phenomenological analysis, or a priori coding. They may use various other terms, such as grounded theory analysis, discourse analysis, narrative analysis, or framework analysis, to name a few. Regardless of the terminology used, you must consider that qualitative analysis has a great degree of flexibility, so it is less about the terminology and more about the detailed description of the process. At this step, consider if the description makes sense. Do the authors describe how they transformed the narrative data into meaningful themes or categories? Was the process organized and reflective? Reflectivity can be demonstrated by keeping a journal or field notes. How many researchers were involved in the process? Were participants involved? Having a team of researchers who process the data and challenge each other to consider other perspectives can limit bias and promote more accurate results. Likewise, involving participants through member checking can support features of trustworthiness. Additionally, did the researchers include a diagram or narratively describe their decision-making process (audit trail)? These are the details you should capture in the first column, allowing you to answer the questions in the appraisal column of Table 9-2. Be sure to include any missing information or concerns in the last column.

### Trustworthiness

Recall that trustworthiness, the degree of confidence you have in the study's methods and findings, comprises four components—credibility, transferability, dependability, and confirmability. In this section of your appraisal, revisit the details of the study design, data collection, and data analysis methods to further assess the study's quality or overall rigor. This is where the details you recorded earlier in Table 9-2 will be valuable. You should also review Table 9-1 and compare the suggested strategies to address each component of trustworthiness to those present in the study being appraised. Using Table 9-2, summarize the evidence available to support each component of trustworthiness and indicate your appraisal. If you have potential concerns, be sure to describe them in the last column of this section. While it is not essential that a qualitative study address all components of trustworthiness or use multiple strategies to address each singular component, it is important to ensure that sufficient efforts were taken in designing and carrying out the study such that the results are relevant and meaningful to others as intended (Stahl & King, 2020).

**TIPS & INSPIRATION**

- A good rule of thumb is that at least one strategy should be used to address at least two or three of the components of trustworthiness. Of course, using more strategies only increases your confidence in the results, but considering this minimum can be helpful in quickly identifying qualitative research that warrants further scrutiny.
- As you appraise a study, do not hesitate to contact the authors if you have questions. The authors' contact information is often included in the article or readily available through an online search. Most authors are more than willing to assist others interested in their area of study.

### Resultant Themes

Qualitative research articles usually include a *Results* or *Outcomes* section, where the study results are shared in narrative form. The results typically include emergent themes, which may be further explained or substantiated with participant quotes, responses, or behavioral descriptions. Qualitative results are not reported in terms of statistical significance since the data include detailed descriptions rather than ratings or scores that can be analyzed statistically. Occasionally, you may find the themes summarized and substantiated in table format. A quality *Results* section should allow you to easily understand how the authors arrived at the final themes and how those themes are connected to or were derived from the data. An accurate appraisal of the results hinges on your ability to understand the study's results and summarize them in layperson's terms. Reviewing the *Discussion* section of the article can also be helpful in processing what the results mean and understanding limitations that may have impacted them. Note your concerns and any limitations in the last column of Table 9-2.

### Conclusions

The study's conclusions represent the "take-home message," and the researchers frequently offer practical implications of the research or recommendations for future inquiries. After you summarize the study's conclusions, now is the time to consider your appraisal of all other study components. Are the conclusions appropriate given these other details? It may be helpful to consider these key aspects:

- **Does the qualitative level of evidence align with the study's conclusions?** Recall that many qualitative studies do not lend themselves to generalizability beyond the study participants. Be wary of qualitative studies conducted with very small samples, and those that explore new topics or have weak theoretical foundations that advocate for the generalization of the outcomes. While these studies have distinct value, generalization is not usually appropriate. If the study's results apply only to the direct participant group or site, the authors should still clearly summarize the value of this information for this group.
- **For level I qualitative studies, do the authors specifically address how the results can be applied to other sites or groups?** If the generalization of outcomes is appropriate, the authors should cite additional literature and provide a thorough rationale to support their recommendations.
- **Did the authors acknowledge limitations in the study?** Remember that all research is flawed, and the authors' recognition of the limitations/potential biases signifies ethical research practices. Outcomes and conclusions of a study with no reported limitations or biases should be considered circumspect. It is also entirely possible that you might consider limitations beyond those explicitly stated by the authors.

### Applicability

Finally, you must consider how this appraised study specifically applies to your purpose, population, or practice setting. Whether you are conducting an evidence-based practice project or a research study, now is the time to determine if and how the study information will be useful to you. In the last section of Table 9-2, check all items that apply. For example, the study may provide useful background information, including establishing the theoretical background or need for your inquiry or defining key terms. This information could be useful in drafting your literature review if you plan to conduct a formal inquiry. The qualitative study may support positive outcomes related to the phenomena under study. Unlike quantitative studies, qualitative studies usually do not confirm the effectiveness of a planned practice intervention since these designs focus on naturally occurring conditions rather than manipulating variables or circumstances to test interventions. The study may also provide insight into appropriate study procedures, data collection methods and tools, and data analysis methods. This information could be helpful in designing your own inquiry procedures, including making decisions about the timing, duration, and other inquiry logistics. If you derive other useful information from a study not encompassed by these categories, an additional section is included for you to provide clarification. As you consider the usefulness of a qualitative study to your purposes, you must compare the study setting and population to your own to determine whether they are similar enough for the information to be applicable. Additionally, you should use caution in applying a qualitative study if you have concerns related to 50% or more of the study components.

## TIPS & INSPIRATION

- When considering the conclusions and application of a study, always consider if the topic falls within your scope of practice.
- Be aware of your preconceived ideas as you complete your appraisal. Looking for only studies that support your ideas may result in a flawed rationale, a poorly designed inquiry, or worse yet, the application of inappropriate information to your clients and setting. Be fully open to discovering the best evidence on your topic.

## CHAPTER SUMMARY

1. State the importance of critical appraisal.
    - Critical appraisal is the process of assessing the quality of an individual study.
    - Critical appraisal can help you make informed decisions about applying existing research to current practice, justify the need for an inquiry, and understand and avoid methodological issues in your own research.
2. Describe reliability and validity in qualitative research.
    - Validity refers to the soundness of the data collection methods and the consistency between the data and the results.
    - Reliability relates to the use of consistent and precise research procedures.
3. Identify the four components of trustworthiness and potential strategies to address each component.
    - Four components of trustworthiness (the degree of confidence in the study methods and findings) can be used to assess the reliability and validity of a qualitative study. Table 9-1 includes strategies that can be used to address each of the four components.
    - Credibility is the confidence that the results are "true" or accurate.
    - Transferability is the confidence that the results can be applied to similar contexts and situations.
    - Dependability is the confidence that the data are consistent with the results.
    - Confirmability is the confidence that steps are taken to limit bias.
4. Critically appraise the components of a qualitative research study.
    - Table 9-2 provides a comprehensive template for appraising a qualitative research study by component.
    - A quality appraisal includes a summary of relevant study details (column 1), the appraisal or determination if the study components are sufficient, appropriate, and of good quality (column 2), and the identification of potential biases or limitations (column 3).
    - The chapter details each component of a qualitative research study to guide you through an appraisal.
    - Qualitative research can be classified into levels of evidence (I to IV, with level I being the most likely generalizable to those beyond the sample and level IV being the least) based on the design features of a study. Levels of evidence cannot be used definitively to assess the quality of a study; aspects of trustworthiness must also be considered. These levels of evidence also do not apply to qualitative studies focused on theory generation.
    - After an appraisal is complete, you must consider if and how the study information applies to your purpose, population, and setting. Exercise caution in applying studies where concerns were noted related to 50% or more of the study components.

## TEST YOUR KNOWLEDGE

1. Which strategy would BEST promote credibility in a qualitative study?
   a. Confirming the participants are invested in the study before it begins
   b. Having a peer compare your data and results
   c. Keeping a reflective journal as you conduct the study
   d. Collecting data via observations and a focus group
2. Which of the following BEST describes dependability?
   a. Confidence that the results can be applied to a similar group of people
   b. Confidence that the results are accurate
   c. Confidence that the data are consistent with the results
   d. Confidence that bias was controlled in the study
3. Which of the following is TRUE about level I qualitative studies?
   a. They are most likely to be generalizable to similar settings or samples.
   b. They are the only level of qualitative evidence that should be applied to practice.
   c. They are like level I quantitative studies, requiring randomization and a control group.
   d. They usually provide insight into new topics or cases.
4. According to the qualitative level of evidence hierarchy in Table 9-3, what level of evidence is a study primarily reporting participants' perspectives on a healthcare experience without connection to a theoretical perspective?
   a. Level I
   b. Level II
   c. Levell III
   d. Level IV
5. Which of the following should be the primary focus of the *Results* section in a qualitative research article?
   a. Statistical significance of the results
   b. The resultant themes and connection to the data
   c. The theoretical perspective and *p* values
   d. The researcher's affiliations and assumptions

Answer key appears at the end of this text.

## NEXT STEPS

1. Locate a qualitative inquiry on a topic of interest. Review the study and identify what strategies were used to address each of the four components of trustworthiness. Explain how this information impacts your acceptance of the study's conclusions.
2. Try to locate two qualitative inquiries on a topic of interest at DIFFERENT levels of qualitative evidence (for example, a level I study and a level IV study). Compare the design features and purpose of each study. How do they differ, and what unique information results from each one? Is one more beneficial for your purposes? Explain why.
3. Locate a qualitative inquiry on a topic of interest and use Table 9-2 to complete a full appraisal. Use the text to guide you through this process.

## REFERENCES

Cypress, B. S. (2017). Rigor or reliability and validity in qualitative research: Perspectives, strategies, reconceptualization, and recommendations. *Dimensions of Critical Care Nursing, 36*(4), 253–263. https://doi.org/10.1097/dcc.0000000000000253

Daly, J., Willis, K., Small, R., Green, J., Welch, N., Kealy, M., & Hughes, E. (2007). A hierarchy of evidence for assessing qualitative health research. *Journal of Clinical Epidemiology, 60*(1), 43–49. https://doi.org/10.1016/j.jclinepi.2006.03.014

Golafshani, N. (2003). Understanding reliability and validity in qualitative research. *Qualitative Report, 8*(4), 597–607. https://doi.org/10.46743/2160-3715/2003.1870

Jackson, S. F., Fazal, N., & Giesbrecht, N. (2010). A hierarchy of evidence: Which intervention has the strongest evidence of effectiveness? *Canadian Best Practices Portal.* https://www.researchgate.net/profile/Suzanne-Jackson-2/publication/242760598_A_Hierarchy_of_Evidence_Which_Intervention_Has_the_Strongest_Evidence_of_Effectiveness

Lincoln, Y. S., & Guba, E. G. (1985). *Naturalistic inquiry*. SAGE Publications.

Lumsden, K. (2019, July 31). A kick in the teeth?: The problems with "hierarchies of qualitative research" for policy-making and evidence-based policing. *The Qualitative Researcher.* https://qualitativetraining.com/2019/07/31/another-kick-in-the-teeth-for-qualitative-research-the-problems-and-dangers-of-a-hierarchy-of-qualitative-research-for-policy-making-and-evidence-based-policing

Noble, H., & Smith, J. (2015). Issues of validity and reliability in qualitative research. *Evidence-Based Nursing, 18*(2), 34–35. https://doi.org/10.1136/eb-2015-102054

O'Connor, D., Lynch, H., & Boyle, B. (2021). A qualitative study of child participation in decision-making: Exploring rights-based approaches in pediatric occupational therapy. *PLoS One, 16*(12), e0260975. https://doi.org/10.1371/journal.pone.0260975

Stahl, N. A., & King, J. R. (2020). Expanding approaches in research: Understanding and using trustworthiness in qualitative research. *Journal of Developmental Education, 44*(1), 26–28. https://files.eric.ed.gov/fulltext/EJ1320570.pdf

Chapter 10

# Critical Appraisal of Mixed Methods Research and Systematic Reviews

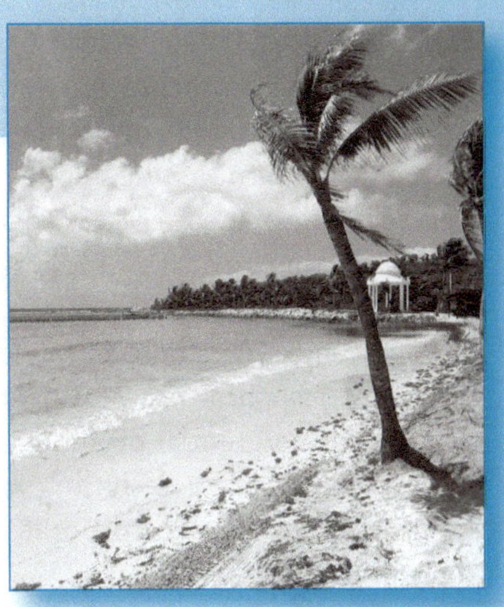

LEARNING OUTCOMES

*The information provided in this chapter will assist you to:*

10.1 Describe the value and challenges of mixed methods research.

10.2 Identify the three primary mixed methods research designs.

10.3 Recall components of reliability and validity in mixed methods research.

10.4 Critically appraise the components of a mixed methods research study.

10.5 Differentiate systematic reviews and literature reviews.

10.6 State the steps for conducting a systematic review.

10.7 Describe the benefits of systematic reviews.

10.8 Critically appraise the components of a systematic review.

## Value of Mixed Methods Research

**Mixed methods research** incorporates quantitative and qualitative research designs and procedures within a single inquiry (Creswell & Plano Clark, 2018). When combined, these distinct methods are viewed as complementary. They are believed to result in a greater understanding of the inquiry phenomena than when quantitative and qualitative methods are used in isolation (Creswell & Plano Clark, 2018; Fetters & Freshwater, 2015). That is not to say that mixed methods studies are preferred over purely quantitative or qualitative designs. It is a matter of considering the aims of an inquiry and whether combining both design approaches is justified and adds value to the inquiry (Creswell & Plano Clark, 2018; Moorley & Cathala, 2019). Justification for mixed methods studies is addressed later in this chapter.

Another benefit of mixed methods designs is **triangulation**, which involves using multiple data collection methods to validate the results and your interpretation of them. For example, you could collect data via a standardized resilience scale (quantitative) and in-depth interviews (qualitative) in a study exploring a structured program to increase resiliency in allied healthcare students. If the data from both methods confirm improvements in resiliency, you can have increased confidence in the results (Creswell & Plano Clark, 2018; O'Cathain et al., 2010).

You can also use mixed methods designs to explain or explore the phenomena you are studying. Using the prior example, if the resiliency scores did not improve, the interview data may *explain* why

Kantenah Beach, Riveria Maya, Mexico.

(O'Cathain et al., 2010). Perhaps students had competing time commitments that impacted their participation in the program, or the recommended coping strategies were too cumbersome to integrate into their schedules. In either case, this is valuable information as you consider future research or programming. To avoid results like this, you could consider using a qualitative approach first, such as a focus group to *explore* healthcare students' perspectives on resiliency and potential programming to address it. By doing this before designing and implementing the program, you can incorporate their suggestions to promote program success.

Finally, mixed methods designs may lead to new ideas for future inquiries (O'Cathain et al., 2010). Integrating the quantitative and qualitative data may uncover nuances not previously considered or garnered from looking at the differing data separately. Engaging in mixed methods inquiries is also an excellent way to hone your skills in both research approaches (Creswell & Plano Clark, 2018).

### Challenges in Mixed Methods Research

Despite the value of mixed methods designs, they may require more time, skills, and resources (Dawadi et al., 2021; Hafsa, 2019; Halcomb, 2018). Some mixed methods studies involve multiple phases, likely translating into longer study durations. Because varying data are collected, the analysis may be cumbersome and time-consuming. Those undertaking mixed methods research should have skills in quantitative and qualitative design; when expertise is lacking, additional resources (financial or personnel) may be needed to support the design and data analysis. In fact, a team of people may be necessary to conduct high-quality, mixed methods studies (Fetters, 2018). These challenges can be addressed with careful planning and consideration of the available supports in the design phase.

#### TIPS & INSPIRATION

- Some mixed methods studies may be explicitly identified as such in the title or abstract. Otherwise, you should read the *Methods* section of the article. If you identify a combination of quantitative and qualitative methods, you can conclude that the study is mixed methods.
- Engaging in a mixed methods inquiry can be an excellent way to develop skills in both research approaches. However, if you are a novice researcher, you may need the support of an instructor or mentor because of the challenges noted.

## Mixed Methods Designs

The primary mixed methods research designs are exploratory sequential, explanatory sequential, and concurrent. Each design is categorized by the purpose and planned order of the quantitative and qualitative approaches. Sequential designs, in which quantitative and qualitative approaches are used in succession, are best when you need or expect to uncover something in the first approach that will inform the next. A concurrent design, also called a convergent design, is appropriate if you want to comprehensively explore phenomena at one point in time. Table 10-1 includes the three mixed methods designs, the steps involved, and an example of each.

#### TIPS & INSPIRATION

- Take a few moments to locate one or more of the studies in Table 10-1. Review the methods sections to help you better understand the designs.
- Be aware that sometimes a mixed methods study is not published in its entirety in one article or source. Journals have page and word limits, which may be challenging to adhere to when multiple methods are involved. Particularly with sequential designs, authors may choose to publish each phase as a separate article with reference to the associated works. If you find a study like this, you should retrieve each article to fully grasp the study's scope and results.

## Validity and Reliability in Mixed Methods Research

The validity and reliability of quantitative and qualitative research are discussed in Chapters 6 and 9, respectively. Strategies to improve the validity and reliability,

**TABLE 10-1 ■ Mixed Methods Designs**

| Mixed Methods Design | Steps (Dawadi et al., 2021; Hafsa, 2019; Moorley & Cathala, 2019) | Study | Synopsis |
|---|---|---|---|
| Exploratory sequential | 1. Qualitative method (findings may inform the next step)<br>2. Quantitative method to confirm qualitative results | Pamungkas et al., 2021 | Pamungkas et al. (2021) used a two-phase study to explore using a health-based coaching program to promote diabetes self-management in adults.<br>**Phase 1** (qualitative) included interviews and focus groups with clients with diabetes and their caregivers, healthcare providers, and volunteers. This phase investigated current knowledge about self-management strategies, challenges in using the strategies, and the feasibility of a coaching program.<br>**Phase 2** (quantitative) was a quasi-experimental pretest-posttest design and involved implementing a coaching program based on data from Phase 1 of the study to an experimental group. A control group received the usual care. Improvements in knowledge, use of self-management strategies, and laboratory values were greater in the experimental group than in the control group. |
| Explanatory sequential | 1. Quantitative method (findings may inform the next step)<br>2. Qualitative method used to explain quantitative results | Siette et al., 2021 | Siette et al. (2021) investigated the impact of an organized social outing program on the quality of life of older adults through a two-phase study.<br>**Phase 1** (quantitative) involved administering a quality-of-life scale to older adults before and after participating in the outings for 6 months. Results indicated significant increases in quality of life after participation in the program.<br>**Phase 2** (qualitative) included in-depth interviews with older adults participating in the outings, their caregivers, and program staff. The qualitative data were used to explain the quantitative findings and uncover the program features that may contribute to its success. |
| Concurrent (or convergent) design | 1. Quantitative and qualitative methods co-occur.<br>2. Integration of results | Tsai et al., 2022 | Tsai et al. (2022) explored the spirituality of elders who recently transitioned to long-term care through the administration of the *Spirituality Well-Being Scale* (quantitative) and interviews (qualitative). The quantitative and qualitative data were analyzed separately but then integrated to create a comprehensive view of the role of spirituality in elder transitions. This information may inform future occupational therapy interventions that target this population. |

or overall rigor, of *both* aspects of the inquiry should be incorporated into mixed methods research. Quantitative approaches should involve carefully designing the inquiry procedures, selecting valid and reliable data collection tools, and using sound data collection and analysis methods to limit bias. Qualitative designs should incorporate design features that promote the components of trustworthiness: credibility, transferability, dependability, and confirmability. However, when appraising mixed methods research, you must also consider the methods and extent to which the findings from both approaches are integrated.

**Integration** in mixed methods research is the explicit combining of the quantitative and qualitative components of the inquiry. Depending on the inquiry aims, this may occur in the design, data collection and analysis, or interpretation phases (or all three; Creswell & Plano Clark, 2018; Fetters et al., 2013). As you review mixed methods studies, you need to know how to spot integration. Figure 10-1 outlines examples of integration at each inquiry phase.

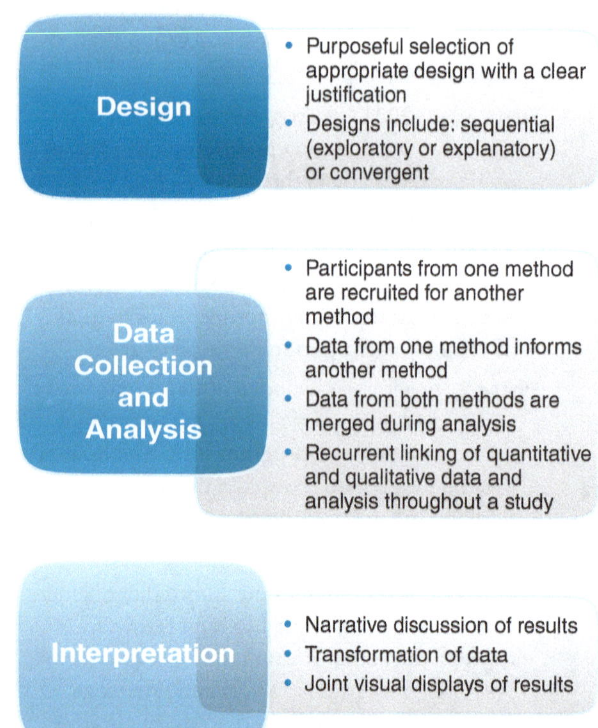


Figure 10-1 Evidence of integration at each inquiry phase in mixed methods research (Fetters et al., 2013; O'Cathain et al., 2010).

Integration at the design phase of an inquiry involves selecting and justifying an appropriate mixed methods design. This information may be provided in an article's *Abstract*, *Introduction*, or *Methods* section. There are several options for integration at the data collection and analysis phase of a study. For example, data collected from a focus group (qualitative) could inform the development of an intervention later explored in a pretest-posttest study (quantitative). Another example would be a multistage study in which data collection and analysis from both methods are embedded and linked throughout the study phases. For example, qualitative data could be collected in multiple phases to inform a later intervention, assess intervention outcomes, and evaluate the long-term carryover of the intervention. Quantitative data could be collected in the intervention phase and analyzed with the qualitative data for triangulation. You can usually find data collection and analysis details in an article's *Procedures*, *Data Collection*, or *Data Analysis* sections.

Evidence of integration in the interpretation of results can take one of three forms, all of which would typically be found in an article's *Results* or *Discussion* sections. First, the results could be presented narratively, either by weaving the quantitative and qualitative results together or discussing them sequentially if that mirrors the study design. Second, all the data could be converted to the same format and presented. Most commonly, this involves content analysis (discussed in Chapter 8), in which qualitative data are quantified by recording the frequency of words, phrases, or themes (Elo & Kyngäs, 2008; Vaismoradi et al., 2013). After conversion, the qualitative data are analyzed together with the quantitative data. Lastly, integration can occur through joint visual displays of quantitative and qualitative results, such as tables or graphs.

The validity and reliability of a mixed methods study are confirmed by examining the quantitative and qualitative study components and determining whether these components are effectively integrated. Effective integration means the quantitative and qualitative components have been purposefully combined at multiple points in a study with reasonable justification, resulting in valuable insights that would not have been generated from independent qualitative and quantitative studies. Without effective integration, the findings are likely no better than those from separate studies (Fetters & Freshwater, 2015; Fetters, 2018; O'Cathain et al., 2010).

**BOX 10-1 ■ Guidelines for Good Reporting of A Mixed Methods Study (GRAMMS)**

1. Justification for using a mixed methods design
2. Description of the specific mixed methods design type
3. Description of sampling, data collection, and data analysis for quantitative and qualitative components
4. Explanation of where integration occurred
5. Report of limitations associated with mixed methods design
6. Outcomes resulting from integration (O'Cathain et al., 2008)

## Components of Mixed Methods Research Critical Appraisal

In Chapters 6 and 9, you reviewed how to individually appraise quantitative and qualitative research. Appraisal of a mixed methods study essentially requires appraisal of the quantitative and qualitative aspects of the study, along with a few other components specific to mixed methods research. These additional components include whether the mixed methods design is justified, if integration occurred, and the insights gained relative to the mixed methods. It is important to note that the rigor or quality of a mixed methods design "cannot exceed the quality of its weakest component" (Hong, Pluye et al., 2018, p. 7). In other words, if you detect many biases or limitations in one component (for example, the qualitative aspect) of a mixed methods study, even if the other component (quantitative) is strong, the entire study's quality is compromised.

There are conflicting views on the best approach to appraising mixed methods studies, but there is agreement that the appraisal can be cumbersome and challenging because of the integration of multiple design features (Fàbregues & Molina-Azorin, 2017; Haile, 2022; Halcomb, 2018; Hong, Pluye et al., 2018; Moorley & Cathala, 2019; O'Cathain et al., 2008; Olaghere et al., 2023; Pluye et al., 2009). Researchers have proposed guidelines for quality reporting of mixed methods studies, provided in Box 10-1, that you can consider when appraising these designs (O'Cathain et al., 2008). These guidelines are called GRAMMS (Good Reporting of A Mixed Methods Study).

While many authors suggest how to appraise mixed methods studies, only one tool or template is currently provided in the literature. The Mixed Methods Appraisal Tool (MMAT) can be used to assess the quality of various quantitative and qualitative studies, including those with combined methods; research is ongoing to improve this tool (Hong, Pluye et al., 2018; Hong, Gonzalez-Reyes et al., 2018; Hong et al., 2019). The MMAT includes clear instructions and streamlined criteria, but it may be challenging to use. If you are new to appraising quantitative and qualitative research (or mixed methods designs), you may benefit from a more detailed template (see Table 10-2) to prompt you to assess key aspects of the study. The template provided in Table 10-2 includes four columns for completion:

1. **Study Details:** where you will summarize information about the mixed methods study being reviewed
2. **Appraisal of Quantitative and Qualitative Methods:** where you will appraise the study components (Is the information provided in the study sufficient, appropriate, and of good quality?)
3. **Appraisal of Mixed Methods:** where you will appraise the integration of quantitative and qualitative components
4. **Potential Biases/Limitations:** where you will clearly outline your concerns related to each "No" response under the Appraisal columns

**TABLE 10-2 ■ Critical Appraisal of Mixed Methods Study Template**

***Study Reference:*** (insert reference for the study being appraised here)

| Study Components | Study Details | Appraisal of Quantitative and Qualitative Methods* | Appraisal of Mixed Methods* | Potential Biases/ Limitations |
|---|---|---|---|---|
| **Purpose** | **Study's purpose:** | **Purpose was clearly stated:**<br>☐ Yes—If yes, indicate where: ________<br>☐ No | | |
| **Literature review** | **Main points of the literature review:** | **Sufficient literature on the topic was reviewed:**<br>☐ Yes ☐ No | | |
| | **Need for the study:** | **Need for the study is clear:**<br>☐ Yes ☐ No | | |
| | **Theoretical perspective:** | **A theoretical perspective was identified:**<br>☐ Yes ☐ No | | |
| **Setting** | **Setting type** (e.g., inpatient rehab unit, rural community with limited health-care access, drug and alcohol clinic, community senior housing complex, support group for those with breast cancer): | **The setting is sufficiently described:**<br>☐ Yes ☐ No<br>**Setting applies to your purpose:**<br>☐ Yes ☐ No | | |
| | **Geographic location** where the study took place (e.g., United States, Australia, rural/urban): | | | |
| **Sampling and recruitment** | **Sampling method(s):**<br>Nonprobability (convenience, quota, purposive, snowball);<br>Probability (simple random, stratified random sampling, systematic random sampling, cluster): | **Quantitative sample size:** ________<br>**Qualitative sample size:** ________<br>**Sample sizes are justified:**<br>☐ Yes ☐ No | | |
| | **Recruitment method(s):** | **Sampling methods are appropriate for study purpose:**<br>☐ Yes ☐ No | | |
| | **Description of participants** (include pertinent demographics such as age, diagnoses): | **Recruitment methods are appropriate for study purpose:**<br>☐ Yes ☐ No | | |

*Continued*

**TABLE 10-2 ■ Critical Appraisal of Mixed Methods Study Template—cont'd**

***Study Reference:*** (insert reference for the study being appraised here)

| Study Components | Study Details | Appraisal of Quantitative and Qualitative Methods* | Appraisal of Mixed Methods* | Potential Biases/ Limitations |
|---|---|---|---|---|
| | | **Samples are sufficiently described:**<br>☐ Yes ☐ No<br>**Sample applies to your purpose:**<br>☐ Yes ☐ No | | |
| **Design and levels of evidence** | Describe the **quantitative study design** (e.g., randomized controlled trial, two-group pretest-posttest, one-group pretest-posttest, time series, repeated measures, cohort design, case study, correlational):<br>Describe the **qualitative study design** (e.g., ethnography, phenomenology, grounded theory, participatory action research, qualitative case study, historical design): | **Quantitative level of evidence:**<br>☐ I ☐ II ☐ III ☐ IV ☐ V<br>**Qualitative level of evidence:**<br>☐ I ☐ II ☐ III ☐ IV ☐ N/A<br>**Institutional Review Board approval/exemption:**<br>☐ Yes ☐ No ☐ Unsure | Describe the **mixed methods design** (exploratory sequential, explanatory sequential, or concurrent/convergent):<br>**Mixed methods design is justified and aligns with the study purpose:**<br>☐ Yes<br>☐ No | |
| **Procedures** | Briefly summarize the methodology or what the researchers did in the study. Be sure to include any interventions as well as who carried them out. Describe how the mixed methods were integrated into the procedures: | **Procedures are sufficiently described to allow replication:**<br>☐ Yes ☐ No<br>**Those carrying out the procedures have sufficient training or experience in the subject area:**<br>☐ Yes ☐ No ☐ Unsure<br>**Procedures avoided contamination:**<br>☐ Yes ☐ No ☐ Unsure<br>☐ N/A<br>**Procedures avoided cointervention:**<br>☐ Yes ☐ No ☐ Unsure<br>☐ N/A | **Mixed methods procedures are complementary and support the study purpose:**<br>☐ Yes<br>☐ No<br>☐ Unsure | |

*Continued*

**TABLE 10-2 ■ Critical Appraisal of Mixed Methods Study Template—cont'd**

***Study Reference:*** (insert reference for the study being appraised here)

| Study Components | Study Details | Appraisal of Quantitative and Qualitative Methods* | Appraisal of Mixed Methods* | Potential Biases/ Limitations |
|---|---|---|---|---|
| **Data collection tools and methods** | Describe the **data collection tools and methods** (e.g., standardized and non-standardized tools, observations, interviews, focus groups, or record/ artifact review). Describe how the data was collected and by whom: | **Data collection methods are sufficiently described:**<br>☐ Yes ☐ No<br>**Efforts were made to use data collection tools with adequate validity and reliability:**<br>☐ Yes ☐ No ☐ Unsure<br>**Those carrying out the data collection have sufficient training or experience in the subject area:**<br>☐ Yes ☐ No ☐ Unsure<br>**The role of the researcher(s) and their relationship to the participants are adequately described:**<br>☐ Yes ☐ No ☐ Unsure<br>☐ N/A<br>**The theoretical perspective, assumptions, and potential biases of the researcher(s) are described:**<br>☐ Yes ☐ No ☐ Unsure | **Evidence of integration in data collection present:**<br>☐ Yes<br>☐ No<br>☐ Unsure<br>**If yes, indicate how** (check all that apply):<br>☐ Participants from one method are recruited for another method<br>☐ Data collection from one method informs another method | |
| **Data analysis** | Describe the **quantitative data analysis methods**: (e.g., statistical methods) | **Data analysis methods are adequately described:**<br>☐ Yes ☐ No | **Evidence of integration in data analysis present:**<br>☐ Yes<br>☐ No<br>☐ Unsure | |
| | Describe the **qualitative data analysis methods** (e.g., thematic analysis, content analysis, constant comparative analysis, interpretive phenomenological analysis, a priori coding): | **Data analysis methods are appropriate for the resulting data:**<br>☐ Yes ☐ No | | |
| **Trustworthiness** | Describe evidence of **credibility** (confidence results are "true" or accurate): | **Credibility present:**<br>☐ Yes ☐ No | | |

*Continued*

**TABLE 10-2 ■ Critical Appraisal of Mixed Methods Study Template—cont'd**

***Study Reference:*** (insert reference for the study being appraised here)

| Study Components | Study Details | Appraisal of Quantitative and Qualitative Methods* | Appraisal of Mixed Methods* | Potential Biases/ Limitations |
|---|---|---|---|---|
| | Describe evidence of **transferability** (confidence results can be applied to similar contexts or situations): | **Transferability present:** ☐ Yes ☐ No | X | |
| | Describe evidence of **dependability** (confidence data are consistent with the results): | **Dependability present:** ☐ Yes ☐ No | X | |
| | Describe evidence of **confirmability** (confidence steps were taken to limit bias): | **Confirmability present:** ☐ Yes ☐ No | X | |
| **Results and discussion** | Describe the study's quantitative and qualitative results: | **Quantitative results are statistically significant:** ☐ Yes ☐ No ☐ N/A<br>**Quantitative results are clinically significant/meaningful:** ☐ Yes ☐ No ☐ N/A<br>**Qualitative results are consistent with the data collected:** ☐ Yes ☐ No | **Quantitative and qualitative results are effectively integrated:**<br>☐ Yes<br>☐ No<br>**If yes, indicate how** (check all that apply):<br>☐ Narrative discussion<br>☐ Transformation of data<br>☐ Joint visual display of data | |
| **Conclusions** | Concisely summarize the **study conclusions**: | **Conclusions are appropriate given the study information provided:** ☐ Yes ☐ No | **Acknowledgment of limitations related to mixed methods design present:**<br>☐ Yes<br>☐ No | |
| **Applicability (Check all that apply)** | ☐ Background information (justifies a need, defines key terms, establishes theoretical background)<br>☐ Shows the effectiveness of or support for a proposed intervention<br>☐ Supports methodology (may include procedures, data collection methods or tools, data analysis)<br>☐ Other: | | | |

*For each "No" response, indicate the potential biases/concerns (for example, researcher bias, sampling bias, inadequate description, missing information) in the corresponding far-right column. Exercise caution in applying mixed methods research with 50% or greater "No" responses, and *if evidence of integration is absent in multiple phases.*

Some information in this table may look familiar since it combines information from Table 6-1 (Critical Appraisal of Quantitative Study Template) and Table 9-2 (Critical Appraisal of Qualitative Study Template). Table 10-2 is reviewed in greater detail throughout this chapter with emphasis on aspects of mixed methods design. If you need further clarification about specific quantitative or qualitative components, you should return to Chapters 6 and 9, respectively.

### TIPS & INSPIRATION

- If you have not learned to appraise quantitative and qualitative studies in isolation, it is recommended that you go to Chapters 6 and 9 to review this information before appraising a mixed methods study.
- If you have already learned to appraise quantitative and qualitative studies separately, you are well prepared to move forward. You should be able to confidently appraise mixed methods studies with attention to just a few extra details.
- Take a few moments to locate one of the studies in Table 10-1. Keep the article close by as you review how to appraise a mixed methods study. For each study component, examine the sample article to see if you can locate the required information. It can be challenging to appraise quantitative and qualitative methods simultaneously, and the concepts often make more sense when looking at an actual study.

### Study Purpose

The purpose is the guiding principle for the entire study. It may be stated in the article's *Abstract* or *Introduction* section or provided in a PIO or PICO (population, intervention, comparison intervention [if applicable], and outcomes) question. If the components of a mixed methods study are sequential, the study may have multiple purposes. For example, in an exploratory sequential design, the purpose of the qualitative component may be to gather perspectives on a particular topic to inform the later quantitative component. The purpose of the quantitative aspect could include determining the efficacy of an intervention.

### Literature Review

As discussed in Chapter 3, the literature review should effectively summarize the existing literature on a topic and identify the need for the present study. The literature review for a mixed methods study may be longer than one for a single design approach. More literature may be included if the study includes multiple purposes. Most studies have a dedicated *Literature Review* or *Background* section.

### Setting

The setting, including the setting type and geographic location, helps determine whether the study's outcomes can be reasonably generalized to your facility or location. The components of a mixed methods study may occur in the same or different settings. A sufficient description includes all relevant details to place the study within context. The setting description is often found in an article's *Methods, Procedures*, or *Participants* sections.

### Sampling and Recruitment

Appraising a mixed methods study's sampling and recruitment methods involves the same considerations as the single designs, with one addition. Samples may differ for the qualitative and quantitative components of a mixed methods study (Dawadi et al., 2021). This may be especially common in sequential mixed methods designs. For example, imagine that you first use a quantitative design to determine any significant improvements in function due to participation in a specialized rehabilitation program. This sample includes 80 clients who engaged in the program and completed the outcome measures. Next, you solicit a subset of these 80 patients (perhaps 20 of them) to participate in the qualitative portion of the study, which includes several focus groups to discuss their perspectives on the rehabilitation program. Each sample size should be adequately justified and connected to the study's purpose. If this is accomplished, the difference in sample sizes would not be concerning (Creswell & Plano Clark, 2018). For concurrent designs, the sample size is usually the same for both study components. The sampling and recruitment methods are often found within an article's *Sample, Procedures*, or *Methods* sections.

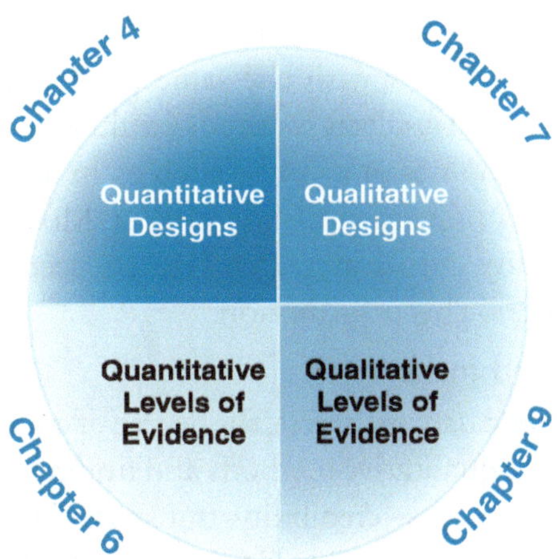


Figure 10-2 Location of quantitative and qualitative designs and levels of evidence.

## Design and Level of Evidence

When appraising mixed methods research, first consider the quantitative and qualitative designs singularly and then in combination. This text has reviewed common quantitative and qualitative research designs and evidence levels. Figure 10-2 summarizes where to locate this information if you need a refresher.

At this point in your appraisal, you should identify the design and the level of evidence for the quantitative and qualitative strands of the study. You might locate the study design in the article's *Abstract, Design,* or *Methods* section or determine it based on the aims and other study features. You should assign the level of evidence based on the specific design features.

Next, you should focus on appraising the mixed methods (or combined) design. Start by identifying the type of mixed methods design. Recall from earlier in this chapter that there are three basic mixed methods designs: exploratory sequential, explanatory sequential, and concurrent/convergent. More often than not, you will determine this by reading through the procedures rather than finding this information explicitly stated. A quality mixed methods design purposefully incorporates quantitative and qualitative methods to promote a greater understanding of the inquiry phenomena than when quantitative or qualitative methods are used separately (Creswell & Plano Clark, 2018; Fetters & Freshwater, 2015).

### BOX 10-2 ■ Justification for Mixed Methods Designs

To confirm study results

- Using both methods can result in triangulation of results.

To expand knowledge on a topic

- Using both methods can provide a more holistic view of the inquiry phenomena.

To address design flaws

- Using both methods may improve rigor since both methods have different strengths and challenges.

To use one method to inform another

- This rationale may apply to sequential designs, wherein the data from the first method informs the second method.

(Dawadi et al., 2021; Plano Clark, 2010)

The authors should justify their choice of a mixed methods design. Box 10-2 summarizes the most common reasons for using a mixed methods design. Ultimately, there should be a clear rationale for each method and for combining both methods within the same study.

## Procedures

A study's procedures include any interventions, who provided the interventions, what materials were used, and any other pertinent action steps. This information is typically found in an article's *Procedures* or *Methods* section. In addition to appraising the quantitative and qualitative procedures separately, you should assess for integration of the study procedures. This involves purposeful sequencing or combining of procedures to complement each other. For example, quantitative methods are best for determining cause and effect and establishing treatment protocols that can be generalized to larger populations. However, these methods are ineffective for understanding unique cases or the contextual factors that impact treatment. This is where qualitative methods are a good choice. The procedures are complementary if you can explain why they occur in the order they do and how they align with the study's purpose.

### TIPS & INSPIRATION

- As you appraise a study, do not hesitate to contact the authors if you have questions. The authors' contact information is often included in the article or readily available through an online search. Most authors are more than willing to assist others interested in their area of study.

### Data Collection Tools and Methods

Mixed methods research typically involves multiple data collection tools and methods. Depending on the study's aims and design, these may be used simultaneously or sequentially. You should consider each tool and method in regard to validity, reliability, expertise of the researchers, and their relationship to the study participants. A consideration specific to the mixed methods design is whether there is evidence of integration in data collection. This might include recruiting participants from one method to participate in a subsequent method or using data from an earlier method to inform a later one. Integration in the data collection phase of a study is common in sequential designs. The absence of integration in this phase is not cause for concern as long as integration is present in other study phases. Information on data collection is often embedded in an article's *Methods* or *Procedures* section but might also be found in a separate section for outcome measures.

### Data Analysis

A disadvantage of mixed methods designs is that data analysis can be cumbersome owing to varying types of data and the need for multiple analysis methods. As you read a mixed methods study, you should identify the separate analysis methods and then consider if there is evidence of integration. Recall that this could include merging data from both analysis methods. For example, quantitative and qualitative data collected from each participant could be analyzed collectively. Objective responses from a survey could be compared to in-depth qualitative responses from an interview with the same participant. Data collection and analysis methods could also be linked at various points in a study, such as in a sequential design or one with multiple phases. Most research articles have a dedicated *Data Analysis* section where you can find this information.

### Trustworthiness

Recall that trustworthiness, the degree of confidence in the study's qualitative methods and findings, includes four components—credibility, transferability, dependability, and confirmability. You should revisit the study design, data collection, and data analysis methods to make your assessment in this section of Table 10-2.

### Results and Discussion

Quantitative results may be reported in narrative, tables, and figures. Qualitative results are commonly reported narratively as themes and linked to participant responses or quotes. A quality mixed methods study should effectively integrate the results from both methods. Integration at this phase may include a narrative discussion, the transformation of data, or joint visual displays of data. The absence of the integration of results should raise concerns about the value of the research. Look for this information in an article's *Results*, *Outcomes*, or *Discussion* sections.

In mixed methods designs, conflicting results are relatively common (Creswell & Plano Clark, 2018). It is essential to explore the discrepancies and attempt to explain them. Conflicting results could be related to data collection and analysis flaws, the impact of assumptions or biases of participants or researchers, or the influence of one method on the other. For example, if participants are given a survey in the quantitative phase of a study, the type of questions and the content of the survey could impact responses to qualitative focus group questions in a later study phase. Ethical research practice calls for acknowledgment of discrepancies and effort to explain them so that others can decide whether to apply the findings or how to avoid similar issues in future inquiries.

### Conclusions

The study's conclusions represent the "take-home message" and may include practical implications of the research or recommendations for future inquiries.

This is where you will consider your appraisal of all other study aspects. Are the conclusions appropriate given these other details? In addition, the limitations of the study should be acknowledged.

### Applicability

Finally, consider how this appraised study specifically applies to your purpose, population, or practice setting. Whether you are conducting evidence-based practice or a formal research study, now is the time to determine if and how the study information will be useful to you. In the last section of Table 10-2, check all items that apply. Compare the study setting and population to your own to determine if they are similar enough for the information to be applicable. Additionally, you should use caution in applying a mixed methods study if you have concerns related to 50% or more of the study components or if evidence of integration does not exist in multiple phases.

## Systematic Reviews

A **systematic review** (SR) is a type of study that summarizes multiple individual research studies on a particular topic. Unlike the traditional literature review discussed in Chapter 3, systematic reviews involve precise methods to locate, appraise, synthesize, and disseminate literature on a focused question or topic (Higgins et al., 2023). Some differences between literature and systematic reviews are further delineated in Table 10-3.

### Systematic Review Process

While detailed instructions on conducting a systematic review are beyond the scope of this text, understanding the basic steps can be helpful as you read and appraise existing systematic reviews. The general steps are as follows:

1. Formulate a research question.
2. Develop a precise search protocol, including the search strategies, inclusion and exclusion criteria for individual study selection, and data extraction and synthesis methods.
3. Conduct a comprehensive and exhaustive literature search using the predetermined protocol.
4. Screen and select relevant studies.
5. Assess selected studies' quality and risk of bias using established assessment tools.
6. Extract relevant data from selected studies, including study characteristics, participant details, interventions, outcomes, and key results.

**TABLE 10-3 ■ Comparison of Literature Review and Systematic Review**

| Features | Systematic Review | Literature Review |
|---|---|---|
| Aim | Answers a focused question | Provides an overview of a topic, often to identify a gap in literature for future study; may include a specific question |
| Search criteria and strategies | Involves a precise protocol including:<br>■ Well-defined criteria for article inclusion<br>■ Search strategies are intentional to promote a comprehensive and exhaustive search. | No protocol is necessary.<br>■ Criteria may be vague or based on the author's familiarity with the topic.<br>■ Search strategies are likely unplanned and may not result in an exhaustive search. |
| Quality of included studies | Comprehensive evaluation of the quality of included studies | May or may not include evaluation of quality of included studies |
| Results | Synthesis of quality studies on the topic may involve meta-analysis. May be used to develop clinical practice guidelines. | Thematic summary of individual studies |
| Completion timeline | Months to years | Weeks to months |
| Publication | Follows established reporting guidelines | May be presented in varying formats |

(AOTA, 2020; Davis, 2016; Higgins et al., 2023)

7. Synthesize and interpret findings from selected studies. If appropriate, conduct a meta-analysis, a statistical procedure used to determine the collective effect size from the selected studies. Pooling the results from multiple individual studies allows for more robust conclusions than what can be garnered from each study.
8. Write the systematic review following established reporting guidelines, such as PRISMA guidelines (Preferred Reporting Items for Systematic Reviews and Meta-Analyses, 2024), and submit it to an appropriate scholarly journal for publication. PRISMA guidelines offer a checklist of items that should be reported when publishing systematic reviews and meta-analyses (American Occupational Therapy Association, 2020; Davis, 2016; Higgins et al., 2023; Khan et al., 2003).

Because of the volume of work and to limit bias, most systematic reviews are conducted by a team of people. Strict adherence to the predetermined protocol and transparency throughout the process are crucial to ensuring the credibility of the systematic review. Box 10-3 provides an example of a systematic review.

### BOX 10-3 ■ Example of a Systematic Review

Tofani et al. (2020) used a systematic review with meta-analysis to investigate the effectiveness of occupational therapy interventions in enhancing the quality of life for patients with Parkinson's disease.

After establishing their focused research question, they identified appropriate search terms and databases. Their search yielded 143 articles, which was pared down to 75 once the duplicates were removed. Next, the remaining articles were screened for relevancy, quality, and bias. They used established tools (Cochrane Collaboration's tool for bias and PEDro scores) to assess bias and quality. Finally, 15 randomized controlled trials met the inclusion criteria, and the results from these studies were synthesized and compared. Four of these studies, which used similar interventions and measured similar outcomes, were used to conduct a meta-analysis. The meta-analysis quantified the collective effect of these study interventions, highlighting occupational therapy's benefits in improving the quality of life for individuals with Parkinson's disease.

### TIPS & INSPIRATION

- **PRISMA** guidelines recommend that systematic reviews and meta-analyses are identified in the article's title. For this reason, you should be able to identify this type of design without much scrutiny.

### Benefits of Systematic Reviews

Systematic reviews offer several benefits related to engaging in research and evidence-based practice. First, a systematic review comprehensively synthesizes existing research by consolidating a large body of evidence into a single, easily accessible source. This lets you quickly grasp the overall state of knowledge on a specific topic and saves significant time. You can always mine the reference list of a systematic review if you want to examine the individual studies more closely. Second, the precise, systematic review process reduces bias and enhances the reliability of the review's conclusions. If a systematic review includes a meta-analysis, there is even more confidence in the findings. Third, systematic reviews often identify gaps in the literature or inconclusive results, which can justify and guide future research. Similarly, practitioners, policymakers, and healthcare professionals can use systematic reviews to inform evidence-based decision-making. The robust evidence from a systematic review can be used in developing clinical practice guidelines, healthcare policies, and evidence-based practice programs to promote health and well-being. Finally, systematic reviews can support your continued professional development by helping you stay updated on the evidence and advancements within your profession and practice area.

## Components of Systematic Review Critical Appraisal

While finding a systematic review on your topic is exciting because of the previously mentioned benefits, you will still need to critically appraise the review to ensure it is of good quality. Table 10-4 provides a

**TABLE 10-4 ■ Critical Appraisal of Systematic Review**

***Study Reference:*** (insert reference for the study being appraised here)

| Study Components | Study Details | Appraisal* | Potential Biases/ Limitations |
|---|---|---|---|
| **Purpose** | **Study's purpose:** | **Purpose was clearly stated:**<br>☐ Yes—If yes, indicate where:<br>______________________<br>☐ No | |
| **Search protocol** | **Databases searched:** | **Searched multiple appropriate databases:**<br>☐ Yes ☐ No | |
| | | **Searched reference lists of selected studies:** | |
| | **Search terms:** | ☐ Yes ☐ No | |
| | **Selection criteria:** | **Contacted topic experts:**<br>☐ Yes ☐ No<br>**Searched grey (unpublished) literature:**<br>☐ Yes ☐ No<br>**Used appropriate search terms:**<br>☐ Yes ☐ No | |
| | **Selection process:** | **Used appropriate selection criteria:**<br>☐ Yes ☐ No<br>**Study selection confirmed by at least two individuals:**<br>☐ Yes ☐ No | |
| **Description of selected studies** | **Study designs of selected studies:** | **No. of articles included:** __________ | |
| | **Description of settings** (e.g., inpatient rehab unit, rural community with limited healthcare access, drug and alcohol clinic, community senior housing complex, support group for those with breast cancer): | **Level of evidence:**<br>☐ I ☐ II<br>☐ Qualitative systematic review | |
| | **Description of geographic locations** (e.g., United States, Australia, rural/urban): | **Settings are sufficiently described:**<br>☐ Yes ☐ No | |
| | **Description of participants** (include pertinent demographics such as age, diagnoses): | **Participants are sufficiently described:**<br>☐ Yes ☐ No | |
| | **Description of interventions, including any comparison interventions:** | **Interventions are sufficiently described:**<br>☐ Yes ☐ No | |
| | **Description of outcomes:** | **Outcomes are sufficiently described:**<br>☐ Yes ☐ No<br>**The selected studies align with the study purpose:**<br>☐ Yes ☐ No | |

*Continued*

**TABLE 10-4 ■ Critical Appraisal of Systematic Review—cont'd**

***Study Reference:*** (insert reference for the study being appraised here)

| Study Components | Study Details | Appraisal* | Potential Biases/ Limitations |
|---|---|---|---|
| **Quality of selected studies** | **Description of how the selected studies were assessed for quality and risk of bias, including the tools used:** | **Appropriate methods were used to assess the quality of selected studies:**<br>☐ Yes ☐ No<br>**Quality of selected studies:**<br>☐ Good ☐ Concerns present | |
| **Results** | **Description of results** (use layperson's terms):<br>**Description of how results are presented** (e.g., narratively, visually in a table/figure/forest plot): | **Results are clearly described:**<br>☐ Yes ☐ No<br>**Results are similar among studies:**<br>☐ Yes ☐ No<br>**If No, are the varying results explained?**<br>☐ Yes ☐ No ☐ N/A | |
| **Conclusions** | Concisely summarize the **study conclusions**: | **Conclusions are appropriate given the study information provided:**<br>☐ Yes ☐ No | |
| **Applicability (Check all that apply** | ☐ Background information (justifies a need, defines key terms, establishes theoretical background)<br>☐ Shows the effectiveness or support for a proposed intervention<br>☐ Supports methodology (may include procedures, data collection methods or tools, data analysis).<br>☐ Other: | | |

*For each "No" response, indicate the potential biases/concerns (for example, limited search strategies, quality of studies not addressed, inadequate description, missing information) in the corresponding far-right column. Exercise caution in applying research with 50% or greater "No" responses.

comprehensive template for appraising a systematic review, and each component is discussed separately here so that you understand what to look for. The template provided in Table 10-4 includes three columns for completion:

1. **Study Details:** where you will summarize information about the systematic review being examined
2. **Appraisal:** where you will appraise the study components (i.e., Is the information provided in the study sufficient, appropriate, and of good quality?)
3. **Potential Biases/Limitations:** where you will clearly outline your concerns related to each "No" response under the Appraisal column

## TIPS & INSPIRATION

- Systematic reviews can be challenging to appraise, and you may be tempted to skip to the conclusions and accept them at face value. However, it is essential to understand and appraise the methodology of the review, which can significantly impact the credibility of the conclusions. Systematic reviews are often the quickest studies to appraise once you grasp the concepts, so definitely keep going!
- Take a few moments to locate Tofani et al.'s (2020) study from Box 10-3. Keep this article close by as you review how to appraise a systematic review. For each study component, examine the sample article to see if you can locate the required information. The concepts often make more sense when looking at an actual study.

### Purpose

A systematic review should have a well-defined purpose, frequently specified in the PICO or PIO question format. As noted previously, these acronyms specify the population, intervention, comparison intervention (if applicable), and outcomes that are the focus of the research. You might find this information in the systematic review's *Title, Abstract*, or *Introduction* sections.

### Search Protocol

Each systematic review should include a comprehensive literature search, including appropriate databases and other search strategies, search terms, selection criteria, and the selection process. The search protocol should be well established before the review begins rather than being developed as the review proceeds. These details are usually found in a systematic review article's *Methods* or *Procedures* section.

Search strategies beyond using appropriate databases may include searching the reference lists of selected studies, contacting topic experts, and searching grey literature. Grey literature, discussed in Chapter 3, is unpublished dissertations, conference proceedings, legal documents, or policy statements (Bonato, 2022), which may be archived in some databases or government or organizational websites. Topic experts may be contacted before the search for guidance in establishing the search protocol or during the search to identify additional relevant sources.

The search terms should align with the review's purpose and incorporate terms synonymous with the population, intervention(s), and outcomes of interest. Ideally, the search terms should include MeSH terms and alternative spellings of words when applicable. For example, if you are interested in behavioral interventions for children with autism, you could search "behavioral" and "behavioural." Use of Boolean operators, truncation, wildcards, phrase searching, and citation tracking, discussed in Chapter 3, are additional indicators of a thorough search.

The selection criteria should be clearly outlined before the search begins. Inclusion criteria are typically based on relevance to the review's purpose or elements of the PIO/PICO question but may also include specific study designs and dates of publication. In the example in Box 10-3, the authors searched for only randomized controlled trials up to 2019 that explored occupational therapy interventions for clients with Parkinson's disease (Tofani et al., 2020). Another criterion that bears mentioning is whether the search included any language restrictions (for example, including only articles published in English). Applying no language restrictions may capture additional relevant sources and minimize language bias. However, it may present challenges in assessing the source due to language barriers and the need for translation. If a language restriction is present, the authors should provide this information and discuss the implications transparently. Tofani et al. (2020) state that they did not limit articles based on the publication language.

The selection process should encompass at least two individuals who independently review the articles from the search to determine if they meet the selection criteria. In Tofani et al.'s (2020) systematic review, two authors independently reviewed the articles to confirm they met the inclusion criteria. When there is a discrepancy between the authors, details should be provided about how the discrepancy was resolved and consensus was reached.

For a search protocol to be considered good quality, enough details should be provided so that you could reasonably replicate the search. The employed search strategies and criteria should be comprehensive enough that relevant studies are unlikely to be missed. Many systematic review articles also include a flowchart that outlines how the articles from the initial search were pared down to those deemed appropriate for inclusion in the review. In the Search Protocol section of Table 10-4, briefly summarize the search details and confirm the presence and appropriateness of the various search strategies and criteria. If you feel the search protocol is lacking, clearly describe the potential biases or limitations in the rightmost column of the table.

#### TIPS & INSPIRATION

- If the authors of a systematic review failed to use one or more of the search strategies discussed here, there may not be cause for concern if other aspects of the search are strong. For example, suppose the authors' search resulted in many articles that met the criteria (by searching appropriate databases and grey literature with appropriate search terms with no language restriction). In that case, their failure to contact topic experts may not be very concerning. You must weigh the impact of this choice to determine if relevant articles could have been missed.

### Description of Selected Studies

A quality systematic review should include clear descriptions of the selected studies, including the total number of studies, their study designs, and relevant details about the settings, participants, interventions, and outcomes. This information may be found in narrative form but is more commonly organized in a table format for ease of review. An example of this table format can be found in Tofani et al.'s (2020) systematic review article. Provided that the search protocol was adequate, the total number of studies can help you judge the scope of literature on the topic. While no set number of articles is required for a systematic review, a relatively low number of articles may indicate a very narrow search or limited research on the topic. Conversely, more articles may indicate a broader search or vast research on a topic.

Identifying the study designs of the selected articles allows you to quickly assess the rigor of the studies. Systematic reviews of high-quality randomized controlled trials are the highest level of evidence (level I), as identified in Figure 6-1. Systematic reviews of smaller-scale randomized controlled trials, cohort studies, case-control studies, pretest-posttest studies, or mixed methods studies are often considered level II evidence (see Figure 6-1). Systematic reviews of quantitative or mixed methods research are more common. However, systematic reviews of qualitative research, which require altered procedures, are gaining traction in understanding perceptions of health and the experiences of healthcare consumers and practitioners (Aromataris et al., 2024).

Enough details about the selected studies should be provided to determine whether they align with the review's purpose and if the findings apply to your purpose. Sufficient descriptions include all relevant details to place the study within context. While you might wish you had more detail in some instances, remember that most journals restrict the length of articles, so authors must prioritize what information to include.

#### TIPS & INSPIRATION

- If you find a systematic review on a topic of interest and plan to conduct your own inquiry, you may want to locate one or more of the selected studies within the review. The finer details about the participants, intervention, and outcome measures may be helpful as you design your inquiry.

### Quality of Selected Studies

The selected studies in a systematic review should be assessed for quality and risk of bias with established assessment tools. The authors should clearly explain the tools used and who performed the assessments. This information may be included in the previously mentioned table format or a separate article section. If you are new to appraising systematic reviews, this area may be confusing because different study designs may require different assessment tools. Each tool is tailored to assess the specific features of the intended design. Table 10-5 includes some of the most common assessment tools and guidelines you may encounter. To determine if the methods used to assess quality were appropriate, compare the study designs to the tools used. Do these align? Having at least two authors independently assess for quality and convene to reach a consensus can also add credibility to the process. As you make your appraisal in this section, indicate if the quality of the selected studies is good or if concerns are present. Include any concerns in the rightmost column of Table 10-4.

#### TIPS & INSPIRATION

- The authors of a systematic review can only include the best literature available on the topic. Concerns about the quality of the selected studies are not a reflection of a poor systematic review but instead

**TABLE 10-5 ■ Quality Assessment Tools for Selected Studies in a Systematic Review**

| Tool | Purpose |
|---|---|
| AMSTAR **(Assessing the Methodological Quality of Systematic Reviews Checklist)** | To assess quality of systematic reviews (Shea et al., 2017) |
| CASP Checklists **(Critical Appraisal Skills Programme Checklists)** | To critically appraise various study designs. Checklists for various designs are available (CASP, 2023). |
| Cochrane RoB 2 Tool **(Version 2 of Cochrane Collaboration Risk of Bias Tool)** | To assess risk of bias in randomized controlled trials (Sterne et al., 2019) |
| Jadad Scale | To assess quality of randomized controlled trials (Jadad et al., 1996) |
| MMAT **(Mixed Methods Appraisal Tool)** | To assess quality of quantitative, qualitative, and mixed methods designs (Hong, Pluye et al., 2018) |
| NOS **(Newcastle-Ottawa Scale)** | To assess quality of non-randomized studies (Wells et al., 2021) |
| PEDro Scale **(Physiotherapy Evidence Database Scale)** | To assess quality of randomized controlled trials in physical rehabilitation (PEDro, 2023) |
| ROBINS-I **(Risk of Bias in Non-Randomized Studies of Interventions Tool)** | To assess bias in in non-randomized interventional studies (Sterne et al., 2016) |
| Quality Reporting Guidelines: | These critical checklists for reporting various study designs may be used to identify missing information and promote quality reporting of study findings.<br>Examples of quality reporting guidelines include: **PRISMA** (guidelines for reporting systematic reviews) and **CONSORT** (guidelines for reporting randomized controlled trials) (Butcher et al., 2022; PRISMA, 2024). |

usually represent the current state of literature on a topic. In other words, the systematic review authors cannot include quality evidence that does not exist. As long as they do not overstate their results, their review can still positively contribute to understanding the topic and may justify future inquiries.

## Results

Systematic review results may be presented in various ways depending on the selected studies' designs and the variability of outcomes. The results may be discussed narratively and organized by key themes, patterns, or outcomes among the individual studies. Results may also be visually displayed in tables or figures. Similar results among individual studies provide more robust support for the conclusions, whereas varied results may prompt further investigation before applying the results. These differences in results, known as **heterogeneity**, can stem from differences in participants, interventions, methods, study quality, or other contextual factors. If heterogeneity exists in a systematic review, the authors should report it and attempt to explain the differences and implications on the conclusions.

Statistical results may be reported if the selected studies have similar quantitative designs and comparable outcomes, which allow the completion of meta-analyses. **Meta-analyses** are statistical procedures to determine the collective effect size from selected studies. The **effect size** describes the magnitude and direction of the outcome being studied. Measures of effect size in a systematic review may include mean difference, Cohen's *d*, odds ratio, risk ratio, or correlation coefficients. Additional information on effect sizes can be found in Chapter 6.

If a meta-analysis is completed, those results may be displayed in a **forest plot**, a graph showing each study's effect size and confidence interval, as well as the combined effect size and confidence interval. An example of a forest plot from Tofani et al.'s (2020) systematic review is shared in Figure 10-3. Statistical tests may also assess heterogeneity; common examples include Cochran's Q test, $I^2$, and $Tau^2$. Some additional resources for understanding forest plots, heterogeneity, and the corresponding statistical tests are provided at the end of this chapter since these details are beyond the scope of this text.

An accurate appraisal of the systematic review results hinges on your ability to understand and accurately summarize the results. While this information is usually found in a dedicated *Results* section, reviewing the *Discussion* section can also help you process what the results mean and understand limitations that may have impacted them.

## TIPS & INSPIRATION

- If a study contains significant heterogeneity, check whether the authors completed additional analysis with subgroups. Breaking the analysis down by population characteristics, interventions, settings, or other factors could be useful in exploring the sources of variation.
- Not all systematic reviews will contain meta-analysis. A meta-analysis may not be feasible or appropriate if there are limited studies on a topic or too much diversity in study designs, interventions, and outcomes. A systematic review without meta-analysis should qualitatively summarize the findings and limitations and may still provide valuable insights for future inquiries or clinical practice.

## Conclusions

The conclusions of a systematic review should highlight the strengths and limitations of the selected studies and may offer recommendations for practice, policy, or future research. In some systematic reviews, an overall rating or GRADE may be given relative to the quality of evidence. GRADE (Grading of Recommendations, Assessment, Development, and Evaluation) is a widely used framework for rating the quality of evidence and strength of recommendations in systematic reviews and clinical practice guidelines (Schunemann et al., 2023). The quality rating, which

| | Experimental | | | Control | | | | Mean Difference | Mean Difference |
|---|---|---|---|---|---|---|---|---|---|
| Study or Subgroup | Mean | SD | Total | Mean | SD | Total | Weight | IV, Random, 95% CI | IV, Random, 95% CI |
| Clarke 2016 | 25.9 | 16.5 | 380 | 25.9 | 16.5 | 377 | 3.3% | 0.00 (-2.35, 2.35) | |
| Tickle Degnen 2010 a | 28.5 | 1 | 37 | 30.6 | 0.9 | 40 | 48.0% | -2.10 (-2.53, -1.67) | |
| Tickle Degnen 2010 b | 28.4 | 1 | 39 | 30.6 | 0.9 | 40 | 48.7% | -2.20 (-2.62, -1.78) | |
| **Total (95% CI)** | | | **456** | | | **456** | **100.0%** | **-2.08 (-2.52, -1.64)** | |

Heterogeneity: $Tau^2 = 0.06$; $Chi^2 = 3.27$, df = 2 ($P = 0.19$); $I^2 = 39\%$
Test for overall effect: $Z = 9.31$ ($P < 0.00001$)



Figure 10-3 This example of a forest plot contains three individual studies (Clarke, 2016; Tickle Degnen, 2010a; Tickle Degnen, 2010b) that assessed quality of life using the Parkinson's Disease Questionnaire-39. This figure shows the statistically significant improvements in quality of life for participants in the experimental groups ($P < 0.00001$) and no heterogeneity ($I^2 = 39\%$). *Tofani, M., Ranieri, A., Fabbrini, G., Berardi, A., Pelosin, E., Valente, D., Fabbrini, A., Costanzo, M., & Galeoto, G. (2020). Efficacy of occupational therapy interventions on quality of life in patients with Parkinson's disease: A systematic review and meta-analysis. Movement Disorders Clinical Practice, 7(8), 898, Figure 2. https://doi.org/10.1002/mdc3.13089*

may be high, moderate, low, or very low, is based on the level of confidence in the outcomes. If the article you are reviewing includes a GRADE rating, you can compare this to the rest of your appraisal. Ultimately, you must decide if the review's conclusions are reasonable given the other study details.

### Applicability

Finally, consider how this systematic review applies to your purpose, population, or practice setting. Whether you are conducting evidence-based practice or a formal research study, now is the time to determine if and how the review information will be helpful to you. In the last section of Table 10-4, check all items that apply. For example, the review may provide useful background information, including establishing the theoretical background or need for your inquiry or defining key terms. This information could be helpful in drafting your literature review if you plan to conduct a formal inquiry. The review may confirm the effectiveness of a planned practice intervention. If you plan to complete an evidence-based practice project, a high- to moderate-quality systematic review can justify your plan. You can also locate some of the selected studies from the review to explore further the study procedures, data collection methods and tools, and data analysis methods. This information could be helpful in designing your inquiry procedures, including making decisions about the timing, duration, and other inquiry logistics. If you derive other useful information from a study not encompassed by these categories, an additional section is included for you to provide clarification.

### TIPS & INSPIRATION

- If you are thinking of completing a systematic review, consider collaborating with a team of at least four or five individuals who are also interested in the topic. A team approach can help you manage the workload and increase the review's credibility.
- Existing systematic reviews may be quickly outdated as new studies are published. If you are conducting an evidence-based practice project, search the literature for new studies since the review. If you are interested in conducting a systematic review and are new to this process, consider updating an existing review with new research on the topic. Doing so will allow you to contribute positively to the literature and avoid some of the challenges associated with a brand-new review.
- Systematic reviews are typically registered by submitting the plan to a database for systematic reviews before completion. Some common examples include PROSPERO (International Prospective Register of Systematic Reviews), the Cochrane Library, OSF (Open Science Framework), and JBI (Joanna Briggs Institute) Systematic Review Register. Registering your systematic review is encouraged to promote adherence to the search protocol, avoid duplication of efforts, reduce bias, and enhance the rigor of the review. If you are appraising an existing systematic review, the authors usually indicate where the review is registered, which is often required for publication.
- When considering the conclusions and application of a systematic review or mixed methods study, always consider if the topic falls within your scope of practice.
- Be aware of your preconceived ideas as you complete your appraisals. Looking for only studies that support your ideas may result in a flawed rationale, a poorly designed inquiry, or the application of inappropriate information to your clients and setting. Be fully open to discovering the best evidence on your topic.

### CHAPTER SUMMARY

1. Describe the value and challenges of mixed methods research.
   - Mixed methods research incorporates quantitative and qualitative research designs and procedures within a single inquiry for greater understanding of the study phenomena than what can be achieved with a purely quantitative or qualitative design.
   - Other benefits of mixed methods research can include the ability to triangulate or confirm results, to better explain or explore the phenomena being studied, to generate ideas for future inquiries, and to hone your skills in quantitative and qualitative approaches.
   - Challenges of mixed methods research may include requiring more time, skills, or resources to conduct.

Continued

2. Identify the three primary mixed methods research designs.
   - Three mixed methods research designs are exploratory sequential, explanatory sequential, and concurrent or convergent. These are further described with examples in Table 10-1.
3. Recall components of reliability and validity in mixed methods research.
   - Mixed methods research should incorporate strategies to improve validity and reliability in quantitative and qualitative research, as well as effective integration.
   - Integration, the explicit combining of the quantitative and qualitative components of the inquiry, can occur in the design, data collection and analysis, or interpretation phases (or all three). Figure 10-1 outlines examples of integration at each inquiry phase.
4. Critically appraise the components of a mixed methods research study.
   - Table 10-2 provides a comprehensive template for appraisal of a mixed methods study by component.
   - A quality mixed methods appraisal includes a summary of relevant study details (column 1), an appraisal of the quantitative and qualitative study components (column 2), an appraisal of the mixed methods (column 3), and the identification of potential biases or limitations (column 4).
   - The chapter details each component of a mixed methods study to guide you through an appraisal.
   - A mixed methods design must be purposefully chosen for one of the following reasons: to confirm study results, expand knowledge on a topic, address design flaws, or use one research method to inform another. Box 10-3 provides further explanation of these justifications.
   - After an appraisal, consider if and how the study information applies to your purpose, population, and setting. Exercise caution in applying studies where concerns were noted related to 50% or more of the study components.
5. Differentiate systematic reviews and literature reviews.
   - A systematic review involves a well-defined search protocol to locate, appraise, synthesize, and disseminate literature on a focused topic or question. The selected studies are evaluated for quality, a meta-analysis may be used to synthesize the results (if appropriate), and publication follows strict reporting guidelines.
   - A literature review may involve unplanned search strategies resulting from the author's familiarity with the topic to generate an overview of a topic. Selected studies may or may not be reviewed for quality. The results are summarized thematically and can be presented in varying formats.
   - Table 10-3 further differentiates systematic and literature reviews.
6. State the steps for conducting a systematic review.
   - Steps for conducting a systematic review are as follows: (1) Formulate a research question, (2) develop a precise search protocol, (3) conduct a literature search with established search protocol, (4) screen and select relevant studies, (5) assess quality and risk of bias in selected studies, (6) extract relevant studies from selected studies, (7) synthesize and interpret findings; conduct a meta-analysis if appropriate, and (8) write the systematic review using PRISMA guidelines.
7. Describe the benefits of systematic reviews.
   - Benefits of systematic reviews include saving time by consolidating a large body of evidence into a single, accessible source, reducing bias and strengthening conclusions, identifying gaps in the literature or inconclusive results, and supporting professional development.
8. Critically appraise the components of a systematic review.
   - Table 10-4 provides a comprehensive template for appraisal of a systematic review by component.
   - A quality systematic review appraisal includes a summary of relevant study details (column 1), an appraisal of review components (column 2), and the identification of potential biases or limitations (column 3).
   - The chapter details each component of a systematic review to guide you through an appraisal.
   - Systematic reviews of high-quality randomized controlled trials are the highest level of evidence (level I); systematic reviews of smaller-scale randomized controlled trials, cohort studies, case-control studies, pretest-posttest studies, or mixed methods studies are considered level II evidence. Systematic reviews of qualitative studies may also be completed with altered procedures.
   - Table 10-5 includes some of the most common tools for assessing the quality of the selected studies in a systematic review.

- Heterogeneity refers to variance in results among studies in a systematic review, which may stem from differences in participants, interventions, methods, study quality, or other contextual factors. Similar results among individual studies provide more robust support for the conclusions.
- A meta-analysis, a statistical procedure to determine the collective effect size from selected studies, may be completed in a systematic review if the selected studies have similar quantitative designs and comparable outcomes. The effect size describes the magnitude and direction of the outcome. Results of a meta-analysis may be displayed on a forest plot, a graph showing each study's effect size and confidence interval and the combined effect size and confidence interval.
- After an appraisal, consider if and how the study information applies to your purpose, population, and setting. Exercise caution in applying studies where concerns were noted related to 50% or more of the study components.

## TEST YOUR KNOWLEDGE

1. What is one advantage of mixed methods research designs?
   a. They are easier to appraise than other research designs.
   b. They are quicker to conduct in real-world settings.
   c. They require fewer resources than other research designs.
   d. They can increase confidence in the study's results.
2. A researcher conducts a focus group with community-dwelling seniors to explore their perspectives on aging in place. The focus group data is then used to develop an education program to promote successful aging in place. Members of a local senior center are invited to participate in the program and are surveyed before and after the program to assess changes in knowledge and confidence. This is an example of what type of mixed methods design?
   a. Convergent
   b. Explanatory sequential
   c. Exploratory sequential
   d. Explicit sequential
3. Which of the following is an example of integration in a mixed methods study?
   a. Using a standardized measure to collect data
   b. Using a bar graph to illustrate the quantitative outcomes
   c. Recruiting participants from one method for another method
   d. Publishing the results in multiple articles
4. The sample sizes for the qualitative and quantitative components of a mixed methods study should be relatively equal. True or false?
5. Which of the following would BEST justify using a mixed methods design?
   a. A mixed methods design was used to address design flaws with the singular methods.
   b. A mixed methods design was used to increase the chances of publication.
   c. A mixed methods design was used because prior studies only used quantitative methods.
   d. A mixed methods design was used to allow for tests of statistical significance.
6. Which of the following is TRUE of systematic reviews?
   a. They can be completed in a few weeks.
   b. They provide a general overview of a topic.
   c. They require precise search protocols.
   d. They can be published in varying formats.
7. In which of the following scenarios would you have more confidence in the results of a systematic review?
   a. A meta-analysis was completed with at least half of the studies in the review.
   b. Heterogeneity is present among the selected studies.
   c. A forest plot indicates homogeneous results among studies.
   d. The GRADE rating is low for the review.

Answer key appears at the end of this text.

## NEXT STEPS

1. Locate a mixed methods study on a topic of interest. Review the study and use Table 10-1 to identify the integration points. Is the integration sufficient to justify the mixed methods design and generate information that singular designs could not uncover? Why or why not?
2. Locate a mixed methods study on a topic of interest and use Table 10-2 to complete a full appraisal. Use the text to guide you through this process.

3. Scrutinize the search protocol from an existing systematic review in an area of interest. What search strategies or criteria are missing? What challenges exist in addressing the shortcomings? If you found the search thorough, what supports likely contributed to this?
4. Locate two systematic reviews on a topic of interest—one with and one without meta-analysis. Compare how the data is synthesized and presented in the two articles. Compare the design features and purpose of each review. How do they differ, and what unique information results from each one? Is one more beneficial for your purposes? Explain why.
5. Locate a systematic review on a topic of interest and use Table 10-4 to complete a full appraisal. Use the text to guide you through this process.

## REFERENCES


American Occupational Therapy Association. (2020). *Guidelines for systematic reviews.* Author. https://research.aota.org/DocumentLibrary/AOTA_AJOT_systematic%20reviews%20instructions.pdf

Aromataris, E., Lockwood, C., Porritt, K., Pilla, B., & Jordan, Z. (Eds.). (2024). *JBI manual for evidence synthesis.* JBI. https://doi.org/10.46658/JBIMES-20-01

Bonato, S. (2022). Grey literature searching. In M. J. Foster & S. T. Jewell (Eds.), *Piecing together systematic reviews and other evidence syntheses* (pp. 111–128). The Medical Library Association.

Butcher, N. J., Monsour, A., Mew, E. J., Chan, A-W., Mohar, D., Mayo-Wilson, E., Terwee, C. B., Chee-A-Tow, A., Baba, A., Gavin, F., Grimshaw, J. M., Kelly, L. E., Saeed, L., Thabane, L., Askie, L., Smith, M., Farid-Kapadia, M., Williamson, P. R., Szatmari, P.,...Offringa, M. (2022). Guidelines for reporting outcomes in trial reports: The CONSORT-Outcomes 2022 extension. *Journal of the American Medical Association, 328*(22), 2252–2264. https://doi.org/10.1001/jama.2022.21022

Creswell, J. W., & Plano Clark, V. L. (2018). *Designing and conducting mixed methods research* (3rd ed.). SAGE Publications.

Critical Appraisal Skills Programme. (2023). *CASP checklists.* https://casp-uk.net/casp-tools-checklists

Davis, D. (2016). A practical overview of how to conduct a systematic review. *Nursing Standard, 31*(12), 60–70. https://doi.org/10.7748/ns.2016.e10316

Dawadi, S., Shrestha, S., & Giri, R. A. (2021). Mixed-methods research: A discussion on its types, challenges, and criticisms. *Journal of Practical Studies in Education, 2*(2), 25–36. https://doi.org/10.46809/jpse.v2i2.20

Elo, S., & Kyngäs, H. (2008). The qualitative content analysis process. *Journal of Advanced Nursing, 62*(1), 107–115. https://doi.org/10.1111/j.1365-2648.2007.04569.x

Fàbregues, S., & Molina-Azorin, J. F. (2017). Addressing quality in mixed methods research: A review and recommendations for a future agenda. *Quality & Quantity, 51*(6), 2847–2863. https://doi.org/10.1007/s11135-016-0449-4

Fetters, M. D. (2018). Six equations to help conceptualize the field of mixed methods. *Journal of Mixed Methods Research, 12*(3), 262–267. https://doi.org/10.1177/1558689818779433

Fetters, M. D., Curry, L. A., & Creswell, J. W. (2013). Achieving integration in mixed methods designs—Principles and practices. *Health Services Research, 48*(6 Pt. 2), 2134–2156. https://doi.org/10.1111/1475-6773.12117

Fetters, M. D., & Freshwater, D. (2015). The 1 + 1 = 3 integration challenge. *Journal of Mixed Methods Research, 9*(2), 115–117. https://doi.org/10.1177/1558689815581222

Hafsa, N. (2019). Mixed methods research: An overview for beginner researchers. *Journal of Literature, Languages and Linguistics, 58*(1), 45–48. https://doi.org/10.7176/JLLL/58-05

Haile, Z. T. (2022). Critical appraisal tools and reporting guidelines. *Journal of Human Lactation, 38*(1), 21–27. https://doi.org/10.1177/08903344211058374

Halcomb, E. J. (2018). Mixed methods research: The issues beyond combining methods. *Journal of Advanced Nursing, 75*(3), 499–501. https://doi.org/10.1111/jan.13877

Higgins, J. P. T., Thomas, J., Chandler, J., Cumpston, M., Li, T., Page, M. J., & Welch, V. A. (Eds.). (2023, August). *Cochrane handbook for systematic reviews of interventions.* Version 6.4. Cochrane. https://training.cochrane.org/handbook/current

Hong, Q. N., Gonzalez-Reyes, A., & Pluye, P. (2018). Improving the usefulness of a tool for appraising the quality of qualitative, quantitative and mixed methods studies, the Mixed Methods Appraisal Tool (MMAT). *Journal of Evaluation in Clinical Practice, 24*(3), 459–467. https://doi.org/10.1111/jep.12884

Hong, Q. N., Pluye, P., Fàbregues, S., Bartlett, G., Boardman, F., Cargo, M., Dagenais, P., Gagnon, M-P., Griffiths, F., Nicolau, B., O'Cathain, A., Rousseau, M-C., & Vedel, I. (2018). *Mixed Methods Appraisal Tool (MMAT), version 2018.* Registration of Copyright (#1148552), Canadian Intellectual Property Office, Industry Canada. http://mixedmethodsappraisaltoolpublic.pbworks.com/w/file/fetch/127916259/MMAT_2018_criteria-manual_2018-08-01_ENG.pdf

Hong, Q. N., Pluye, P., Fàbregues, S., Bartlett, G., Boardman, F., Cargo, M., Dagenais, P., Gagnon, M-P., Griffiths, F., Nicolau, B., O'Cathain, A., Rousseau, M-C., & Vedel, I. (2019). Improving the content validity of the mixed methods appraisal tool: A modified e-Delphi study. *Journal of Clinical Epidemiology, 111,* 49–59. https://doi.org/10.1016/j.jclinepi.2019.03.008

Jadad, A. R., Moore, R. A., Carroll, D., Jenkinson, C., Reynolds, D. J. M., Gavaghan, D. J., & McQuay, H. J. (1996). Assessing the quality of reports of randomized clinical trials: Is blinding necessary? *Controlled Clinical Trials, 17*(1), 1–12. https://doi.org/10.1016/0197-2456(95)00134-4

Khan, K. S., Kunz, R., Kleijnen, J., & Antes, G. (2003). Five steps to conducting a systematic review. *Journal of the Royal Society of Medicine, 96,* 118–121. https://doi.org/10.1177/014107680309600304

Moorley, C., & Cathala, X. (2019). How to appraise mixed methods research. *Evidence-Based Nursing, 22*(2), 38–41. http://doi.org/10.1136/ebnurs-2019-103076

O'Cathain, A., Murphy, E., & Nicholl, J. (2008). The quality of mixed methods studies in health services research. *Journal of Health Services Research & Policy, 13*(2), 92–98. https://doi.org/10.1258/jhsrp.2007.007074

O'Cathain, A., Murphy, E., & Nicholl, J. (2010). Three techniques for integrating data in mixed methods studies. *British Medical Journal, 341,* c4587. https://doi.org/10.1136/bmj.c4587

Olaghere, A., Wilson, D. B., & Kimbrell, C. (2023). Inclusive critical appraisal of qualitative and quantitative findings in evidence synthesis. *Research Synthesis Methods, 14*(6), 847–852. https://doi.org/10.1002/jrsm.1659

Pamungkas, R. A., Chamroonsawasdi, K., Charupoonphol, P., & Vatanasomboon, P. (2021). A health-based coaching program for diabetes self-management (DSM) practice: A sequential exploratory mixed-methods approach. *Endocrinología, Diabetes y Nutrición, 68*(7), 489–500. https://doi.org/10.1016/j.endinu.2020.07.010

Physiotherapy Evidence Database. (2023). *Welcome to PEDro, the physiotherapy evidence database.* https://pedro.org.au

Plano Clark, V. L. (2010). The adoption and practice of mixed methods: U.S. trends in federally funded health-related research. *Qualitative Inquiry, 16*(6), 428–440. https://doi.org/10.1177/1077800410364609

Pluye, P., Gagnon, M-P., Griffiths, F., & Johnson-Lafleur, J. (2009). A scoring system for appraising mixed methods research, and concomitantly appraising qualitative, quantitative, and mixed methods primary studies in mixed study reviews. *International Journal of Nursing Studies, 46*(4), 529–546. https://doi.org/10.1016/j.ijnurstu.2009.01.009

PRISMA. (2024). *Welcome to the new preferred reporting items for systematic reviews and meta-analyses (PRISMA) website.* http://www.prisma-statement.org

Schunemann, H. J., Brennan, S., Akl, E. A., Hultcrantz, M., Alonso-Coello, P., Xia, J., Davoli, M., Rojas, M. X., Meerpohl, J. J., Flottorp, S., Guyatt, G., Mustafa, R. A., Langendam, M, & Dahm, P. (2023). The development methods of official GRADE articles and requirements for claiming the use of GRADE—A statement by the GRADE guidance group. *Journal of Clinical Epidemiology, 159,* 79–84. https://doi.org/10.1016/j.jclinepi.2023.05.010

Shea, B. J., Reeves, B. C., Wells, G., Thuku, M., Hamel, C., Moran, J., Moher, D., Tugwell, P., Welch, V., Kristjansson, E., & Henry, D. A. (2017). AMSTAR 2: A critical appraisal tool for systematic reviews that include randomised or non-randomised studies of healthcare interventions, or both. *British Medical Journal, 358,* j4008. https://doi.org/10.1136/bmj.j4008

Siette, J., Jorgensen, M., Nguyen, A., Knaggs, G., Miller, S., & Westbrook, J. I. (2021). A mixed-methods study evaluating the impact of an excursion-based social group on quality of life of older adults. *BMC Geriatrics, 21*(1), 356. https://doi.org/10.1186/s12877-021-02295-7

Sterne, J. A. C., Hernán, M. A., Reeves, B. C., Savović, J., Berkman, N. D., Viswanathan, M., Henry, D., Altman, D. G., Ansari, M. T., Boutron, I., Carpenter, J. R., Chan, A. W., Churchill, R., Deeks, J. J., Hróbjartsson, A., Kirkham, J., Jüni, P., Loke, Y. K., Pigott, T. D.,... Higgins, J. P. T. (2016). ROBINS-I: A tool for assessing risk of bias in non-randomized studies of interventions. *British Medical Journal, 355,* i4919. https://doi.org/10.1136/bmj.i4919

Sterne, J. A. C., Savović, J., Page, M. J., Elbers, R. G., Blencowe, N. S., Boutron, I., Cates, C. J., Cheng, H-Y., Corbett, M. S., Eldridge, S. M., Emberson, J. R., Hernán, M. A., Hopewell, S., Hróbjartsson, A., Junqueira, D. R., Jüni, P., Kirkham, J. J., Lasserson, T., Li, T., ... Higgins, J. P. T. (2019). RoB 2: A revised tool for assessing risk of bias in randomised trials. *BMJ, 366,* l4898. https://doi.org/10.1136/bmj.l4898

Tofani, M., Ranieri, A., Fabbrini, G., Berardi, A., Pelosin, E., Valente, D., Fabbrini, A., Costanzo, M., & Galeoto, G. (2020). Efficacy of occupational therapy interventions on quality of life in patients with Parkinson's disease: A systematic review and meta-analysis. *Movement Disorders Clinical Practice, 7*(8), 891–901. https://doi.org/10.1002/mdc3.13089

Tsai, K., Chang, P. J., Mathew, A. J., Richard, C., Davidson, H. A., & Hersch, G. I. (2022). Exploring spirituality of elders relocating into long-term care facilities. *The Open Journal of Occupational Therapy, 10*(2), 1–11. https://doi.org/10.15453/2168-6408.1959

Vaismoradi, M., Turunen, H., & Bondas, T. (2013). Content analysis and thematic analysis: Implications for conducting a qualitative descriptive study. *Nursing & Health Sciences, 15*(3), 263–405. https://doi.org/10.1111/nhs.12048

Wells, G. A., Shea, B., O'Connell, D., Peterson, J., Welch, V., Losos, M., & Tugwell, P. (2021). *The Newcastle-Ottawa Scale (NOS) for assessing the quality of nonrandomized studies in meta-analyses.* The Ottawa Hospital. https://www.ohri.ca/programs/clinical_epidemiology/oxford.asp

## RESOURCES FOR APPRAISING SYSTEMATIC REVIEWS

Dettori, J. R., Norvell, D. C., & Chapman, J. R. (2021). Seeing the forest by looking at the trees: How to interpret a meta-analysis forest plot. *Global Spine Journal, 11*(4), 614–616. https://doi.org/10.1177%2F21925682211003889

Shaneyfelt, T. (2013, March 25). *How to interpret a forest plot.* [Video]. YouTube. https://youtu.be/py-L8DvJmDc?si=6WFQYR68OtMG-g2R

Shaneyfelt, T. (2013, March 30). *What is heterogeneity?* [Video]. YouTube. https://youtu.be/KSKCTXciGjI?si=_W0z1lzng38_wAJv

# Section 3

# Designing Your Inquiry

Section 3 (Chapters 11–13) of this text reviews important steps in designing an inquiry. Specifically, Chapter 11 covers how to choose an inquiry design, draft an inquiry plan, and select or create quality data collection tools for an inquiry. Ethics is also a primary consideration in designing any inquiry, so Chapter 12 discusses the function of ethics committees and components of an inquiry proposal that meets ethical standards. Finally, Chapter 13 discusses the steps of program development and funding of your inquiry including types and sources of grants. Additional guidance is provided to help you choose an appropriate grant and draft a grant proposal worthy of funding. The tasks discussed in this section of the text require thoughtful consideration, attention to detail, and a willingness to accept constructive feedback to make your inquiry a reality. Let's begin with choosing your inquiry design.

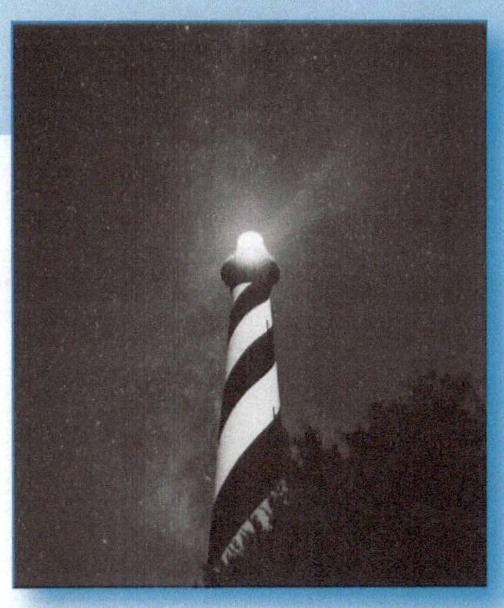

Chapter 11

# Developing Your Inquiry Plan

**LEARNING OUTCOMES**

*The information provided in this chapter will assist you to:*

11.1 Choose an appropriate inquiry design.
11.2 Differentiate pilot studies and feasibility studies.
11.3 Identify possible aims of evidence-based practice inquiries.
11.4 Develop an inquiry plan.
11.5 Describe considerations in choosing data collection tools.
11.6 Distinguish closed-ended and open-ended survey and interview questions.
11.7 Explain how to organize survey and interview questions to promote quality data collection.

## Choosing an Inquiry Design

The inquiry design dictates the methodology for investigating a particular inquiry question or problem. In this text, we have discussed quantitative designs (Chapter 4), qualitative designs (Chapter 7), and mixed methods designs (Chapter 10). The selection of an inquiry design hinges on various factors, including the nature of the inquiry problem, the available time and resources, and the desired depth of understanding. The chosen inquiry design shapes the sampling methods, procedures, and data collection and analysis methods. It is, therefore, a decision that demands careful consideration and alignment with the inquiry's purpose. For example, your purpose might include exploring a new topic, describing a particular phenomenon, explaining cause-and-effect relationships, determining the effectiveness of an intervention, or evaluating the success of a quality improvement program. Figure 11-1 includes a decision tree to help you choose an appropriate inquiry design.

Quantitative designs are most appropriate if you have a hypothesis you want to test, if you want to determine cause-and-effect relationships or the effectiveness of an intervention, or if you are interested in the relationships between variables. Many quantitative designs involve providing an experimental intervention or treatment to one or more groups of people. However, these designs can also include observation or data collection without an intervention. Quantitative designs are also best if you plan to do something experimental. In other words, if there is little to no support in the literature for what you plan to do, a quantitative research design may be most appropriate to investigate the phenomena.

Cape Hatteras Lighthouse, Buxton, North Carolina.

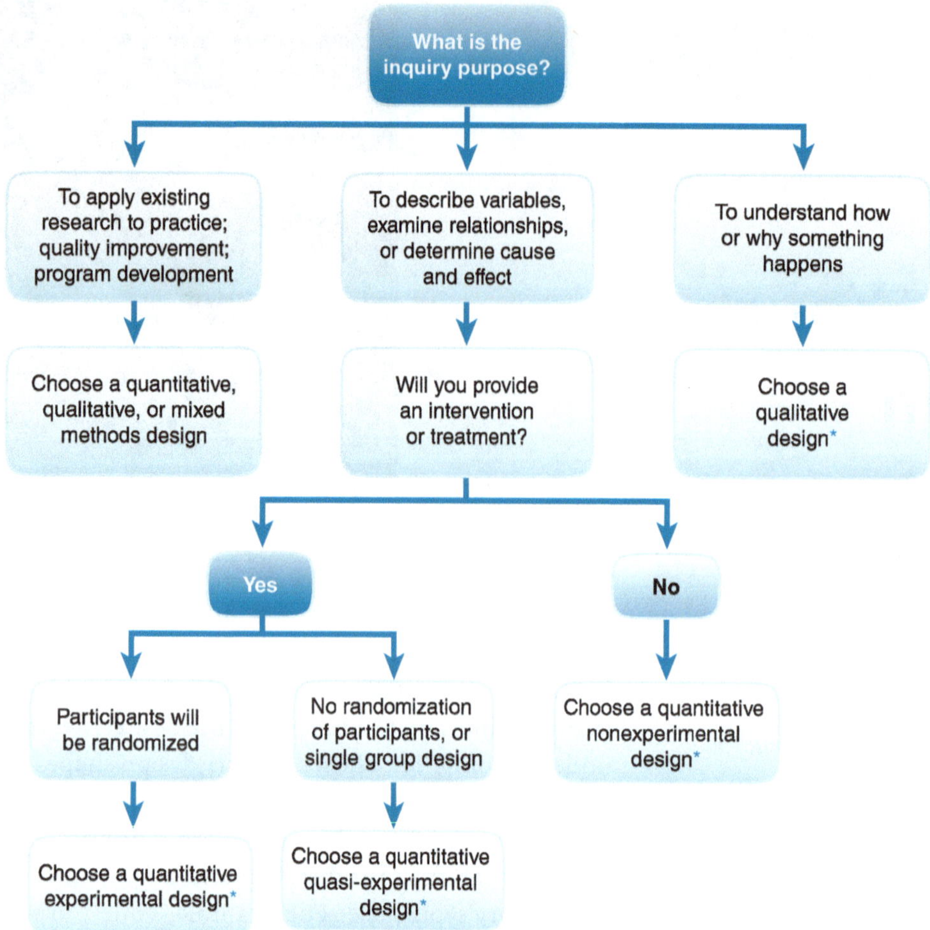


*If you want to incorporate quantitative and qualitative methods to triangulate results or use one method to inform another, consider using a mixed methods design.

Figure 11-1 Choosing an inquiry design.

Conversely, qualitative designs are most suitable if you want to know how or why something happened; if you want to explore the perspectives, meanings, or values of others; or if you want to generate a new theory or hypothesis for later testing. While qualitative designs may involve providing an intervention, most focus on stories and narratives that emerge from naturally occurring events or settings. Therefore, these designs are more common if you have access to naturalistic settings and plan to spend large amounts of time there gathering data from individuals, groups, or records.

A mixed methods design perhaps represents the best of both worlds by combining quantitative and qualitative methods within a single inquiry. However, integrating these methods should be purposefully chosen to triangulate results, promote a greater understanding of a topic, or use one method to inform or support the other. If you choose a mixed methods design, you still need to commit to specific individual quantitative and qualitative designs. A mixed methods design can be challenging because of the advanced knowledge, skills, and time required. If you have limited experience with mixed methods design, you might choose a singular quantitative or qualitative design instead or seek assistance from an instructor or mentor.

## Pilot and Feasibility Studies

In some instances, quantitative, qualitative, or mixed methods designs may also be classified as pilot or feasibility studies. Some researchers argue that pilot and feasibility studies are synonymous, while others believe they have distinct purposes (Abbott, 2014; Eldridge et al., 2016; Whitehead et al., 2014). These differing beliefs result in confusion when studies are classified and published inconsistently. Pilot and feasibility studies are both preliminary investigations conducted before larger, more comprehensive inquiries, but there is a growing consensus that these designs are not the same (Eldridge et al., 2016; Kolenic, 2018). Therefore, pilot and feasibility studies will be further differentiated here.

**Pilot studies** are preliminary investigations that help refine the inquiry methods before the full-scale inquiry (Abbott, 2014; Eldridge et al., 2016). Conducting a pilot study may be valuable when there are uncertainties or complexities in the inquiry design, procedures, or data collection and analysis methods. You should consider a pilot study if you want to test the reliability and validity of your data collection tools or identify potential procedural issues. For example, is the recruitment process efficient? Is the process of randomizing participants to study groups effective? Is the intervention of the appropriate duration and intensity to elicit change and retain participants? A well-planned pilot can help you fine-tune your inquiry methods so that the larger, comprehensive inquiry proceeds smoothly and produces meaningful, reliable results. Box 11-1 gives an example of a pilot study.

In contrast, a **feasibility study** is a preliminary investigation used to determine whether a full-scale inquiry is viable and practical—in other words, is a larger inquiry worth pursuing (Eldridge et al., 2016; Kolenic, 2018)? A feasibility study primarily looks at logistical, financial, and organizational factors to determine if the inquiry can be carried out successfully. Specific aspects of feasibility may also include the availability of necessary equipment, resources, and personnel, interest of potential participants in the intervention, practicality of conducting the procedures under the current conditions, and alignment with operational procedures of the inquiry site. Box 11-2 provides an example of a feasibility study.

While a pilot study focuses on doing a mini version of a full-scale inquiry to test and refine the procedures, a feasibility study focuses on exploring whether a full-scale inquiry is even appropriate. Combining these designs is also possible, and sometimes researchers conduct both types of studies to ensure the success of their later research. If you are contemplating choosing one of these designs, you

### BOX 11-1 ■ Example of a Pilot Study

Kemp et al. (2018) conducted a pilot study to refine the methods for a future randomized controlled trial investigating the impact of a physical therapy program after hip replacement surgery. In the pilot, 17 patients were randomized into two groups—one that received education (control) and another that received a combination of exercises, manual therapy, and education. The authors justified the pilot design, citing the high cost of conducting randomized controlled trials, the fact that this intervention had not been previously investigated with this population, and the need to hone the research design. Recommendations to improve the design include offering more physical therapy appointments and supervised exercise sessions and involving more surgeons to ensure the recruitment of enough participants.

### BOX 11-2 ■ Example of a Feasibility Study

While literature consistently supports stress management programming to decrease stress in college students, Morin and Lape (2023) located only one study incorporating foster youth as participants. Therefore, they used a pretest-posttest design to explore the feasibility of a future study with this population. Three foster youth participated in weekly individualized occupational therapy sessions aimed at reducing their perceived stress. While the program was found to be feasible in terms of need, favorable outcomes, and cost, significant challenges experienced or anticipated included difficulty scheduling sessions, poor time management of participants, and the need for a program facilitator trained in trauma-informed care. Therefore, a full-scale study with this population may not be feasible.

should also be aware of some common misconceptions about them:

1. Studies with a small sample size represent a pilot or feasibility study.
   *False:* While many pilot or feasibility studies have small samples, this is not a requirement (Abbott, 2014).
2. Pilot and feasibility studies can be used to test hypotheses or determine the effectiveness of interventions.
   *False:* While the impact of an intervention in a pilot or feasibility study may be reported, the design is not rigorous enough to prove anything. At best, these designs might provide preliminary support for the intervention. Their primary purpose is to identify problems and refine the inquiry methods before conducting a full-scale inquiry (Abbott, 2014; Kistin & Silverstein, 2015).
3. Pilot and feasibility studies require less time and effort than other designs.
   *False:* These designs still require careful planning and attention to the data collection and analysis methods to uncover potential challenges.
4. Pilot and feasibility designs should only be used to explore new topics.
   *False:* These designs can be used to refine the methods for exploring well-researched topics. They can also be used in **implementation research**, which focuses on translating rigorous research into real-world practice scenarios (Pearson et al., 2020).

### TIPS & INSPIRATION

- Until now, you have likely spent much time learning about the inquiry process, searching and appraising the literature, and dreaming about what your inquiry might look like. Reward yourself for the small successes that have gotten you to this point in your journey. You are well prepared for this next step!
- Identify what design you are considering and why. Discuss your ideas with your peers, advisors, or other professionals in your field. This feedback can help you choose the best design before planning the details.

## Evidence-Based Practice Projects and Knowledge Translation

Recall that the purpose of a formal evidence-based practice project is to apply existing research to practice for quality improvement purposes (highlighted at the left of Figure 11-1). Evidence-based practice projects can incorporate quantitative, qualitative, or mixed methods designs, depending on the topic and outcomes. These projects often involve only single-group designs because the aim is to implement the best or most effective intervention rather than to test out and compare interventions as you would in a research study. However, in some evidence-based practice scenarios, you might gather data from more than one group of participants who both experienced the *same* intervention. For example, suppose you implemented a training program supported by current literature for stroke survivors and their primary caregivers. In this case, you might assess both groups' knowledge and confidence to evaluate the program's success.

The purpose of collecting data in an evidence-based practice project is not to generate new knowledge but to evaluate the success of applying existing research to practice. In other words, did the client outcomes improve because of the intervention or program as expected? What are the clients' perspectives about the intervention or program? Does the data support continuing the intervention or program at the site? Assessing the outcomes can inform future practice decisions and justify the need for personnel, equipment, or other resources.

Even though the results of a formal evidence-based practice project may not be generalizable beyond the implementation setting, they might be disseminated to a broader audience to facilitate knowledge translation. **Knowledge translation** involves implementing existing research, evaluating the outcomes, identifying supports and challenges in applying research to practice, and disseminating the findings to promote better clinical outcomes (Chan et al., 2023; Wensing & Grol, 2019). Knowledge translation goes beyond the mere application of existing evidence to practice (evidence-based practice) to sharing the outcomes with others so that they might also benefit from this information. In other words, individuals

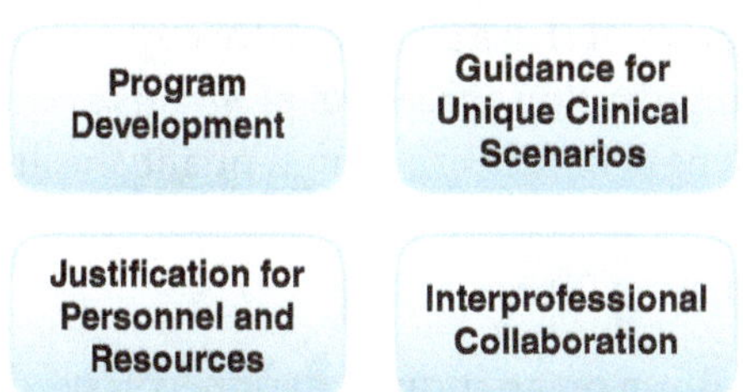


Figure 11-2 Examples of knowledge translation through evidence-based practice.

applying existing research can help others to navigate the challenges and improve clinical outcomes and experiences. Therefore, formal evidence-based practice inquiries may help translate research into practice and improve healthcare quality. Examples of knowledge translation through evidence-based practice are provided in Figure 11-2 and discussed further in this chapter. This information might help spark your ideas for addressing clinical problems through a formal evidence-based practice project.

### Program Development

**Program development**, covered in depth in Chapter 13, is the process of planning, implementing, and evaluating a new program, service, or practice protocol or improving or expanding an existing one. Many evidence-based practice projects take the form of program development.

### Guidance for Unique Clinical Scenarios

While programs typically impact larger groups of people, smaller inquiries can guide clinical decision-making for unique or complex client cases. For example, a client diagnosed with Issacs syndrome, a rare neuromuscular disorder characterized by continual muscle contractions, joint stiffness, and pain, visits a massage therapist for pain management (National Institute of Neurological Disorders and Stroke, 2023). The massage therapist is unfamiliar with this diagnosis but searches the literature for guidance.

Since the condition is rare, limited research exists. The existing literature, which includes two single-case examples, supports using range of motion, exercise, and deep tissue massage to manage the symptoms and decrease pain. These findings align with the therapist's experiences treating clients with other conditions involving muscle spasticity. The therapist uses the information to collaborate with the client to decide the best course of action. If a massage protocol is established and implemented, the therapist might consider collecting data about the client's pain level and perceptions of the intervention. The outcomes could be shared with others to add to the evidence about this rare condition.

### Justification for Personnel and Resources

Evidence-based practice inquiries can justify additional personnel, equipment, and resources for quality health services or programming. For example, a high school hires a new athletic trainer who soon realizes the available training equipment is outdated and poses safety risks. She searches for research on the most effective equipment to address these concerns. Her search reveals that various types of budget-friendly equipment, including therapy balls and resistive bands, are as effective as more costly weight-lifting machines. The literature also supports that the current free weights and outdated equipment pose serious risks to athletes with continued use. The athletic trainer uses this information to support her request to the school board for new equipment. She proposes obtaining this new equipment in phases throughout the school year and provides a plan for data collection to support the continued need for additional equipment. In cases like this, the evidence often speaks louder than any words. Although the district needs to be mindful of its spending, the board may find it difficult to deny the request when safety is on the line. This same procedure can be used to justify additional personnel or equipment in a hospital rehabilitation clinic, a clinical laboratory, or an academic setting. Although you may know the needs firsthand, the literature can provide more objective support.

Clients, families, third-party payors, grant funders, and policymakers may also demand proof of efficacy for your interventions or programs. You can present the evidence to validate using specific assessments or interventions, to appeal denials of payment for services provided, to justify funding needs, and to establish effective healthcare programs. Disseminating your outcomes from these efforts can also improve knowledge translation.

### *Interprofessional Collaboration*

Interprofessional collaboration occurs when "multiple health workers from different professional backgrounds work together with patients, families, carers and communities to deliver the highest quality of care" (World Health Organization, 2010, p. 7). Collaboration among professionals is necessary to effectively address clients' needs, improve client outcomes, and enable knowledge translation (Brandt et al., 2014; Newhouse & Spring, 2010; Reeves et al., 2017). Evidence-based inquiries may involve healthcare professionals or students from different disciplines collaborating to explore the literature on a common topic and developing a program or clinical practice guideline for implementation in the setting. This scenario allows everyone to have a voice in creating the program or protocol and the opportunity to apply the evidence under real-world conditions. Sharing the outcomes of these collaborative inquiries can help other teams develop successful programs and navigate the challenges in delivering high-quality healthcare.

## Developing Your Plan

After deciding on an inquiry design, you need to outline your detailed plan for carrying out the inquiry. This plan should include everything from recruiting, selecting, and consenting participants to delivering the intervention and collecting and analyzing your data. Table 11-1 summarizes the considerations in developing your plan and includes design suggestions and where to find more information on some inquiry elements.

### Inquiry Procedures

The steps of the program or intervention should be laid out in enough detail so that they could

**TABLE 11-1 ■ Considerations in Developing Your Inquiry Plan**

| Elements of Inquiry Plan | Considerations | Suggestions and More Information |
|---|---|---|
| Inquiry title | ■ What title best describes all aspects of your inquiry? | ■ Use a concise yet descriptive title for your inquiry that includes the population, intervention or topic, and outcome of focus. |
| Investigators | ■ Who will conduct the phases of inquiry? | ■ Include individuals who will obtain consent from participants, conduct the intervention, and collect or analyze data. |
| Participant criteria | ■ What participant inclusion and exclusion criteria align with your purpose? | ■ Ensure criteria are sufficiently focused for your purpose but not so restrictive that you will have trouble getting enough participants. |
| Recruitment and selection | ■ Who will recruit the participants?<br>■ What methods and places will be most effective for recruiting your target population?<br>■ Will all participants who respond to recruitment efforts be included in the inquiry, or will you use established groups or a screening to select participants?<br>■ Will participants be allocated to different inquiry groups? If so, will this be random? Purposeful? Convenience?<br>■ What is your anticipated sample size and why? | ■ Avoid self-recruitment, if possible, to limit the risk of coercion.<br>■ Consider using flyers, email, social media, phone calls, letters, or verbal scripts to recruit participants.<br>■ Be realistic about the sites, groups, and individuals you have access to when making decisions about your sample.<br>■ *For more information, see:*<br>  ■ Chapter 12 (recruitment)<br>  ■ Chapter 5 (sampling—quantitative inquiries<br>  ■ Chapter 8 (sampling—qualitative inquiries) |

*Continued*

**TABLE 11-1 ■ Considerations in Developing Your Inquiry Plan—cont'd**

| Elements of Inquiry Plan | Considerations | Suggestions and More Information |
|---|---|---|
| Consent process | ■ Will participants need to provide informed consent to participate in the inquiry?<br>■ If consent is required, how will consent be conducted and by whom? | ■ Use an electronic consent process if your inquiry is virtual or if participants have adequate technological skills and devices. Otherwise, consider a paper consent process.<br>■ A member of the inquiry team is usually the best person to obtain consent from participants because that person can answer participants' questions about the procedures.<br>■ *For more information, see:*<br>■ Chapter 12 (consenting) |
| Procedures | ■ What will you expect participants to do if they are part of the inquiry? What activities or interventions will they engage in? Where will these take place, and when?<br>■ Will you use a commercially available program or materials? If so, you may need permission to use the materials in your inquiry.<br>■ What is the time commitment that is required? | ■ Consider individual sessions or interventions in a private space for sensitive topics.<br>■ List the detailed steps in chronological order to draft your initial plan.<br>■ Ensure the time commitment is sufficient to address your topic but not so cumbersome that it deters participation. |
| Data collection tools | ■ What data collection tools will you use to assess your outcomes?<br>■ Will you use standardized assessments or assessments designed by others?<br>■ Will you use assessments that are within the public domain?<br>■ Will you design your own data collection tool (survey or interview questions)?<br>■ If you plan to use a self-designed tool, do you have a strong justification for doing so (for example, no appropriate tools currently exist)? | ■ Look to your literature review for guidance on the best outcome measure for your purpose. Consider how your outcomes have been measured in prior studies.<br>■ Request permission to use standardized assessments.<br>■ For assessments in the public domain, provide documentation that supports use without additional permissions.<br>■ If you will design your own survey or interview, consider having experts in survey design or the topic review it for quality, and pilot the tool with individuals similar to your anticipated participants.<br>■ *For more information, see:*<br>■ Chapter 5 (quantitative data collection)<br>■ Chapter 8 (qualitative data collection)<br>■ Chapter 11 (survey development) |
| Materials and equipment | ■ What materials and equipment are necessary to conduct your inquiry successfully? | ■ Consider items needed to recruit participants and obtain their consent, carry out the intervention, and assess outcomes. |

reasonably be implemented by someone else with the same instructions. Using a table or figure to outline these steps can help convey your ideas to an administrator, instructor, or research committee who must approve your inquiry before you can implement it. Similarly, a simplified table can make the expectations overwhelmingly clear to prospective participants. Table 11-2 provides an example of an inquiry procedure table for a pretest-posttest quantitative inquiry targeting college students with high stress. The planned intervention includes providing stress management education in a group format over 6 weeks. The table consists of four columns—one for each session (or week), one for the educational topics covered, one for the assessments administered, and one for the time commitment. This table could be altered to fit the needs of your inquiry. For example, if your inquiry involves an intervention with children but parents (or caregivers) are also involved or surveyed at specific points, you could include additional columns for the parent activities, assessments, and time commitment. You can add or delete rows to align with the intervention duration and add additional assessments for repeated measure designs or those with follow-up assessments.

For inquiries with multiple study groups, a flow diagram could be used to delineate the separate procedures for each group. The prior inquiry example could be expanded to a two-group experimental design with follow-up, as depicted in Figure 11-3.

### TIPS & INSPIRATION

- You likely began this journey motivated to address a problem, make a practice change, or investigate a new topic. Developing your inquiry procedures will bring you one step closer to achieving your goal. Take time to imagine your future success and the positive impact on your participants or clients. Your only limit is the one you set for yourself!

## Choosing Data Collection Tools

Your chosen data collection tools (or outcome measures) should align with your inquiry purpose, design, and the phenomena you are investigating. Appropriate tools for quantitative and qualitative inquiries were reviewed in Chapters 5 and 8, respectively. It is essential to consider the reliability

**TABLE 11-2 ■ Example Inquiry Procedure Table**

| Week | Intervention Topics | Assessments | Time Commitment for Participants |
|---|---|---|---|
| *1* | Introduction to the program; causes of stress | Administration of the Perceived Stress Scale | 1.5 hours |
| *2* | Education on guided imagery (group session) | – | 2 hours |
| *3* | Education on progressive muscle relaxation (group session) | – | 2 hours |
| *4* | Education on mindfulness (group session) | – | 2 hours |
| *5* | Education on breathing exercises and physical activity (group session) | – | 2 hours |
| *6* | Development of individual stress management plans; program wrap-up (group session) | Readministration of the Perceived Stress Scale | 1.5 hours |
| Total time commitment for each participant: | | | 11 hours |

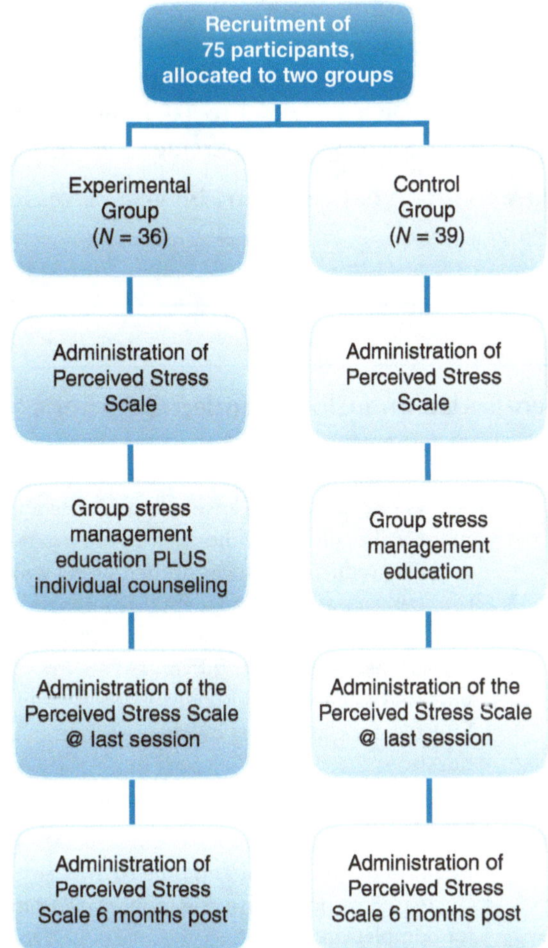


Figure 11-3 Example of an inquiry flow diagram.

and validity of the chosen tools to ensure they accurately measure the intended constructs. Other considerations include the tool's availability, the ease of administration and interpretation, and the cost or additional training required to use it. Some inquiries may rely on a single data collection tool, whereas others may employ multiple tools to triangulate results. If you choose multiple data collection tools, you should ensure that each has a distinct purpose related to your inquiry.

Outcome measures that are well established and widely used are preferred if they align with your inquiry purpose, but often, no appropriate tools are available. In this situation, you might develop a tool tailored to your inquiry purpose, such as a survey or interview. Guidance for question construction and organization is offered next.

## TIPS & INSPIRATION

- If this is your first or second inquiry, consider focusing on a singular outcome and choose only one or two quality data collection tools. Novice researchers and evidence-based practitioners often make the mistake of using too many outcome measures, which can overwhelm participants and complicate the data analysis. More data is not always better.
- Review the studies in your literature portfolio to see what tools the authors used to assess outcomes similar to yours. If multiple studies used the same standardized assessment or an author-generated survey to assess a specific outcome, this may justify you doing the same.
- If you are considering using an existing tool, carefully review its manual, intended audience, and test items or questions to determine if they align with your inquiry purpose and participant population.
- If a prior study used an author-generated tool that you are interested in, consider contacting the authors to see if you can gain access to the tool, use it in your inquiry, or modify it for your purposes.

## Question Construction

Questions for surveys and interviews can be formatted as closed-ended or open-ended. **Closed-ended questions** have predetermined response choices, such as "yes/no" or multiple-choice options. Closed-ended questions yield data that can be easily quantified for comparison across respondents. In contrast, **open-ended questions** allow respondents to provide detailed answers in their own words. Open-ended questions, which generate qualitative data, allow respondents to elaborate on a closed-ended question or share more detailed perspectives. Box 11-3 includes examples of closed-ended and open-ended questions. Closed-ended and open-ended questions are often used in the same survey or interview, as they each have distinct advantages and disadvantages, which are described in Table 11-3.

### *Closed-Ended Questions*

One of the most common closed-ended question formats is multiple choice. **Multiple-choice questions** can collect demographic information,

### BOX 11-3 ■ Examples of Closed-Ended and Open-Ended Questions

**Closed-ended:** Do you teach clinical reasoning skills to your therapy students? Yes _____ No _____

**Open-ended used to elaborate on the prior question:** If yes, please explain how and at what point in the curriculum:

**Closed-ended:** On a scale of 1 to 10, how stressed are you (1 = no stress; 10 = extreme stress)?

**Open-ended:** What is your biggest stressor and why?

### TABLE 11-3 ■ Advantages and Disadvantages of Open-Ended and Closed-Ended Questions

| | Closed-Ended Questions | Open-Ended Questions |
|---|---|---|
| Advantages | ■ Easy and fast for respondents to answer<br>■ Good response rates due to ease of answering<br>■ Yields quantitative data that can be easily analyzed<br>■ Best for gathering data from large samples | ■ Allows respondents to answer in any style and manner they choose without giving them suggestions, reducing chances of their giving what they perceive as socially acceptable answers<br>■ Best for addressing complicated or sensitive topics where even slight differences are important to know<br>■ Effective for elaborating on closed-ended questions<br>■ Provides detailed information on the inquiry topic |
| Disadvantages | ■ Does not provide detailed information<br>■ Response choices could be suggestive or may not represent all possible responses<br>■ May force responses even if the options do not fit a respondent<br>■ May provide less useful data for a small sample | ■ Requires more thought and time to answer<br>■ Decreased response rate due to increased time for completion<br>■ Primarily yields qualitative data that is more time-consuming to analyze<br>■ Challenging to use with large samples |

assess knowledge or understanding, or gather opinions. Fixed response items can help you describe your participants regarding gender, age, diagnoses, or other relevant factors. Multiple-choice questions crafted with one correct answer for each question could be used to assess your participants' knowledge before and after an educational session or intervention. Finally, you might use multiple-choice items to gather perspectives on select topics where you can reasonably generate the most plausible response choices.

Response choices for multiple-choice questions should be mutually exclusive, meaning that a respondent should be able to reliably select just one option (unless you ask them to check all responses that apply). Box 11-4 includes a poorly constructed closed-ended demographic question. In this example, a respondent who is 24 years old could select option a or b. Efforts should also be made to include all possible response options in a closed-ended question. In this example, there would be no appropriate response

### BOX 11-4 ■ Example of a Poor Closed-Ended Question

What is your age?

a. 18–24 years
b. 24–35 years
c. 36–45 years
d. Over 45 years

**TABLE 11-4 ■ Examples of Likert Scale Questions**

**Instructions:** Please rate your level of agreement with each statement.

| Statements | Strongly Agree | Agree | Neither Agree nor Disagree (Neutral) | Disagree | Strongly Disagree |
|---|---|---|---|---|---|
| I am knowledgeable of strategies to promote wound healing. | 5 | 4 | 3 | 2 | 1 |
| I am confident in selecting appropriate interventions for clients with chronic wounds. | 5 | 4 | 3 | 2 | 1 |
| I am comfortable using physical agent modalities for wound care. | 5 | 4 | 3 | 2 | 1 |
| I can positively impact the quality of life of clients I treat. | 5 | 4 | 3 | 2 | 1 |

choice if respondents younger than 18 were included in the inquiry. This scenario could force an inaccurate response. For instances where it might be impossible to include all response choices, you might consider providing the most likely responses and an "other" option. "Other" can be a standalone response, or you might include space for the respondent to provide clarification. The questions at the end of this chapter (Test Your Knowledge) are examples of quality multiple-choice questions.

**Likert scale questions** are a type of rating scale widely used to measure perceptions or attitudes related to the inquiry topic. In these questions, respondents are presented with a series of statements and asked to indicate their level of agreement with each statement, typically on a five-point or seven-point scale (Likert, 1932). The scale usually ranges from "Strongly Agree" to "Strongly Disagree," as shown in Table 11-4. These questions are commonly organized in a table format for ease of completion, regardless of whether they are completed on paper or electronically. Likert scale questions are valuable since they quantify perceptions and attitudes for analysis and comparison of responses across a sample.

In yes/no and Likert scale questions, there are differing opinions on whether to include "I don't know," "undecided," and neutral response options (Sturgis et al., 2014; Wetzelhütter, 2020). Since someone may have no opinion about a topic or be undecided, offering these alternatives can improve the accuracy of responses. However, respondents who are fatigued or disinterested in the survey may choose an alternative option because it is easier and quicker, though the response may be inaccurate. Additionally, eliminating alternative response options could force respondents into a positive or negative answer, which is beneficial only if the response is accurate. Removing a neutral option on a Likert scale requires a respondent to agree or disagree, even if they have no opinion about the statement. Ultimately, you must consider the item content and your inquiry participants to decide if any alternative response choices should be offered. Unlike in surveys, when Likert scale questions are used in interviews, the interviewer may be able to ask additional probing questions to clarify responses if necessary.

## TIPS & INSPIRATION

- Depending on the topic of Likert scale items, you may want to offer *both* a neutral option and an "I don't know" option since they are distinctly different. Many Likert scale items omit the "I don't know" option, which may force respondents to choose the neutral option even if they hold no opinion. This scenario, known as the "hidden don't know" response, can lead to inaccurate interpretations of the data (Sturgis et al., 2014, pp. 17–18).

Various other **rating scales** can also be used to gather data from inquiry participants. Rating scales require respondents to rate or rank items within categories or on a continuum. Examples of additional rating scale questions are included in Table 11-5.

### *Open-Ended Questions*

Open-ended questions may be formatted as short- or long-response questions. **Short-response questions** usually restrict answers to a few words or less. They are most suited for gathering straightforward information on topics for which fixed response choices are inappropriate. For example, what is one word you would use to describe your recent course of occupational therapy? In this example, it would be impossible to generate all plausible choices. Short-response items usually have higher response rates compared to items requesting longer answers. These items are also less cumbersome to analyze, especially when you anticipate a larger sample.

**Long-response questions** require lengthier responses ranging from a few sentences to paragraphs, depending on the topic and purpose. These questions require greater investment from the respondents to provide thorough answers. Less motivated respondents may skip these questions or answer very quickly. For this reason, you should carefully consider if a long-response, open-ended question will enhance the information gained from the closed-ended questions. Including at least one long-response question might be customary, but if you cannot explain why you need this data and how you will analyze it, you should omit the question (Decorte et al., 2019). Long-response questions are the

**TABLE 11-5 ■ Examples of Other Rating Scale Questions**

| Question Type | Example |
|---|---|
| Semantic differential: Uses ratings along a continuum of opposing adjectives (Osgood et al., 1967) | Please rate your instructor on the following traits:<br>Disorganized ① ② ③ ④ ⑤ Organized<br>Unfair ① ② ③ ④ ⑤ Fair<br>Inaccessible ① ② ③ ④ ⑤ Accessible<br>Ineffective ① ② ③ ④ ⑤ Effective |
| Numerical rating scale: Uses numbers to rate feelings or experiences | Please rate your confidence in designing a research study on a scale of 1-10, where 1 = not confident at all, and 10 = extremely confident. |
| Frequency scale: Uses descriptors or numbers to rate how often an event or behavior occurs | How often do you follow the recommendations of your doctor?<br>a. Never<br>b. Seldom<br>c. Sometimes<br>d. Frequently<br>e. Always |
| Rank-order scale: Uses numbers to rate the value or importance of items against one another | Please rank the following features of a healthcare facility in order of importance to you, 1 being the MOST important, and 5 being the LEAST important.<br>Quality of care ________<br>Location ________<br>Cost ________<br>Ease of scheduling ________<br>Availability of online portal ________ |

primary question type used in interviews, where many of the previously noted challenges are not a concern since the interviewer can prompt for greater depth of response as necessary.

### TIPS & INSPIRATION

- Carefully consider the need for open-ended questions in your survey. A good rule is to include no more than five open-ended questions within one survey. Use fewer, if possible, to promote a good response rate and thorough responses.

## Question Organization

Every survey or interview should begin with an introduction clarifying the purpose of the questions, how the data will be used and kept confidential, instructions for respondents, and whether the option to skip questions or stop the survey or interview exists. The questions should be sequenced logically, beginning with general questions and proceeding to more complex ones. Early questions might include demographic or closed-ended questions that require little cognitive effort and keep the respondent interested. Questions regarding sensitive topics, those that take more thought, or open-ended questions should be sequenced later in the survey or interview. Multiple questions of the same format in succession, such as multiple yes/no questions or rating scale questions, should be limited to avoid respondents "straightlining" or clicking the same response for each question in the series (Kim et al., 2019, p. 214). Breaking these questions up with questions of different formats can deter this practice.

Another option to better organize your survey or interview is branching or skip logic. This design feature allows you to customize the sequence of questions for a respondent based on their prior answers. For example, a respondent who answers "yes" to the question "Do you exercise at least once per week?" could be directed to another question asking about the type of exercise they engage in. Those who answer "no" to the first question would not be asked the second question because it is not applicable. This feature is most effective in interviews or electronic surveys, where the irrelevant questions are not even available to respondents. For paper surveys, the second question would be phrased: "If yes, indicate your preferred exercise," and the respondent would have to follow the directions to determine whether they should respond.

Additional considerations for survey organization include the visual layout, ease of navigation, accessibility, and features to promote completion. These elements are discussed primarily for electronic surveys since this is the most common survey distribution method, though many of the concepts can also be incorporated with paper surveys. To improve readability, incorporate a consistent color scheme, font, and adequate white space in the visual layout. The survey should be easy to navigate with clear instructions and easily identifiable fields or response buttons. You should also consider if your survey will be accessible and understood by all potential respondents, particularly those with varying linguistic and health literacy levels, those for whom English is their second language (ESL), or those from diverse cultures. For electronic surveys, accessibility can be improved by ensuring your survey functions well on mobile devices or integrates with a screen reader for individuals with visual deficits. Surveys completed on paper could be made available in large print or read to a respondent.

Several other design features can be used to promote survey completion. First, the survey should be kept to a reasonable length. Sources estimate that the time respondents will devote to electronic surveys is between 7 and 8 minutes (Chudoba, 2023). Shorter or longer surveys may be justified based on your inquiry respondents, their commitment to the topic, and the aims of the inquiry. Second, you should consider when the survey is administered or delivered. Surveys administered during inquiry procedures often have higher completion rates since respondents are present when time is allotted for survey completion. If electronic surveys are delivered separately from other inquiry activities, you should consider the routines and preferences of your respondents. Generally, surveys sent during regular working hours on a weekday will garner higher response rates than those sent after hours or on weekends. Finally, presenting just one question at a time in electronic surveys can decrease participant overload. Providing a progress bar to indicate the percentage of the survey remaining can also be helpful.

## TIPS & INSPIRATION

- When designing a survey or interview, consider the participants' language, cultural norms, and linguistic and health literacy to ensure their understanding of the questions. Avoid abbreviations, professional jargon, and potentially biased wording. You can use readability formulas (discussed in Chapter 14), available in most word processing software, to determine the average sentence and word length used in your survey or interview. This information translates to an educational grade level to ensure you are writing at a level appropriate for your participants.
- Use two levels of review to improve the quality of a survey or interview before you administer it.
  - Expert review: Have experts in your topic area and/or those skilled in survey and interview design examine your tool to identify any content or methodological issues.
  - Pilot testing: Administer the tool to a small group of people similar to your inquiry participants. Analyze their responses to identify issues with the wording of the questions, response options, and data analysis.

## CHAPTER SUMMARY

1. Choose an appropriate inquiry design.
   - An inquiry design should be based on the inquiry problem, available time and resources, and the desired depth of understanding. Figure 11-1 can help you choose a design.
   - Quantitative designs are most appropriate if you have a hypothesis you want to test, if you want to determine cause-and-effect relationships or the effectiveness of an intervention, or if you are interested in the relationships between variables.
   - Qualitative designs are most suitable if you want to know how or why something happened; if you want to explore the perspectives, meaning, and values of others; or if you want to generate a new theory or hypothesis for later testing.
   - Mixed methods designs incorporate quantitative and qualitative methods within a single inquiry.
   - Quantitative, qualitative, or mixed methods evidence-based practice projects can be used to apply existing research to practice.
2. Differentiate pilot studies and feasibility studies.
   - Pilot studies are preliminary investigations that help refine the inquiry methods before the full-scale inquiry.
   - Feasibility studies are preliminary investigations that primarily look at logistical, financial, and organizational factors to determine if a full-scale inquiry is viable and practical—in other words, is a larger inquiry worth pursuing?
3. Identify possible aims of evidence-based practice inquiries.
   - Evidence-based practice inquiries evaluate the success of applying existing research to practice.
   - Knowledge translation goes beyond applying existing evidence to practice to disseminating outcomes, experiences, successes, and challenges to promote better clinical outcomes.
   - Evidence-based inquiries may serve several purposes: (1) program development, (2) guidance for unique clinical scenarios, (3) justification for personnel or resources, and (4) interprofessional collaboration.
4. Develop an inquiry plan.
   - An inquiry plan should include the inquiry title, investigators, participant criteria, recruitment, selection, and consent strategies, inquiry procedures, data collection tools, and required materials and equipment. Table 11-1 further describes each required element.
   - The procedures should be described in enough detail that they could be replicated by someone else. Consider using a table or figure to outline the inquiry procedures. Examples are provided in Table 11-2 and Figure 11-3.
5. Describe considerations in choosing data collection tools.
   - Chosen data collection tools should align with the inquiry purpose, design, and phenomena being investigated. While using multiple tools can triangulate results, too many can overwhelm participants and complicate data analysis.

- When selecting an existing tool, consider the reliability and validity, the availability of the tool, the ease of administration, any costs or training required to use it, and whether it is appropriate for your purpose. If no appropriate tool exists, consider creating your own.

6. Distinguish closed-ended and open-ended survey and interview questions.
   - Closed-ended questions have predetermined response choices, such as "yes/no" or multiple-choice options.
     - Closed-ended questions include multiple-choice questions, Likert scale items, and various other rating scales (semantic differential, numerical rating scale, frequency scale, and rank-order scale). Examples are provided in Tables 11-4 and 11-5.
     - Closed-ended questions yield quantitative data, require less time for completion, and are easier to analyze.
   - Open-ended questions allow respondents to provide detailed responses in their own words.
     - Open-ended questions include short-response and long-response questions.
     - Open-ended questions yield qualitative data, require more time for completion, and are best for addressing complicated or sensitive topics or elaborating on closed-ended questions.
7. Explain how to organize survey and interview questions to promote quality data collection.
   - Surveys and interviews should include an introduction to clarify the purpose, instructions, how the data will be used, and if survey or interview questions can be skipped or terminated.
   - Questions should proceed from general to more complex. Open-ended questions should be sequenced later.
   - Limit multiple questions of the same format in succession to avoid "straightlining" (respondents clicking the same response for all questions in a series).
   - Use branching or skip logic to eliminate respondents having to weed through irrelevant questions to get to those that apply to them.
   - Other survey design considerations include the visual layout, ease of navigation, accessibility, survey length, timing of administration, and progress indicators.

## TEST YOUR KNOWLEDGE

1. Which of the following BEST describes the criteria for choosing an inquiry design?
   a. Select a design that aligns with the inquiry purpose.
   b. Select a design based on the anticipated sample size.
   c. Select a design that will be least time-consuming to implement.
   d. Select a design that is the most rigorous.
2. A practitioner plans to investigate the efficacy of an experimental intervention for improving range of motion in clients post-stroke. What is the MOST suitable inquiry design?
   a. An evidence-based practice project
   b. A qualitative design
   c. A quantitative design
   d. A mixed methods design
3. A feasibility study would be appropriate in which of the following scenarios?
   a. An individual is researching historical events that shaped practice trends in nursing.
   b. A group of researchers want to refine their methods before conducting a large-scale randomized controlled trial.
   c. A faculty member wants to assess the practicality of a weekend study program for nontraditional students.
   d. A therapist wants to distribute an anonymous satisfaction survey to recently discharged clients.
4. Which statement BEST describes the relationship between evidence-based practice and knowledge translation?
   a. Knowledge translation is a precursor to evidence-based practice.
   b. Knowledge translation involves appraising the evidence to be applied in evidence-based practice.
   c. Knowledge translation is theoretical, whereas evidence-based practice is practical.
   d. Knowledge translation extends evidence-based practice by disseminating outcomes to improve healthcare.
5. An inquiry plan should include which of the following?
   a. Procedures similar to an existing study on the topic
   b. Procedures that can be reasonably replicated and align with the inquiry purpose
   c. Procedures to thoroughly investigate all aspects of the topic
   d. Procedures that are most efficient regardless of data quality

6. Which of the following is an open-ended question?
   a. Have you received occupational therapy services at this facility?
   b. Can you describe your experience of participating in the support group?
   c. Have you earned your geriatric specialty certification?
   d. How would you rate your pain on a scale of 0 to 10, where 0 is no pain, and 10 is extreme pain?
7. You are planning an inquiry to investigate using an educational intervention to improve teachers' knowledge and confidence in implementing social-emotional learning strategies in their classrooms. Your anticipated sample size is 350 teachers across 12 schools in an urban school district. What is the most appropriate data collection tool?
   a. An author-generated survey with primarily open-ended questions
   b. Individualized qualitative interviews with each teacher
   c. An author-generated survey composed of primarily closed-ended questions
   d. One virtual focus group that includes a sample of 45 teachers
8. Which strategy could increase the response rate and accuracy of data from an electronic survey?
   a. Including multiple questions of the same format consecutively
   b. Distributing the survey on a Saturday evening
   c. Piloting the survey with family and friends
   d. Customizing the sequence of questions based on a respondent's prior answers

Answer key appears at the end of this text.

## NEXT STEPS

1. Using the information in this chapter, identify a potential inquiry design to explore a topic of interest. Make a list of reasons this design is appropriate. You might consider your inquiry purpose, participants, intended outcome(s), your knowledge and experience in conducting inquiries, and the social, situational, and financial supports available. Share your list with others before making your final decision.
2. Create a table like Table 11-2 to summarize your proposed inquiry procedures. Are the plans logical and in alignment with the inquiry purpose? Is the time commitment for participants realistic? Discuss this table with others to identify any challenges with your plan.
3. Outline a plan for developing a survey or interview for a potential inquiry. Clarify the outcome(s) you want to assess, the relevant characteristics of your potential respondents (for example, literacy level, prior knowledge of the topic, age), the distribution method, and what steps you will take to improve the tool after initially drafting the questions. Justify your decisions before moving forward with question development.
4. Practice drafting three closed-ended and three open-ended questions for a potential survey or interview. Experiment with varying question formats to hone your skills in constructing quality questions.

## REFERENCES

Abbott, J. H. (2014). The distinction between randomized clinical trials (RCTs) and preliminary feasibility and pilot studies: What they are and are not. *Journal of Orthopaedic & Sports Physical Therapy, 44*(8), 555–558. https://doi.org/10.2519/jospt.2014.0110

Brandt, B., Lutfiyya, M. N., King, J. A., & Chioreso, C. (2014). A scoping review of interprofessional collaborative practice and education using the lens of the Triple Aim. *Journal of Interprofessional Care, 28*(5), 393–399. https://doi.org/10.3109/13561820.2014.906391

Chan, R. J., Knowles, R., Hunter, S., Conroy, T., Tieu, M., & Kitson, A. (2023). From evidence-based practice to knowledge translation: What is the difference? What are the roles of nurse leaders? *Seminars in Oncology Nursing, 39*(1), 151363. https://doi.org/10.1016/j.soncn.2022.151363

Chudoba, B. (2023). *How much time are respondents willing to spend on your survey?* SurveyMonkey website. https://www.surveymonkey.com/curiosity/survey_completion_times

Decorte, T., Malm, A., Sznitman, S. R., Hakkarainen, P., Barratt, M. J., Potter, G. R., Werse, B., Kamphausen, G., Lenton, S., & Frank, V. A. (2019). The challenges and benefits of analyzing feedback comments in surveys: Lessons from a cross-national online survey of small-scale cannabis growers. *Methodological Innovations, 12*(1), 1–16. https://doi.org/10.1177/2059799119825606

Eldridge, S. M., Lancaster, G. A., Campbell, M. J., Thabane, L., Hopewell, S., Coleman, C. L., & Bond, C. M. (2016). Defining feasibility and pilot studies in preparation for randomised controlled trials: Development of a conceptual framework. *PLoS One, 11*(3), e0150202. https://doi.org/10.1371%2Fjournal.pone.0150205

Kemp, J., Moore, K., Fransen, M., Russell, T., Freke, M, & Crossley, K. M. (2018). A pilot randomised clinical trial of physiotherapy (manual therapy, exercise, and education) for early-onset hip osteoarthritis post-hip arthroplasty. *Pilot and Feasibility Studies, 4*(1), 1–9. https://doi.org/10.1186%2Fs40814-017-0157-4

Kim, Y., Dykema, J., Stevenson, J., Black, P., & Moberg, D. P. (2019). Straightlining: Overview of measurement, comparison of indicators, and effects in mail-web mixed-mode surveys. *Social Science Computer Review, 37*(2), 214–233. https://doi.org/10.1177/0894439317752406

Kistin, C., & Silverstein, M. (2015). Pilot studies: A critical but potentially misused component of interventional research. *Journal of the American Medical Association, 314*(15), 1561–1562. https://doi.org/10.1001%2Fjama.2015.10962

Kolenic, A. M. (2018). Feasibility studies: What they are, how they are done, and what we can learn from them. *Oncology Nursing Forum, 45*(5), 572–574. https://doi.org/10.1188/18.onf.572-574

Likert, R. (1932). A technique for the measurement of attitudes. *Archives of Psychology, 22*(140), 5–55.

Morin, A. M. F., & Lape, J. E. (2023). Feasibility of a stress reduction program among foster youth in college. *The Open Journal of Occupational Therapy, 11*(3), 1–11. https://doi.org/10.15453/2168-6408.2050

National Institute of Neurological Disorders and Stroke. (2023). *Isaacs syndrome.* National Institutes of Health. https://www.ninds.nih.gov/health-information/disorders/isaacs-syndrome

Newhouse, R. P., & Spring, B. (2010). Interdisciplinary evidence-based practice: Moving from silos to synergy. *Nursing Outlook, 58*(6), 309–317. https://doi.org/10.1016%2Fj.outlook.2010.09.001

Osgood, C. E., Suci, G. J., & Tannenbaum, P. H. (1967). *The measurement of meaning.* University of Illinois Press.

Pearson, N., Naylor, P-J., Ashe, M. C., Fernandez, M., Yoong, S. L., & Wolfenden, L. (2020). Guidance for conducting feasibility and pilot studies for implementation trials. *Pilot and Feasibility Studies, 6*(1), 167. https://doi.org/10.1186/s40814-020-00634-w

Reeves, S., Pelone, R., Harrison, R., Goldman, J., & Zwarenstein, M. (2017). Interprofessional collaboration to improve professional practice and healthcare outcomes. *Cochrane Database of Systematic Reviews, 2017*(6), CD000072. https://doi.org/10.1002/14651858.CD000072.pub3

Sturgis, P., Roberts, C., & Smith, P. (2014). Middle alternatives revisited: How the neither/nor response acts as a way of saying "I don't know"? *Sociological Methods & Research, 43*(1), 15–38. https://doi.org/10.1177/0049124112452527

Wensing, M., & Grol, R. (2019). Knowledge translation in health: How implementation science could contribute more. *BMC Medicine, 17*(1), 1–6. https://doi.org/10.1186/s12916-019-1322-9

Wetzelhütter, D. (2020). "Scale-sensitive response behavior!? Consequences of offering versus omitting a 'don't know' option and/or a middle category." *Survey Practice, 13*(1). https://doi.org/10.29115/SP-2020-0012

Whitehead, A. L., Sully, B. G. O., & Campbell, M. J. (2014). Pilot and feasibility studies: Is there a difference from each other and from a randomised controlled trial? *Contemporary Clinical Trials, 38*(1), 130–133. https://doi.org/10.1016/j.cct.2014.04.001

World Health Organization. (2010). *Framework for action on interprofessional education & collaborative practice.* Author. https://iris.who.int/handle/10665/70185

## Chapter 12

# Protecting of Human Subjects or Participants

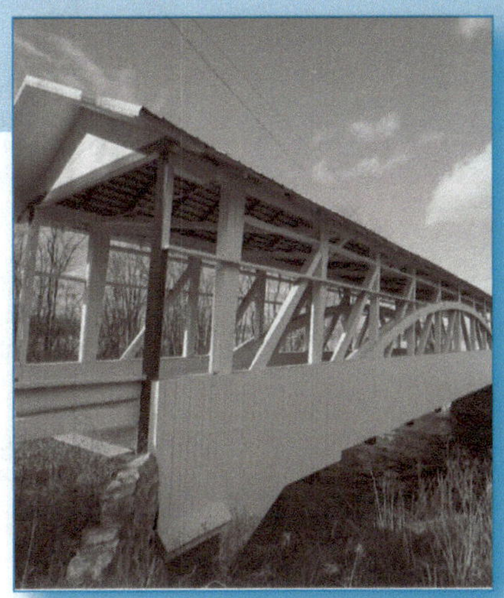

LEARNING OUTCOMES

*The information provided in this chapter will assist you to:*

12.1 Define a code of ethics and its application to conducting an inquiry.

12.2 Outline the history of legislation related to protecting human subjects or participants.

12.3 Explain the function of an Institutional Review Board (IRB) and the levels of review.

12.4 Describe the need for IRB oversight of an evidence-based practice project.

12.5 Identify key features of a quality IRB proposal.

12.6 Differentiate confidentiality, anonymity, and privacy.

## Ethics in Healthcare

Healthcare professionals and students are expected to behave professionally and ethically in all situations, including during their engagement in research and evidence-based practice. Each healthcare profession has published ethical standards that can be readily obtained through its national organization. These standards, often referred to as a **code of ethics**, outline the core values, principles, and standards of conduct expected of practitioners or those studying to become a practitioner within that profession. Figure 12-1 provides brief excerpts of ethical standards related to conducting research among several healthcare disciplines. Researchers must show integrity in the inquiry process, which includes respecting the rights of participants, abiding by the research design, and reporting results accurately and truthfully.

### Subjects Versus Participants

As noted in Chapter 1, the terms "subjects" and "participants" are often used interchangeably to refer to individuals being studied. However, the use of "participants" has gained traction in recent years to emphasize the autonomy of these individuals. Historical legislation incorporates "subjects," and some institutional review boards (discussed in this chapter) still rely on this term. Both terms have been purposefully incorporated into this chapter to represent what you might encounter on your journey. The choice of terminology for your own inquiry may be based on your specific discipline, publication or academic requirements, or your preference.

## History of the Protection of Human Subjects

While the ethical standards of each profession support ethical research practices and moral treatment

Hall's Mill Covered Bridge, Bedford County, Pennsylvania.

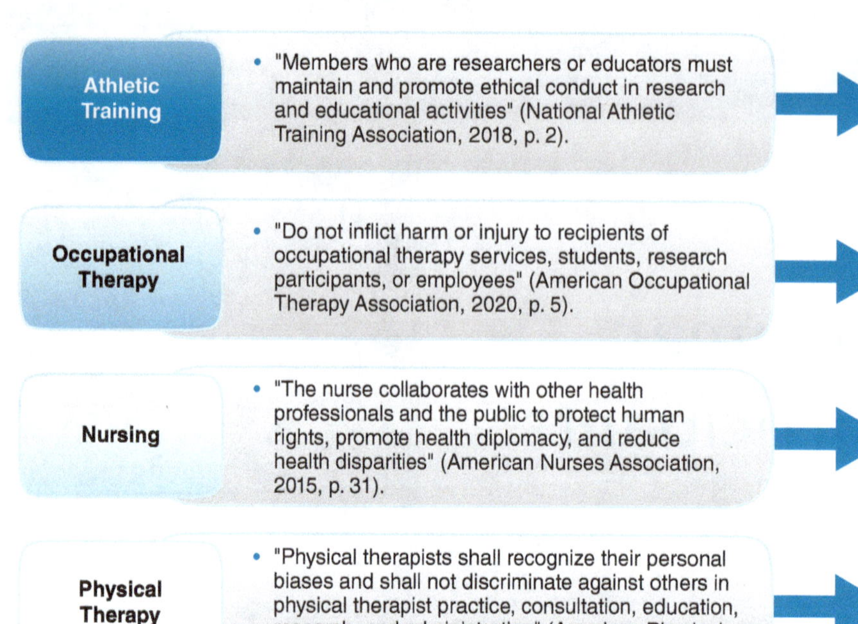


Figure 12-1 Excerpts of professional ethical standards.

of human subjects or participants, additional guidelines for conducting research were established beginning in the early 1900s; these gained traction between the 1940s and 1970s and are continually updated today (Ghooi, 2011). Various examples of abusive and unethical research practices prompted these guidelines. For instance, around the time of World War II, a series of medical experiments were conducted on prisoners in concentration camps, including adults and children who did not provide consent, and often resulted in trauma, death, disability, or illness (Weindling et al., 2016). Another common example is the Tuskegee syphilis study performed on African American men with the disease to better understand its progression when untreated. This study was performed between 1932 and 1972 and resulted in the death of many subjects who did not receive penicillin as treatment, even though it was widely available and shown to be effective by the 1940s (Duff-Brown, 2017). Legislation has led to the current parameters around acceptable research procedures, informed consent, and the review and approval of research protocols by an independent committee:

- **Berlin Code of 1900** is the first known regulation to govern research, enacted by the Prussian Minister of Religious, Educational and Medical Affairs after evidence of unethical experiments was discovered (Vollmann & Winau, 1996).
- **Nuremberg Code of 1947** consists of 10 principles of ethical research, including voluntary informed consent of subjects, use of adequately trained and skilled investigators/researchers, and elimination of unnecessary risks to subjects (U.S. Department of Health and Human Services [DHHS], 2015).
- **Declaration of Helsinki**, adopted in 1964 and continually updated today, outlines ethical research principles, including the requirement of a research proposal describing the planned procedures to be reviewed and approved by an independent ethics committee before a study can begin. Approval of a research proposal is also required for dissemination of study outcomes (World Medical Association, 2023).
- **National Research Act** (1974), enacted by U.S. lawmakers, promoted high-quality research and the protection of human subjects by establishing the *National Commission for the Protection of Human Subjects of Biomedical and Behavioral Research*. This commission was the first national group tasked with oversight of research ethics whose work resulted in the Belmont Report (DHHS, 2022).

- **Belmont Report** (1979) solidified previous legislation and explicitly defined three ethical principles: respect for persons, beneficence, and justice (National Commission for the Protection of Human Subjects of Biomedical and Behavioral Research, 1979).
  1. **Respect for persons** supports one's right to autonomy or the ability to make decisions about their lives. This principle also describes groups such as children or prisoners that represent vulnerable populations, who lack the capacity to make their own decisions (children) or may feel pressured to decide in a particular way (prisoners). In these instances, care should be taken to avoid coercion in research procedures and to involve legally appointed guardians in the decision-making process when necessary.
  2. **Beneficence** involves avoiding harm, maximizing benefits, and minimizing risks in research procedures. Researchers should carefully consider the possible benefits of the research and ensure they outweigh the risks.
  3. **Justice** refers to the fair distribution of research benefits and risks. In other words, discriminatory practices in recruiting and selecting research participants must be avoided. Participant inclusion criteria should be based on the inquiry topic and justified in the research proposal.
- **The Federal Policy for the Protection of Human Subjects**, better known as the **Common Rule**, was issued in 1991 and revised most recently in 2018. This policy outlines standards for federally funded research, though most U.S. academic and medical institutions enforce this policy regardless of funding. The policy specifies the function of institutional review boards (discussed next), informed consent requirements, research approval criteria, and additional protections for pregnant women, human fetuses, neonates, prisoners, and children (DHHS, 2019).

## Institutional Review Board

As a result of the legislation just discussed, if you plan to conduct an inquiry, you will likely be required to draft and submit a proposal outlining your planned procedures to an Institutional Review Board. An **Institutional Review Board (IRB)**, also referred to as an independent ethics committee (IEC), research ethics committee (REC), or ethical review board (ERB), is a group of people with varied backgrounds who are tasked with thoroughly reviewing research proposals to ensure the procedures meet all ethical standards. In most cases, you cannot begin an inquiry without having your proposal reviewed by an IRB. IRB approval or exemption is also required to publish or disseminate inquiry outcomes. The rest of this chapter walks you through the components of an IRB proposal to help you navigate the process.

An IRB comprises at least five members and typically meets at scheduled intervals to review proposals and issue decisions as to whether the inquiry may proceed. A decision is based on the need for and perceived benefits of the investigation, the quality of the inquiry procedures, the level of risk to the participants, and the qualifications of the researchers (i.e., do they have the skills, expertise, and resources to complete the research ethically and successfully?). After a committee reviews a proposal, they can accept it if it represents sound and ethical research practices. A proposal can be rejected immediately if it lacks required information or fails to adequately address all ethical standards. The most likely response to an initial proposal is a request for additional information or clarification on potential points of concern. For this reason, sufficient time should be allotted for the initial review and response, as well as multiple revisions as needed to gain final approval.

Most academic institutions have their own IRB that reviews the proposals of the faculty and students. Similarly, many healthcare systems and facilities also have their own IRB to oversee research conducted by health professionals and students who are affiliated there. Most commonly, research proposals are reviewed by the institution where the research will occur, if a board exists there. For example, if you are a student planning to complete a study at a hospital, you will likely submit your proposal to the hospital's IRB. If the hospital does not have an IRB, then you would submit to the IRB at your academic institution. Likewise, research in community-based settings such as a senior center or fitness facility may undergo review by an academic institution since most community settings do not have IRBs. In some instances, you may be required to gain dual approvals from your academic institution and clinical or community facility. Discussing the requirements early can help you best prepare for the review.

## TIPS & INSPIRATION

- Identify if the site where you will conduct your inquiry has an IRB or if you must submit your inquiry proposal to your academic institution or both. Reach out to the appropriate board(s) early to confirm deadlines for submission. Deadlines are aligned with their meeting schedule, so if you miss a deadline, your proposal review may be delayed until the next time the board convenes.
- Do not underestimate the time needed to gain approval from an IRB. This process can range from 1 to 6 months, depending on the frequency of board meetings and whether all materials have been submitted correctly and completely. If the proposal needs to be revised, it may take even longer. You cannot start your inquiry until the board approves or exempts your proposal.

### Levels of Review

There are three potential levels of review for a research (or IRB) proposal—exempt, expedited, or full review. The level of review is determined by the IRB (not the researcher) and corresponds primarily to the anticipated level of risk, the sensitivity of the topic under study, and whether vulnerable populations are involved. An inquiry can be categorized as minimal risk or greater than minimal risk. With **minimal risk**, "the probability and magnitude of harm or discomfort anticipated in the research are not greater, in and of themselves, than those ordinarily encountered in daily life or during the performance of routine physical or psychological examinations or tests" (DHHS, 2019, §46.102 j). **Vulnerable populations** may include children under 18 years of age, pregnant persons, prisoners, individuals who are economically or educationally disadvantaged, or those with impaired decision-making capacity (such as persons with dementia). Proposals requiring exempt and expedited reviews involve no more than minimal risk and avoid sensitive topics and vulnerable populations. Proposals requiring full (or convened) reviews may entail more than minimal risk, sensitive topics, and vulnerable populations. Table 12-1 describes the levels of review with examples and the review process for each level.

## TIPS & INSPIRATION

- Many IRBs have specific templates for each level of review. While the final decision about the level of review rests with the board, they typically provide some guidelines to help you prepare the required information. Sometimes, the board may be willing to discuss your potential inquiry with you and provide further directions before submission. Do not be afraid to reach out and ask questions. The better prepared you are, the smoother the review will be for the board.
- If you are working through this process with co-investigators or a faculty advisor, or if the IRB requires electronic submission of your proposal, it can be beneficial to download the required forms or templates and create a "working draft" of your IRB proposal. It is quite common to make multiple rounds of revisions before submission, and this working draft can support collaboration for the creation of a sound proposal.

### Ethics, IRB, and Evidence-Based Practice Projects

Up to this point, we have been discussing ethics and IRB review in terms of research, but you may also be required to undergo an IRB review when completing a formal evidence-based practice project. You might be confused by this requirement because clinicians apply the principles of evidence-based practice in their everyday work, including evaluating the needs of their clients, establishing evidence-based plans, and collecting data on those clients (likely in the form of tests and measures documented in clients' medical records)—all without approval from an IRB. The difference with a formal evidence-based practice project is that you

**TABLE 12-1 ■ Levels of Institutional Review Board (IRB) Review**

| Level of Review | Definition | Examples | Review Process |
|---|---|---|---|
| **Exempt** | Inquiries involving no more than minimal risk and any of the following:<br>■ Research in educational settings that involve normal educational practices<br>■ Research using *only* educational tests, surveys, observation, or interviews<br>■ Benign behavioral interventions with adults (must be brief, harmless, not upsetting or physically invasive)<br>■ Analysis of data or specimens previously collected for another purpose, with no contact between participants and the investigators<br>■ Research through federal departments or agencies to evaluate programs<br>■ Taste and food quality studies | ■ A study comparing the outcomes of a new curriculum to the outcomes of a former one<br>■ A focus group with nurses about their motivation for returning to school<br>■ An anonymous survey about exercise habits<br>■ A study on the impact of brief education or provision of educational materials on healthy eating<br>■ Analysis of fall risk data within a facility over multiple years, including review of medical records and facility reports | ■ The IRB chairperson or a designated committee member reviews the proposal to determine if it qualifies for exemption.<br>■ If a proposal is determined to be exempt (by the IRB member), it does not require further review before beginning the inquiry. |
| **Expedited** | Inquiries involving no more than minimal risk that do *not* meet the exempt criteria. Inquiries requiring expedited review may include the following:<br>■ Research on individual or group characteristics or behavior or research using surveys, interviews, oral history, focus groups, program evaluation, or quality assurance methods<br>■ Collecting data through voice, video, digital, or image recordings<br>■ Collection of data through noninvasive routine clinical practice procedures<br>■ Analysis of data, documents, records, or specimens previously collected or those that will be collected for nonresearch purposes<br>■ Prospective collection of biological specimens or blood samples by noninvasive means<br>■ Clinical studies of drugs or medical devices under specific conditions | ■ Research on the impact of a balance training program for healthy adults<br>■ A study on the effectiveness of a wrist splint in decreasing pain related to carpal tunnel syndrome<br>■ Use of video recordings to analyze gait patterns in patients following bilateral knee replacement<br>■ Use of a mindfulness program to decrease stress in college students<br>■ Education on aging in place for cognitively intact community-dwelling seniors | ■ The IRB chairperson or one or more qualified members review the proposal.<br>■ These reviews are not necessarily quicker, as the name implies, but fewer people review them (compared to full reviews). |

*Continued*

**TABLE 12-1 ■ Levels of Institutional Review Board (IRB) Review—cont'd**

| Level of Review | Definition | Examples | Review Process |
|---|---|---|---|
| **Full (or convened)** | Inquiries that do *not* qualify for exempt or expedited review. Inquiries requiring full review may include the following:<br>■ Inquires with greater than minimal risk, such as those that may cause physical harm or significant emotional distress<br>■ Inquires involving vulnerable populations<br>■ Inquiry topics that are highly sensitive or illegal | ■ A study on the effectiveness of physical therapy in improving motor skills in children with cerebral palsy<br>■ A survey of elementary school children on their attitudes toward online education<br>■ Evaluation of a community reintegration program for prisoners<br>■ Focus groups with survivors of domestic violence<br>■ A study investigating nonpharmacological interventions for nursing home residents with dementia | ■ All members of the IRB review the proposal, meet to discuss it, and vote on the proposal status. |

usually collect data on many participants and share it in de-identified form *outside* the site where the project occurred. This dissemination of your project outcomes could include a presentation at your academic institution, a presentation at a state conference, or a publication in a peer-reviewed journal, as examples. The oversight of an IRB protects you, your participants, and your site, and allows you to disseminate your outcomes to others interested in your topic. Similar to research, an IRB review is required to publish outcomes from an evidence-based practice project.

Additional ethical considerations when conducting an evidence-based practice project include the following:

- Ensuring that the evidence is appraised before using it to guide decision-making. Do not assume that all evidence is good quality or applies to your clients or practice setting.
- Maintaining client-centeredness, which means in some cases, you may not implement interventions found to be most effective in research, particularly if they conflict with the client's values or circumstances.
- Implementing only those interventions that are within your scope of practice and for which you have the required trainings/certifications and resources.

## Considerations in Drafting an IRB Proposal

Owing to federal regulations, the purpose and guidelines for constructing an IRB proposal are similar across institutions and settings. However, the specific format of the proposal, the deadlines, and the expected turnaround times may differ. The information provided in this section should help you understand the key features of a quality IRB proposal so that you can best design your inquiry to protect your participants. Once you identify the IRB you will submit to, you should contact them directly to obtain the necessary forms and guidelines.

### Research Ethics Training

Federal regulations require that anyone submitting an IRB proposal (usually known as the **primary investigator** on the proposal) and any co-investigators who will participate in the inquiry (i.e., those consenting participants, those conducting an intervention, or those analyzing data) complete training on research ethics, confidentiality, and conflicts of interest. This training must be completed before submitting a proposal, and each IRB specifies the required training that meets this standard. One of the most common training programs is the Collaborative Institutional Training Initiative (CITI), which offers initial certification courses as well as refresher courses. CITI Program (n.d.) training courses must be renewed every 3 years. Your training should be active at the time of IRB submission and throughout the completion of your inquiry.

### TIPS & INSPIRATION

- Complete your required research ethics training before starting any IRB proposal. The training information will help you avoid mistakes in your proposal.
- Allow sufficient time to complete your research ethics training, which could take several hours. You can usually break the training into several shorter sessions if necessary. Be sure to save your work before exiting any training.

### Letter of Site Support

A letter of support will likely be needed from the site where you plan to conduct the inquiry. Suppose you plan to conduct an inquiry at a local senior center. The IRB may require a letter of support from the senior center director to confirm that the site agrees with your proposed plan. A letter of support on the site's letterhead should briefly describe the inquiry plans and confirm that additional approval from the site is unnecessary. The dated letter should also include the name, signature, title, and contact information of the site authority providing permission.

### TIPS & INSPIRATION

- You may be asked to draft a letter of site support with the required information. If so, you would provide the draft letter, and the site authority could modify it as necessary, print it on letterhead, and add their signature if they agree. An example letter of site support is provided in Figure 12-2 to help you.

### Recruitment

The IRB proposal should outline how participants will be recruited and by whom, with care taken to avoid concerns about coercion. **Coercion** is the use of excessive influence in recruiting and consenting participants. For example, an investigator who directly approaches participants may be more persuasive because of their investment in the inquiry. Similarly, employees recruited for a study conducted by their boss may feel undue pressure to participate due to fear of retribution. When possible, recruitment should avoid direct contact between potential participants and investigators or between those with a power differential, such as the scenario of employees recruited by their supervisor. Passive recruitment methods, such as flyers, online postings, or mailings, can also eliminate these concerns since potential participants must respond if interested. If you must directly recruit your participants (i.e., if no one else is available), you should draft a clear script of the objective information you will share. You may be asked to submit your recruitment materials, including flyers, online postings, letters, or verbal scripts used for direct recruitment, along with your IRB proposal. Figure 12-3 and Box 12-1 provide examples of a flyer and a recruitment script, respectively.

### TIPS & INSPIRATION

- If you are having difficulty determining the best method of recruitment for your inquiry, consider some of these ideas:
  - Have someone at the inquiry site not associated with the inquiry do the initial outreach. For example, the receptionist at a healthcare facility could read a recruitment script to potential participants when they sign in for their appointment.
  - Post an approved flyer at the inquiry site or on a social media site (or group) that potential participants are likely to frequent.
  - Send a letter to potential participants or their legal guardians inviting them to participate. For example, a letter could be sent home in children's backpacks inviting parents to attend an information session about the inquiry or sign a consent form if they agree to their child's participation.

### Informed Consent

**Informed consent**, one of the most important features of an inquiry involving human participants, is

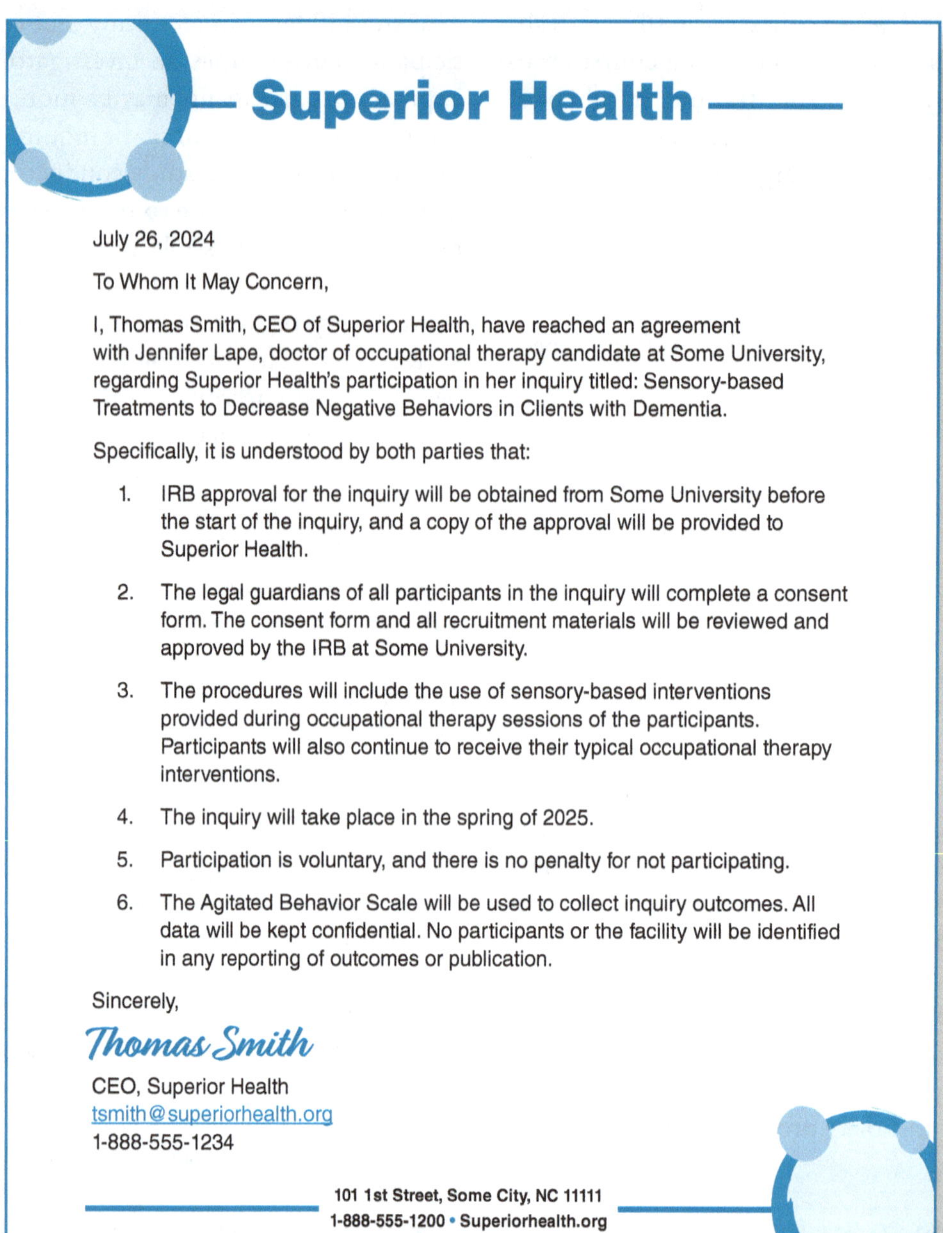

Superior Health

July 26, 2024

To Whom It May Concern,

I, Thomas Smith, CEO of Superior Health, have reached an agreement with Jennifer Lape, doctor of occupational therapy candidate at Some University, regarding Superior Health's participation in her inquiry titled: Sensory-based Treatments to Decrease Negative Behaviors in Clients with Dementia.

Specifically, it is understood by both parties that:

1. IRB approval for the inquiry will be obtained from Some University before the start of the inquiry, and a copy of the approval will be provided to Superior Health.
2. The legal guardians of all participants in the inquiry will complete a consent form. The consent form and all recruitment materials will be reviewed and approved by the IRB at Some University.
3. The procedures will include the use of sensory-based interventions provided during occupational therapy sessions of the participants. Participants will also continue to receive their typical occupational therapy interventions.
4. The inquiry will take place in the spring of 2025.
5. Participation is voluntary, and there is no penalty for not participating.
6. The Agitated Behavior Scale will be used to collect inquiry outcomes. All data will be kept confidential. No participants or the facility will be identified in any reporting of outcomes or publication.

Sincerely,

Thomas Smith

CEO, Superior Health
tsmith@superiorhealth.org
1-888-555-1234

101 1st Street, Some City, NC 11111
1-888-555-1200 • Superiorhealth.org

Figure 12-2 Example letter of site support.

an inquiry participant's agreement to participate, freely given, after full disclosure of the inquiry procedures. In other words, participants must understand the purpose of the inquiry, the inquiry procedures, the potential risks and benefits, how their information will be used and protected, alternatives to participation, and any compensation offered before voluntarily providing their consent. The participants can complete the consent form on paper or electronically, depending on the site's requirements or the inquiry's logistics. The informed consent should appear on the institutional letterhead where the IRB is located; most institutions have a required template for drafting your consent form. Table 12-2 summarizes the

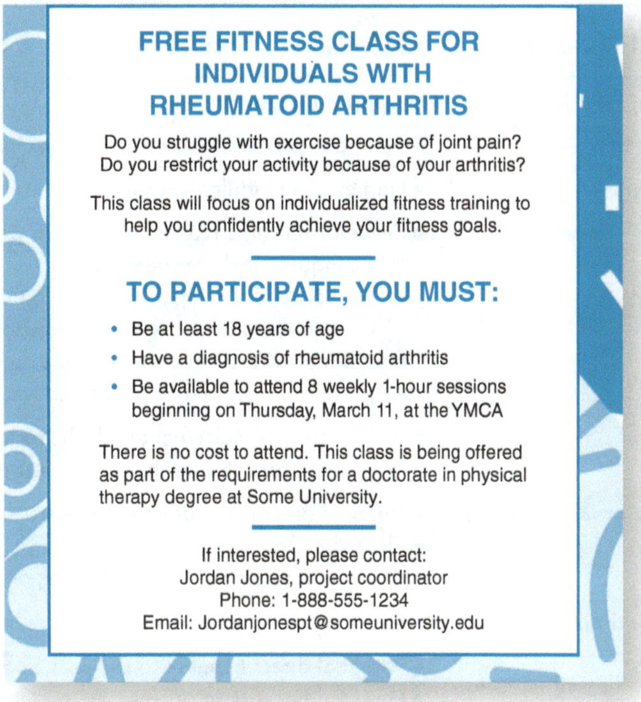

FREE FITNESS CLASS FOR INDIVIDUALS WITH RHEUMATOID ARTHRITIS

Do you struggle with exercise because of joint pain?
Do you restrict your activity because of your arthritis?

This class will focus on individualized fitness training to help you confidently achieve your fitness goals.

TO PARTICIPATE, YOU MUST:

- Be at least 18 years of age
- Have a diagnosis of rheumatoid arthritis
- Be available to attend 8 weekly 1-hour sessions beginning on Thursday, March 11, at the YMCA

There is no cost to attend. This class is being offered as part of the requirements for a doctorate in physical therapy degree at Some University.

If interested, please contact:
Jordan Jones, project coordinator
Phone: 1-888-555-1234
Email: Jordanjonespt@someuniversity.edu

Figure 12-3 Example recruitment flyer.

### BOX 12-1 ■ Example Recruitment Script

Script to be read by the practice receptionist when clients check in for their appointments:

"You are invited to join a study on using specific strategies to decrease pain from arthritis. The study includes three sessions where you would learn the strategies and practice them. These sessions would be separate from your regular occupational therapy sessions. If you want to participate or learn more, you can call the therapist at 333-333-3333."

most common content included in a consent form. It is essential that the consent form be drafted using layperson's terminology and geared toward the potential participants' literacy level and knowledge of the topic.

In select cases, a **waiver of consent** may be appropriate if the inquiry involves minimal risk and will not adversely affect the rights or welfare of participants (DHHS, 2019). Even with a waiver, you may still be required to provide the participants with the consent information, but their signature may not be required. In other instances, the need for informed consent may be waived entirely. The final decision regarding the appropriateness of a waiver rests with the IRB. Here are some scenarios where a waiver may be appropriate:

- The informed consent would be the sole document linking a participant to an inquiry and increasing the potential for a breach of confidentiality. For example, an electronic survey is distributed to healthcare professionals regarding their use of evidence-based practice in their clinics. The information in the survey's introduction explains the survey's purpose, how the data will be used, and that completion of the survey implies participants' consent.
- The inquiry involves minimal risk and procedures where consent is not typically required outside the inquiry process. For example, a school adopts a new handwriting curriculum and wants to assess the impact on students' handwriting legibility of their final projects to determine if other schools in the district should adopt the program. A letter is sent home informing parents about using the handwriting curriculum. However, their

**TABLE 12-2 ■ Informed Consent Content**

| Consent Section | Required Content |
|---|---|
| **Inquiry title** | ■ A concise yet descriptive title for your inquiry |
| **Investigators** | ■ Names of all inquiry investigators |
| **Concise summary** | ■ Key information a reasonable person would want to have to decide whether to participate in the inquiry. Include the following:<br>■ That consent is being sought for voluntary participation in the inquiry<br>■ The inquiry purpose, expected duration of participation, and inquiry procedures<br>■ Reasonably foreseeable risks and potential benefits<br>■ Appropriate alternative procedures or courses of treatment for the participant |
| **Purpose** | ■ A clear purpose statement with the rationale for the inquiry<br>■ The reason for offering the participant the opportunity to participate |
| **Specific procedures** | ■ Detailed description of what the participant is expected to do<br>■ The time commitment required<br>■ Consider inserting a chart, calendar, or chronological list of procedures. |
| **Risks and discomforts** | ■ Summary of potential inconveniences, risks, and discomforts |
| **Benefits** | ■ Potential direct benefits to the participant<br>■ Potential benefits to others |
| **Alternative procedures** | ■ Alternative procedures available. At least one alternative should be offered, if possible. |
| **Confidentiality** | ■ Procedures to ensure participant information will remain confidential during and after the inquiry<br>■ Who will have access to the data<br>■ Where data will be stored, how long it will be retained, and how it will eventually be destroyed (Your site may require you to retain the data for a specific time period.) |
| **Compensation** | ■ If participants will receive financial compensation or other incentives for participation<br>■ Compensation in the form of continuing education, refreshments at a session, or a small gift card drawing may be appropriate to encourage participation. Excessive compensation may raise concerns about coercion.<br>■ Any costs that may be incurred by the participant (for example, medical costs for injuries, registration fees) |
| **Contact information** | ■ Contact information for the investigator(s) for questions about the inquiry<br>■ Contact information for the Institutional Review Board for questions or concerns about their rights as a participant |
| **Voluntary participation and termination statements and signature** | ■ Statement that participation is voluntary<br>■ A statement indicating the participant may withdraw their participation at any point and the decision will have no negative consequences<br>■ Printed names, signatures, and dates for the investigator, participant, and faculty advisor (if you are a student) |

signature is not required since this represents a school-wide curricular change, and no personally identifiable information is being collected from students.

- The inquiry involves minimal risk, and the procedures represent the standard of care in a clinical setting. For example, an evidence-based practice project involves a nursing practice adopting a new screening tool for smoking cessation. The screening tool is adopted as the standard of care in the setting, and the nurses use it to identify patients who might benefit from additional support in this area. The nurses collect data on the number of referrals to specialists as well as the number of smoking cessation prescriptions written in a 2-month period and compare the data to historical data within the practice.

- Retrospective studies, especially those involving the review of many medical records, may qualify for a waiver of consent. At the point of record review, you may no longer have access to the patients to ask for informed consent, or it would be impractical to track them down. Imagine a study investigating the number of rehabilitation sessions and level of independence at discharge by the type of orthopedic surgery completed. This information can be retrieved and analyzed without identifying individual patients and with less than minimal risk.

### Assent

In cases in which a potential participant cannot give informed consent due to impaired decision-making capacity or age, you must obtain consent from the appointed legal guardian or parent. For example, consent from legal guardians or parents would be necessary for inquiries involving individuals with dementia or children under the age of 18. Individuals who cannot provide informed consent but generally understand the inquiry activities should also provide assent before the inquiry begins. **Assent** is agreement with the inquiry procedures by someone unable to legally provide informed consent. So, in an inquiry involving children as participants, informed consent would be obtained from the parents or legal guardians, and the children would also provide assent if they reasonably had the capacity to understand. Federal regulations do not specify a minimum age for assent since consideration must also be given to their mental capacity. However, many IRBs require assent over the age of 6 years without justification for skipping this step. Assent may be completed in written form or verbally completed and documented, depending on the circumstances. A witness may be asked to observe the assent process and attest that the required information was covered, and that assent was provided. Care should be taken to gear assent language toward the children or other populations who will provide assent. See Figures 12-4 and 12-5 for examples of a parental consent form and a child assent form for the same inquiry.

### Volunteer Agreements

An **inquiry volunteer** is an individual who will assist with conducting an inquiry but who is *not* one of the investigators and who you are *not* collecting data from. For example, an occupational therapist is conducting an inquiry in an elementary school on the use of self-regulation strategies within the classroom to improve students' attention. The therapist solicits the help of the classroom teacher to serve as a volunteer in the inquiry; the teacher is provided with education on the planned strategies and asked to implement them 3 days per week to improve carryover and maximize the benefits to students. The therapist models the strategies for the students on the other 2 days per week and collects all inquiry data on the students' attention. In this scenario, no data are collected from the teacher, and the teacher is not collecting or handling any inquiry data. If you have volunteers in your inquiry, you may be required to have them complete a volunteer agreement. If so, the agreement should outline the purpose of the inquiry, what you expect the volunteer to do, and the anticipated time commitment. See Figure 12-6 for an example of a volunteer agreement.

### TIPS & INSPIRATION

- One of the most time-consuming parts of constructing a quality IRB proposal is drafting the informed consent, assent, and volunteer agreements (if needed). It is essential to use layperson's terminology and align the information with the participants' literacy level and knowledge of the topic. Chapter 14 provides information on assessing the reading level of your documents. You should aim for a sixth- to eighth-grade level or lower (Hadden et al., 2017).
- Have multiple people, particularly those similar to the potential participants or volunteers, review your consents, assents, and volunteer agreements to gather feedback on their clarity. For example, suppose you plan to ask fourth graders for their assent in the inquiry. You might ask fourth graders not associated with the inquiry site, who will not be targeted as potential participants, to review the assent beforehand. This is an excellent way to determine if your message is clear.

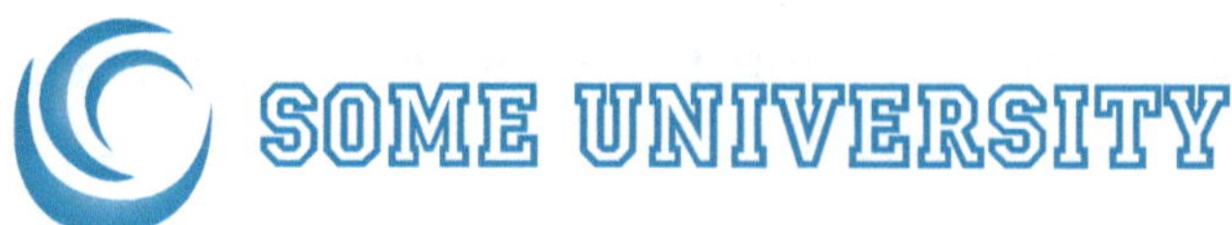


**Parental Consent Form**

**Inquiry Title:** Handwriting Legibility in Elementary School Students

**Primary Investigator:** Joseph Zhang

**Concise Summary:** Your child is invited to participate in an inquiry to assess whether a new handwriting program can improve writing skills for second graders. This form provides you with information about the inquiry activities and the risks and benefits so you can decide if you want your child to participate.

- Your child's participation is voluntary.
- The new handwriting program will be taught in your child's classroom over the next 4 weeks. The program activities will occur for 15 minutes daily during writing class and be taught by the classroom teacher and the occupational therapist. If you agree to your child's participation, they will complete a short handwriting test before and after the program. The occupational therapist will administer the short handwriting tests.
- The risks to participation are no greater than those encountered in daily life as a second-grade student. Participation may improve your child's writing skills, hand strength, and grasp of pencils and crayons.
- If you do not want your child to participate in the handwriting tests, they may still participate in the handwriting program as part of the typical classroom instruction.

**Purpose of the Inquiry:** Your child is invited to participate in this inquiry because they attend second grade at South Elementary School. This year, a new handwriting program with fun games and activities is being used in the second-grade classrooms to teach students to write their upper- and lowercase letters. I want to know whether this new program helps second-grade students write their letters better.

**Specific Procedures:** All second-grade students will participate in the new handwriting program for 15 minutes daily for 4 weeks during writing class (total of 300 minutes over 4 weeks). The program activities will be led by the classroom teacher and the occupational therapist who is the primary investigator. If you choose for your child to participate in the inquiry, in addition to the activities, they will also complete a 10-minute handwriting test before and after the program. The tests will help me learn whether this handwriting program improves your child's writing.

**Risks & Discomforts:** The anticipated risks and discomforts to your child are minimal and no greater than those encountered in daily life as a second-grade student. Your child may be frustrated if the letters are hard to learn, but individual help will be provided if needed. Your child may be uncomfortable sitting during the lessons, but they can take a break or move around if needed. Your child may be nervous about the tests, but they will be reminded that there is no grade for the tests. The tests will occur in a private room with the occupational therapist during writing class, and your child will not miss other classroom activities.

**Benefits:** Participation may improve your child's writing skills, hand strength, and grasp of pencils and crayons. Participation may also help the school choose future handwriting programs for second-grade students.

Figure 12-4 Example of a parental consent form.

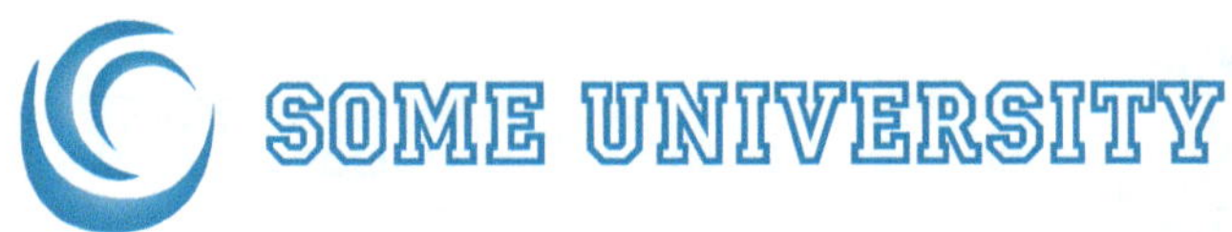


**Alternative Procedures:** If you do not want your child to participate in the handwriting tests, they may still participate in the handwriting games and activities as part of the typical classroom instruction.

**Confidentiality:** All information collected during this inquiry will be kept confidential. Your child's name will not be included on their test. Instead, a code number will be used. Your child will not be individually identified in any presentation or publication of the results. All tests will occur on paper but will be immediately scanned and saved to an electronic file. All electronic files will be stored on the primary investigator's password-protected computer. The paper tests will be shredded immediately after scanning. The electronic files will be saved for 7 years and then deleted. Only the primary investigator and their faculty advisor will have access to the electronic data.

**Compensation:** Neither you nor your child will be compensated for participation in the inquiry. Your child may receive stickers or other small incentives during the writing lessons. Neither Some University, the elementary school, nor any agency funding this inquiry will provide special services, free care, or compensation of injuries resulting from this inquiry. By providing consent, you understand that treatment for such injuries will be at your expense and/or paid through your medical plan.

**Contact Information:** If you have questions about the inquiry, you can contact the primary investigator at j.zhang@someuniversity.edu or 555-555-5555. If you have questions about the rights of inquiry participants, you can contact the chairperson of the Some University Institutional Review Board at IRBchair@someuniversity.edu or 444-444-4444.

**Voluntary Participation & Termination:** I understand that my child's participation in this inquiry is entirely voluntary and that refusal to participate will involve no penalty or loss of benefits to my child or me. I am free to withdraw or refuse consent or discontinue my child's participation in this inquiry at any time without negative consequences or penalties. I voluntarily give my consent for my child to participate in this inquiry. I understand I will be given a copy of this consent form.

**Parent or Guardian's Printed Name:** ______________________________

**Parent or Guardian's Signature & Date:** ______________________________

**Investigator's Printed Name:** ______________________________

**Investigator's Signature & Date:** ______________________________

**Faculty Advisor's Printed Name: (if applicable)** ______________________________

**Faculty Advisor's Signature & Date: (if applicable)** ______________________________

Figure 12-4 cont'd

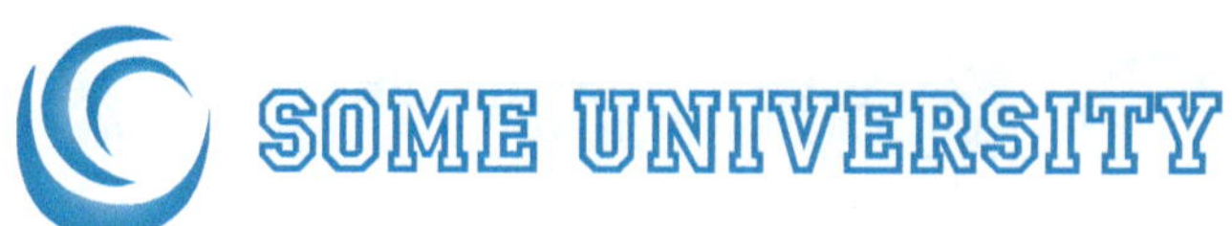


**Child Assent Form**

**Inquiry Title:** Handwriting Legibility in Elementary School Students

**Primary Investigator:** Joseph Zhang

**Introduction:** This letter explains a project I am doing with your teacher. You can decide whether you want to be in the project.

**Reason for the Project:** I want to see whether teaching you how to write upper- and lowercase letters in a new way helps you to write your letters better.

**What You Will Have to Do:** I will be teaching everyone in your class how to write upper- and lowercase letters in a new way. Your teacher will help me teach the letters. You will practice the letters every day for 20 minutes. I will give you a short writing test at the start of the project and at the end to see whether the lessons helped you write better.

**Discomforts/Risks:** Some of the letters might be hard to learn. Your teacher and I will help you with any letters that are hard. It might be hard to sit still for writing time, but you can take a break and move around if you need to. You might be worried about the test. The test is only for the project and is not part of your class grade.

**Confidentiality:** I will put a number on your test instead of your name. I will not tell anyone else how you did on the test.

**Voluntary Agreement:** You can put your name on this form if you want to be in the project. You can stop the project anytime you want.

**Student Printed Name (or signature):** ______________________________

**Witness's Signature & Date:** ______________________________

**Investigator's Signature & Date:** ______________________________

Figure 12-5 Example child assent form.

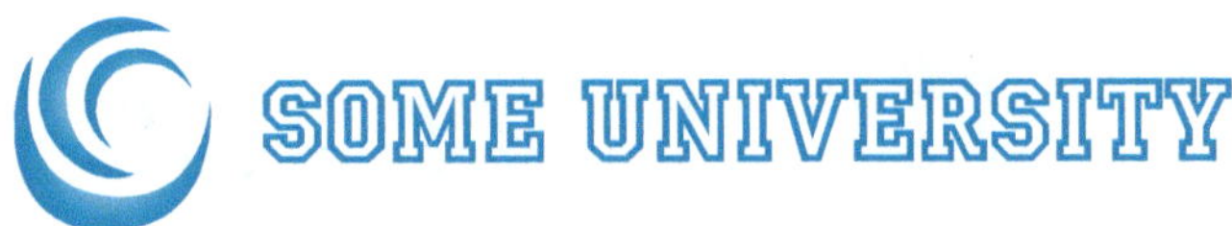


**Volunteer Agreement**

**Inquiry Title:** Use of Self-Regulation Strategies to Improve Students' Attention

**Primary Investigator:** Avett Brooks

**Concise Summary:** You are invited to participate as a volunteer in an inquiry to evaluate whether the consistent use of self-regulation strategies in the classroom can improve attention in first-grade students. This agreement provides you with information about the inquiry, your potential role, and the risks and benefits so that you can decide whether you want to volunteer.

- Your participation as a volunteer is voluntary.
- If you agree to volunteer, you will be asked to attend a training on self-regulation strategies and then implement the strategies within your classroom 3 days per week for 6 weeks.
- The risks to volunteering are no greater than those encountered daily as a teacher at South Elementary School, and no information will be collected directly from you. Your participation may improve the learning environment and the attention of students in your classroom. You may also learn some new strategies for use in the classroom.
- If you choose not to volunteer, you can proceed with your typical classroom activities without negative consequences or penalties.

**Your Tasks as a Volunteer:** You will attend a 30-minute training on self-regulation strategies. Then you will be asked to implement the strategies within your classroom every Monday, Wednesday, and Friday for 6 weeks. The primary investigator will implement the strategies on Tuesdays and Thursdays. The strategies will include short (1–2 minute) stretches, activities, and movement breaks and you can decide when to incorporate them on the 3 days. The primary investigator will assess students' attention at multiple points during the inquiry, but you will not participate in any of the assessments.

**Risks & Discomforts:** The risks to volunteering are no greater than those encountered daily as a teacher at South Elementary School. Attending the training or implementing the strategies in your classroom 3 days per week may be inconvenient. The training will be offered multiple times so you can choose a convenient one. To reduce the burden of implementing the activities, all materials will be supplied by the primary investigator and support will be provided as needed.

**Benefits:** You may learn new strategies you can use with students. Students in your class may show improved attention during seated work, and the learning environment may be improved for all students. The outcomes of the inquiry may inform future programming within the district to improve students' attention.

**Confidentiality:** If you agree to volunteer, you will be asked to sign your name to this volunteer agreement. It will be kept in the locked office of the primary investigator in a locked file cabinet. No other information will be collected from you. Neither you, the school, nor any student participants will be individually identified in any presentation or publication of the results.

Figure 12-6 Example volunteer agreement.

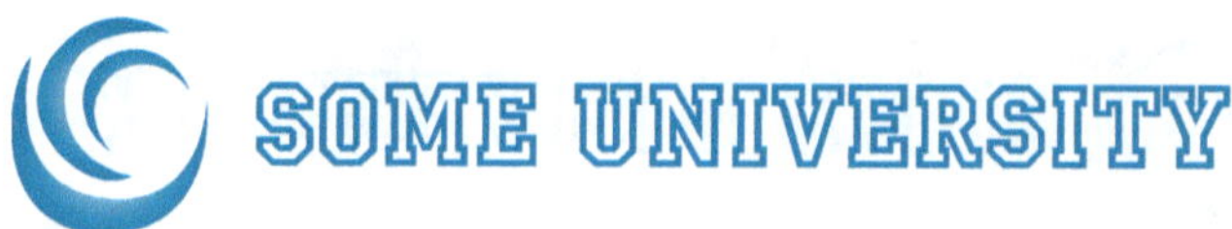


**Compensation:** There is no fee for participation, nor will you be financially compensated for volunteering. A certificate for continuing education units will be offered for your participation, and refreshments will be provided at the training. Neither Some University, the elementary school, nor any agency funding this inquiry will provide special services, free care, or compensation of injuries resulting from this inquiry. By providing consent, you understand that treatment for such injuries will be at your expense and/or paid through your medical plan.

**Contact Information:** If you have questions about the inquiry, you can contact the primary investigator at a.brooks@someuniversity.edu or 555-555-5555. If you have questions about the rights of inquiry participants, you can contact the chairperson of the Some University Institutional Review Board at IRBchair@someuniversity.edu or 444-444-4444.

**Voluntary Participation & Termination:** I understand that my participation in this inquiry is entirely voluntary, and that refusal to volunteer will involve no penalty or loss of benefits to me. I am also free to withdraw or discontinue my participation in this inquiry at any time without negative consequences or penalties. I voluntarily agree to volunteer for this inquiry. I understand I will be given a copy of this volunteer agreement.

**Volunteer's Printed Name:** ______________________________

**Volunteer's Signature & Date:** ______________________________

**Investigator's Printed Name:** ______________________________

**Investigator's Signature & Date:** ______________________________

**Faculty Advisor's Printed Name: (if applicable)** ______________________________

**Faculty Advisor's Signature & Date: (if applicable)** ______________________________

Figure 12-6 cont'd

### Inquiry Procedures

A detailed description of the inquiry procedures is required in the IRB proposal. This includes a clear and concise summary of what participants will be asked to do and the expected time commitment. Including a table, calendar, or chronological list of procedures, such as that included in Table 11-2, can make this information explicit to reviewers. Ultimately, providing a strong rationale for the inquiry, using sound methodology and ethical procedures, and highlighting your qualifications for conducting the inquiry will be necessary for approval. Some other considerations in outlining your procedures are as follows:

- Ensure that your inquiry design aligns with your inquiry purpose. See Chapters 4, 7, and 10 for information on the purpose of various quantitative, qualitative, and mixed method designs.
- Choose appropriate data collection tools and analysis methods for your inquiry's purpose. Chapters 5 and 8 provide additional guidance on appropriate data collection tools and analysis methods for quantitative and qualitative methods, respectively. Chapter 11 includes information on developing your own survey or interview questions.
- Ensure that the benefits of the inquiry outweigh the risks. You should point out all potential inconveniences, discomforts, and risks, even minor ones. Some inquiries might include the inconvenience of time devoted to the inquiry, discomfort from prolonged sitting during educational sessions or from sharing personal feelings or perspectives, or the risk of increased anxiety related to the survey content. After you have pointed out the inconveniences, discomforts, and risks, you should discuss the precautions you will take to minimize them.
- In studies with a control group, acknowledge that treatment will not be withheld. In these cases, the control group can be offered the standard treatment (instead of no treatment), the experimental group can serve as its own control, or the control group can be offered the experimental treatment after the initial phase of the study.
- Be clear about who will complete the various phases of the inquiry and their qualifications. You may be asked to provide proof of your research ethics training, resume or curriculum vitae, or a summary of your credentials related to the inquiry.
- You will also be required to provide written permission to use any data collection tools or intervention programming you did not design that is not in the public domain.
- Disclose any potential or actual conflicts of interest or personal benefits of the inquiry that might reasonably compromise your judgment. This might include affiliations of you or your immediate family.

#### TIPS & INSPIRATION

- Consider that most or all members of the IRB will not be a part of your healthcare discipline. For this reason, avoid discipline-specific jargon in the proposal. Summarizing the information in layperson's terms will decrease requests for clarity.
- Name all documents, data collection tools, processes, and inquiry personnel consistently throughout the proposal. For example, if you name the data collection tool the pretest early in the proposal, keep this same terminology throughout. Switching to the presurvey, the preassessment, or other terminology may cause the reviewer to think these are different tools. Similarly, as the submitter of the proposal, you will typically be identified as the primary investigator, or PI. Use this identifier consistently rather than switching to the project coordinator, the therapist, or another title. Inconsistencies like this can increase the review time and delay your approval.

### Modifications to Your Inquiry Procedures

If you need to modify your inquiry procedures after receiving approval from an IRB, you should contact the board immediately for directions on how to proceed. Sometimes unexpected issues arise that necessitate changes to the design, recruitment methods, inquiry site, data collection tools, or analysis methods. In most cases, you will be required to submit additional documents detailing the changes you want to make, and the board will review the revisions to ensure they still meet all ethical guidelines. While the review of modified procedures often takes less time than the original review, you cannot implement the changes before the board's confirmation. If any changes impact the informed consent signed by the participants, they must also be informed, and a new consent form should be signed.

## Confidentiality, Anonymity, and Privacy

Confidentiality, anonymity, and privacy (see Figure 12-7) must be adequately addressed when designing and conducting an inquiry, but these concepts are frequently confused.

**Confidentiality** refers to protecting private information disclosed by a participant during an inquiry, for example, through their interview or survey responses. As the investigator, you are responsible for collecting, coding, and storing the data such that a breach of confidentiality (or sharing beyond those individuals specified in the IRB proposal and consent form) is minimal. Strategies to promote confidentiality may include the following:

- Storing electronic data on a password-protected computer and encrypted server.
- Storing hard copies of data in a double-locked location (i.e., locked file cabinet within a locked office).
- If data are collected with identifiers (for example, data collected as part of an individual's medical record), de-identify the data for analysis as soon as possible. This involves assigning a benign code to the data and removing all identifiers. A benign code is a series of numbers and/or letters that cannot be connected to an individual (i.e., avoid birthday, Social Security number, medical record number).
- If you need to match assessments or surveys (for example, when you want to match pre- and post-surveys from individual participants for analysis), consider having the participants self-code these items. For the first question on the presurvey, provide an instructive prompt for participants to complete the coding. For example, "Provide a 4-digit code using your mother's birth month and year. If your mother's birthday was March 7, the code would be 0307." If you provide the same instructions on the postsurvey, they should generate the same code, enabling you to match the surveys for analysis.
- When you need to know which survey belongs to each participant, you should create a master list of codes and names. This might be necessary when you plan to follow up the survey with a detailed interview, or when dealing with a sensitive topic and need to provide participants with additional resources or referrals to support services based on their responses.
- Always store the master code list, data, and signed informed consent forms in separate locations.
- Restrict access to the data to as few people as possible. This is usually limited to those on the inquiry team who will be analyzing the data. If you are a student, your faculty advisors would typically have access to the de-identified data.

In an inquiry, **anonymity** is a condition in which data cannot be linked to a participant, even by the

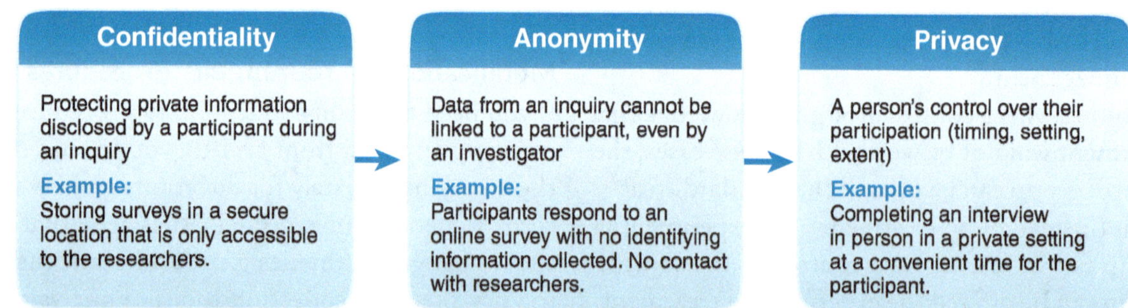


Figure 12-7 Confidentiality, anonymity, and privacy.

investigator. For inquiries that occur face to face, such as those in which an intervention is provided in person or via telehealth, participants are not anonymous because you can see them and may be able to link them to the data. In these cases, you should make every effort to keep the participants' data confidential.

The misconception is that if direct personal identifiers, such as name or Social Security number, are not collected, then the data will be anonymous. However, even with the collection of descriptive demographic data, such as gender, age range, or years in practice, you may be able to identify participants. This is especially true with small sample sizes. For example, a survey exploring perceptions of interprofessional collaboration at one nursing facility includes a demographic question regarding healthcare discipline/department, and only one administrator responds to the survey. In another example, a department of nurses is surveyed about their confidence in applying fall prevention strategies. Most nurses at the facility are female, and only two males respond to the survey. Responses to a combination of demographic questions could also allow you to link participants to their data.

A good example of anonymous data would be responses from a survey distributed to all physical therapists who belong to the *American Physical Therapy Association* on their views and activities related to specialty certification. The survey is likely to garner a decent response rate, and while it includes some demographic questions about age, gender, and primary practice setting, these are unlikely to enable identification of individual members. There is also no direct contact between the investigators and survey respondents.

Confidentiality and anonymity are mutually exclusive. In other words, your data cannot be confidential *and* anonymous within a particular inquiry activity. Anonymous data represent almost no risk to participants, whereas confidential data represent minimal risk. Minimal risk is reasonable in most healthcare inquiries, and employing multiple strategies to promote confidentiality denotes ethical research practice. In your IRB proposal, you must clearly indicate if the data will be anonymous or confidential (not both), where it will be stored, and who will have access to it.

Besides confidentiality (i.e., how you will protect the participants' private information or data), consider participants' privacy as you outline your procedures. **Privacy** is the participants' right to control access to their information or themselves. Strategies to protect participant privacy might include conducting the inquiry procedures in a private room, ensuring participants' bodies are covered to the greatest extent possible during the procedures, or allowing participants to choose the time and location of the interview.

### HIPAA and Confidentiality

Another consideration related to confidentiality is whether the research will involve **protected health information**, or PHI, which includes healthcare data linked to any of the 18 identifiers specified in the Health Insurance Portability and Accountability Act (HIPAA; DHHS, 2017). These identifiers may include name, physical or email address, important dates (birthday, admission date, etc.), phone or fax numbers, Social Security number, medical record number, health plan numbers, account numbers, license numbers, finger or voice prints, photos, or other unique identifiers. HIPAA regulations apply to any inquiry that includes at least one of the following:

- Use of PHI directly from a medical record
- Inquiry data that are also added to a medical record
- Inquiry data that are used to make healthcare decisions

The regulations clarify that for most inquiries involving PHI, participants must authorize any use or disclosure of their medical information. This authorization statement is sometimes incorporated into the informed consent document but may also be presented as a separate document.

#### TIPS & INSPIRATION

- **Provide the** IRB with any additional information **they request** in response to your original submission **and make** plans to celebrate your approval. The IRB **process** is the last step before making your inquiry a **reality**.

## CHAPTER SUMMARY

1. Define a code of ethics and its application to conducting an inquiry.
   - A code of ethics outlines the core values, principles, and standards of conduct for practitioners or students within a profession.
   - Practitioners or students show integrity in the inquiry process, including respecting the rights of participants, adhering to the inquiry design, and reporting results accurately and truthfully.
2. Outline the history of legislation related to protecting human subjects or participants.
   - Berlin Code of 1900 is the first known regulation to govern research, enacted by the Prussian Minister of Religious, Educational and Medical Affairs after evidence of unethical experiments was discovered.
   - Nuremberg Code of 1947 consists of 10 principles of ethical research, including voluntary informed consent of subjects, use of adequately trained and skilled investigators/researchers, and elimination of unnecessary risks to subjects.
   - The Declaration of Helsinki, adopted in 1964 and continually updated today, requires a research proposal to be reviewed and approved by an independent ethics committee before a study can begin or the outcomes can be disseminated.
   - National Research Act (1974) promoted high-quality research and the protection of human subjects by establishing the National Commission for the Protection of Human Subjects of Biomedical and Behavioral Research, the national group that drafted the Belmont Report.
   - Belmont Report (1979) solidified previous legislation and explicitly defined three ethical principles: respect for persons, beneficence, and justice.
   - The Federal Policy for the Protection of Human Subjects, better known as the Common Rule, issued in 1991 and revised in 2018, specifies the function of institutional review boards, informed consent requirements, research approval criteria, and additional protections for pregnant women, human fetuses, neonates, prisoners, and children.
3. Explain the function of an Institutional Review Board (IRB) and the levels of review.
   - An IRB is a group of at least five members who review research proposals to ensure the procedures meet ethical standards.
   - Factors in IRB approval include the need for the inquiry, the benefits of the inquiry, the level of risk to the participants, the quality of the research proposal, and the qualifications of the investigators.
   - There are three potential levels of IRB review—exempt, expedited, and full (or convened). Table 12-1 provides examples and the process of each level of review.
   - Exempt and expedited reviews involve no more than minimal risk and avoid sensitive topics and vulnerable populations.
   - Full reviews may entail more than minimal risk, sensitive topics, and vulnerable populations.
4. Describe the need for IRB oversight of an evidence-based practice project.
   - Evidence-based practice projects may undergo IRB review when dissemination of the outcomes, even if the individual participants or site is not identified, is planned.
5. Identify key features of a quality IRB proposal.
   - Research ethics training is required for anyone participating in an inquiry. Training needs to be completed before submitting an IRB proposal and be active throughout the completion of the inquiry.
   - A letter of site support on the institution's letterhead may be required. The letter should describe the inquiry plans and be signed by the site authority providing permission.
   - Recruitment of participants should avoid coercion and direct contact between potential participants and the investigators to the greatest extent possible. All recruitment materials, including flyers, online postings, letters, or verbal scripts, should be provided in the IRB proposal.
   - Informed consent is the agreement to participate, freely given, by an inquiry participant after investigators have fully disclosed the inquiry procedures. Table 12-2 summarizes the required content of a consent form. A waiver of consent may be appropriate in select scenarios in which the inquiry involves minimal risk and will not adversely affect the rights or welfare of participants.
   - Assent is the agreement with the inquiry procedures by someone unable to legally provide informed consent because of impaired decision-making capacity or age.
   - Volunteer agreements may be required for individuals who are assisting with an inquiry

but who are not one of the investigators and are not persons you are collecting data from. These agreements should outline the purpose of the inquiry, what the volunteer is expected to do, and the anticipated time commitment.
- Inquiry procedures should be clearly summarized using a table, calendar, or chronological list of procedures. You should ensure that the inquiry design, data collection tools, and analysis methods align with the inquiry purpose; the benefits outweigh the risks; necessary treatment is not withheld; all investigators are qualified; written permission is provided for use of any tools or materials you did not create; and conflicts of interest are declared or avoided.
- Modifications to the inquiry procedures after initial IRB approval must be reviewed by the board to confirm that the procedures still meet ethical standards. If changes impact the informed consent, participants must be informed and sign a new consent.

6. Differentiate confidentiality, anonymity, and privacy.
   - Confidentiality is protecting private information disclosed by a participant during an inquiry, whereas anonymity is a condition in which data cannot be linked to a participant, even by the investigator. Your data within an inquiry activity cannot be confidential *and* anonymous.
   - Anonymous data represent almost no risk to participants, while confidential data represent minimal risk.
   - Strategies to promote confidentiality should incorporate secure data storage, coding and de-identifying the data when possible, and limiting who has access to the data.
   - Privacy is the participants' right to control access to their information or themselves. Strategies to protect participant privacy might include conducting the inquiry procedures in a private room, ensuring participants' bodies are covered to the greatest extent possible during the procedures, or allowing participants to choose the time and location of the interview.
   - For most inquiries involving protected health information (PHI), participants must sign an HIPAA authorization for use and disclosure of their medical information in the inquiry.

## TEST YOUR KNOWLEDGE

1. A code of ethics governs clinical and research practice. True or false?
2. Which of the following requires an independent ethics committee to approve research proposals?
   a. Nuremberg Code of 1947
   b. Declaration of Helsinki
   c. National Research Act
   d. Berlin Code of 1900
3. Which legislation specified additional protections for pregnant persons, prisoners, and children?
   a. The Belmont Report
   b. National Research Act
   c. The Nuremberg Code of 1947
   d. The Common Rule
4. Which of the following inquiries would likely undergo a full IRB review?
   a. A focus group with teachers about their preferred instructional methods
   b. A study involving the use of fitness tracking with healthy adults
   c. An anonymous survey of athletic trainers on their work-life balance
   d. A study on the effectiveness of a social-emotional learning program for children with autism
5. Which of the following is a required component of an IRB proposal?
   a. A letter of site support from your advisor
   b. A copy of your recruitment materials
   c. A copy of the research articles that support your inquiry
   d. Written permission to use a data collection tool you created
6. Which of the following is TRUE of an informed consent document?
   a. It must be completed by anyone participating in the inquiry.
   b. It must appear on the letterhead of the inquiry site.
   c. It must explain the inquiry procedures in layperson's terms.
   d. It must be completed in paper form.
7. Which participant would likely be asked to provide assent for an inquiry?
   a. A cognitively intact adult
   b. An 8-year-old child
   c. A 2-year-old child
   d. A child's legal guardian

8. Identify the term (anonymity, confidentiality, privacy) that aligns with each definition.
   a. The protection of private information disclosed by a participant during an inquiry
   b. A participant's right to control access to their information or themselves
   c. A condition in which the data cannot be linked to an inquiry participant

Answer key appears at the end of this text.

## NEXT STEPS

1. Locate the ethical standards or code of ethics for your discipline and review it for any standards that apply directly to conducting an inquiry.
2. Design one tool for recruitment for an inquiry. This could be a flyer, an online post, a letter, or a verbal script. Use the information on readability formulas in Chapter 14 to assess your recruitment tool. Recall that the target is between a sixth- to eighth-grade level or lower, depending on your targeted participants. How does your document measure up? Do you need to make further revisions?
3. Use Table 12-2 to draft an informed consent for your potential participants. Share it with at least one person who is similar to your inquiry participants for feedback. What did you learn? What might you need to revise? You may also consider assessing the readability of your informed consent.
4. If you are conducting an inquiry, identify the IRB that you will submit to. Obtain the required form or template and use the information provided in this chapter to create a working draft of your IRB proposal.

## REFERENCES


American Nurses Association. (2015). *Code of ethics for nurses with interpretative statements.* Author. https://www.nursingworld.org/practice-policy/nursing-excellence/ethics/code-of-ethics-for-nurses

American Occupational Therapy Association. (2020). AOTA 2020 occupational therapy code of ethics. *American Journal of Occupational Therapy, 74*(Suppl. 3), 7413410005p1-7413410005p13. https://doi.org/10.5014/ajot.2020.74S3006

American Physical Therapy Association. (2020). *Code of ethics for the physical therapist.* Author. https://www.apta.org/siteassets/pdfs/policies/codeofethicshods06-20-28-25.pdf

CITI Program. (n.d.). *Get to know CITI Program.* https://about.citiprogram.org/get-to-know-citi-program

Duff-Brown, B. (2017, January 6). *The shameful legacy of Tuskegee syphilis study still impacts African-American men today.* Stanford Health Policy. https://healthpolicy.fsi.stanford.edu/news/researchers-and-students-run-pilot-project-oakland-test-whether-tuskegee-syphilis-trial-last

Ghooi, R. B. (2011). The Nuremberg Code—A critique. *Perspectives in Clinical Research, 2*(2), 72–76. https://doi.org/10.4103/2229-3485.80371

Hadden, K. B., Prince, L. Y., Moore, T. D., James, L. P., Holland, J. R., & Trudeau, C. R. (2017). Improving readability of informed consents for research at an academic medical institution. *Journal of Clinical and Translational Science, 1*(6), 361–365. https://doi.org/10.1017/cts.2017.312

National Athletic Training Association. (2018). *NATA code of ethics.* Author. https://www.nata.org/sites/default/files/nata-code-of-ethics.pdf

National Commission for the Protection of Human Subjects of Biomedical and Behavioral Research. (1979). *The Belmont Report.* Department of Health, Education, and Welfare. https://www.hhs.gov/ohrp/sites/default/files/the-belmont-report-508c_FINAL.pdf

U.S. Department of Health and Human Services. [HHS]. (2015). *The Nuremberg Code.* https://www.hhs.gov/ohrp/regulations-and-policy/archived-materials/index.html

U.S. Department of Health and Human Services. [DHHS]. (2017). *Health information privacy: Research.* https://www.hhs.gov/hipaa/for-professionals/special-topics/research/index.html

U.S. Department of Health and Human Services. [DHHS]. (2019). *Office for human research protections: 2018 Requirements (2018 Common Rule).* https://www.hhs.gov/ohrp/regulations-and-policy/regulations/45-cfr-46/revised-common-rule-regulatory-text/index.html

U.S. Department of Health and Human Services. [DHHS]. (2022). *Office for human research protections: The Belmont Report.* https://www.hhs.gov/ohrp/regulations-and-policy/belmont-report/index.html

Vollmann, J., & Winau, R. (1996). The Prussian Regulation of 1900: Early ethical standards for human experimentation in Germany. *IRB: Ethics & Human Research, 18*(4), 9–11. https://doi.org/10.2307/3564006

Weindling, P., von Villiez, A., Loewenau, A., & Farron, N. (2016). The victims of unethical human experiments and coerced research under national socialism. *Endeavour, 40*(1), 1–6. https://doi.org/10.1016/j.endeavour.2015.10.005

World Medical Association. (2023). *WMA Declaration of Helsinki—Ethical principles for medical research involving human subjects.* https://www.wma.net/policies-post/wma-declaration-of-helsinki-ethical-principles-for-medical-research-involving-human-subjects

## Chapter 13

# Funding Your Inquiry

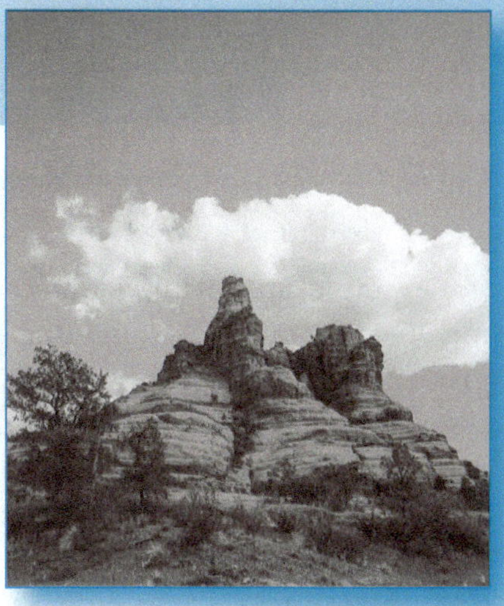

LEARNING OUTCOMES

*The information provided in this chapter will assist you to:*

13.1 Describe the steps of program development.
13.2 Differentiate types of grants.
13.3 Identify potential grant sources.
13.4 Explain how to choose an appropriate grant.
13.5 Recall the primary components of a grant proposal.
13.6 Explore tips for successful grant writing and the potential impact of grant funding.

## Program Development

**Program development** is the process of planning, implementing, and evaluating a new program, service, or practice protocol or improving or expanding an existing one. Many evidence-based practice projects take the form of program development. In designing a program, the aim is to create a plan to benefit larger groups or entire populations rather than individual clients. Developing and implementing new programs often require financial resources. One method of funding programs is through grants, which is discussed later in this chapter. The four steps of program development are illustrated in Figure 13-1 (Braveman, 2001; Grossman & Bortone, 1986).

Let us consider an example of program development as we discuss each step. A skilled nursing facility recently implemented a specialized cardiac program aimed at helping clients with congestive heart failure effectively manage their condition and avoid rehospitalization. This quality improvement program is currently limited to actions nurses and physicians take, such as ordering dietary restrictions or medication changes for clients in the program. However, the administrator has asked the rehabilitation department to be involved. The therapists routinely implement cardiac precautions (i.e., limited use of weights, no reaching overhead during therapeutic activities), monitor blood pressure and oxygen saturation, and educate these clients on energy conservation techniques, but no formal cardiac rehabilitation protocol exists. The needs assessment is the first step of the process.

### Needs Assessment

A **needs assessment** is a systematic process to identify existing supports, challenges, and the *need* for improvement within an organization, setting, or group to guide future decision-making. While you likely have already identified a general area of focus

Bell Rock, Sedona, Arizona.

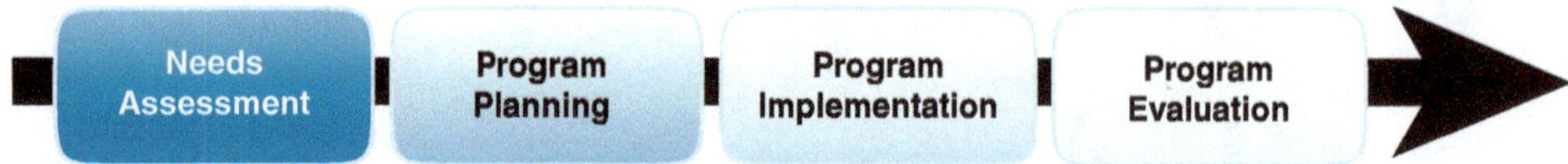


Figure 13-1 Steps of program development.

(for example, improving wound care), a needs assessment helps you understand and prioritize existing problems and can justify the need for additional resources and funding for program development. A needs assessment could incorporate existing data, such as facility reports or satisfaction surveys, but may also include data collected specifically for the needs assessment. Depending on the topic, collecting data from various stakeholders, such as clients, caregivers, or facility staff, might also be necessary. Chapter 2 provides additional information on the needs assessment.

The need for a program may arise out of a quality improvement initiative, as in the example in Box 13-1. Some clients with congestive heart failure were frequently readmitted to the hospital and voiced dissatisfaction with their care at the nursing facility. These events prompted the development of an interdisciplinary cardiac program. Regulatory changes or citations on an agency, state, or national survey may also substantiate a need. For example, a facility that received a citation for failure to prevent or heal pressure ulcers would be required to submit a plan of correction to the surveying body. This plan may include revision of the existing protocol for wound care with additional involvement of all members of the interdisciplinary team to manage diets (dietary), medication (physicians), positioning in and out of bed (therapists, nurse aides), and dressing changes (nurses). The needs assessment format may vary but includes four basic steps.

1. **Plan:** This step involves identifying existing data on the topic, the key stakeholders (who might serve as sources of additional information), and the existing resources for conducting the needs assessment (i.e., how much time, money, or personnel you have).
2. **Develop:** This step entails developing the specific questions and data collection methods to gather needed information. The question format may vary—for example, multiple-choice or open-ended questions. Questions should be purposeful, culturally sensitive, and of the appropriate health literacy level to be easily understood by the targeted individuals. Data collection methods can include surveys, interviews, or focus groups.
3. **Conduct:** Data collection may incorporate multiple data collection methods and involve stakeholders at various levels. In the prior example of the cardiac program, a survey could be deployed to recently discharged clients with congestive heart failure, and a focus group could be conducted with the therapists who routinely treat those clients. The questions would be tailored to each group; gathering multiple perspectives ensures the new program addresses clients' concerns and aligns with therapists' skills and experiences. The SWOT analysis (identifying strengths, weaknesses, opportunities, and threats), discussed in Chapter 2, could also be incorporated during this step.
4. **Analyze:** This step requires synthesizing and sharing the data so that the information can be used to prioritize future actions. What do most stakeholders think? Are there any unique views that do not align with the majority? How is this information helpful? What are the potential next steps, and how can the data be used to identify the highest priorities?

### TIPS & INSPIRATION

- In the planning phase of the needs assessment, do not be afraid to engage colleagues and other key stakeholders in casual conversations. These initial brainstorming sessions can be beneficial in honing your ideas before formal data gathering of the needs assessment begins.

- Collect data from multiple sources or groups of people to ensure your needs assessment is thorough and garners an accurate picture of the situation or setting.
- Use multiple data collection methods in your needs assessment. Your options include surveys, interviews, focus groups, or previously gathered data available through institutional reports or records. Consider the pros and cons of surveys, interviews, and focus groups discussed in Chapters 5 and 8 of this text to help you decide.
- The needs assessment should help you identify and prioritize programming needs. The needs should be considered in tandem with the available resources of the setting. A gap between needs and available resources is where grant funding may be helpful.

**BOX 13-1 ■ Example of a Needs Assessment**

The rehabilitation director conducts a preliminary literature search through the American Physical Therapy Association's website (because she is a member) and Google Scholar using a combination of the following search terms: "cardiac rehabilitation," "cardiac protocols," "congestive heart failure," and "rehab protocols." This search uncovers a plethora of information on client education, evaluation and treatment protocols, assessments, and exercise and ambulation programs. The director realizes the team could be doing more for this client group and solicits the help of three other therapists. The therapists develop specific questions to gather current and past clients' perspectives about the therapy services received. Based on the available resources and client needs, some questions are included in a survey provided to all clients with congestive heart failure. A focus group with a subset of clients is also completed to gather more in-depth information. The clients' lived experiences will be used to inform future cardiac programming.

## Program Planning

**Program planning** is a series of tasks to design a quality program and secure funding for that program when necessary. Funding is covered later in this chapter. Box 13-2 provides an example of program planning. Critical program planning tasks are as follows:

- **Prioritizing needs from the needs assessment:** Often, there are multiple needs, and it may not be feasible to address all of them in one program.
- **Identifying supporting literature and a theoretical base to guide the program:** Prior research that supports the new program is often critical in obtaining approval and securing funding to implement the program. The theoretical base can include existing concepts and theories to guide the program's development and implementation.
- **Setting measurable program goals:** These goals should clearly outline targeted outcomes of the program that are measurable. Goals help keep the program focused and provide a mechanism for documenting outcomes.
- **Defining programmatic roles and timelines:** Multiple individuals in varying positions may be necessary to implement a program successfully. The setting, funders, or other program logistics may dictate implementation timelines.
- **Designing the program, including specific recruitment, marketing, and budgeting plans:** Each program step and the responsible individuals are outlined. Effective, sustainable programming also includes detailed plans for who is eligible to participate, how they are recruited, how the program is promoted, and what financial resources are required. The program design should integrate the best research on the topic and the needs, values, and experiences of the targeted individuals.
- **Developing an evaluation plan:** Programs should have an ongoing evaluation plan to monitor progress toward program goals. Incremental monitoring of progress may support modifications to the program plan to ensure the ability to meet program goals.
- **Obtaining approval and funding for program implementation:** Before program implementation, approval may be required from administration, supervisors, regulatory bodies, or other institutions. Additional funding may also be required to cover the cost of personnel, training, equipment, or resources. The most common funding source is grants, discussed later in this chapter.

### BOX 13-2 ■ Example of Program Planning

During program planning, each therapist conducts a detailed search on a specific area of cardiac rehabilitation. The rehabilitation director searches the literature for evaluation and assessment procedures, and the other therapists delve into patient education, exercise and ambulation programs, and patient activities. They agree to look at literature limited to the last 5 years since the goal is to create a rehabilitation protocol for clients based upon the most current evidence. When the therapists meet again, they appraise the literature to determine whether the information is of sound quality and relevant to their clients. The group uses a concise template like those in Table 6-1, Table 9-2, and Table 10-2 to assess the quality and applicability of the studies. Those studies that are deemed to be the best evidence are retained for incorporation into the new program. Locating multiple articles that support a particular assessment or protocol will add strength to the findings and the subsequent program.

Next, the group uses the best available evidence, their skills and experiences, and the perceived values and circumstances of clients typically encountered in their setting (recall this is evidence-based practice!) to create a rehabilitation protocol for clients with chronic congestive heart failure. The information is organized into a resource binder with tabs for therapist procedures, patient handouts, and exercise and ambulation protocols. Information for therapists includes how and when to monitor blood pressure, oxygen saturation, and perceived client exertion during evaluation and treatment. Protocols for exercise and ambulation are also included to guide therapists' decision-making. Patient education includes information on the use of adaptive equipment, energy conservation and work simplification techniques, stress management, and precautions. The administrator and medical director approve the new program, funding is secured for additional equipment and resources, and all rehab staff are educated on the program before its formal implementation.

### Program Implementation

Once a detailed program plan is established, approval is granted, and funding is secured, program implementation can begin. This phase typically involves collaboration between all individuals with programmatic roles. Frequent communication ensures the program activities are on track and progress is being made toward the program goals. See Box 13-3 for an example of program implementation.

### Program Evaluation

**Program evaluation** is a continuous process throughout a program to determine if program goals are being achieved. While program evaluation is included as the last step in program development, it usually occurs simultaneously with program implementation. Program evaluation involves measuring the projected program outcomes to determine the program's success. This might include tracking the incidence of events, such as the number of referrals to a wound specialist, falls within a specified period, or the average length of stay. Program evaluation may also include using surveys, interviews, or focus groups to collect data on the phenomena of interest. Many programs are designed to be sustainable without a defined endpoint where progress would be evaluated. Similarly, delayed evaluation limits your ability to revise the program to maximize effectiveness. Program evaluation is also a requirement for most grant funding. Box 13-4 provides an example of program evaluation.

### BOX 13-3 ■ Example of Program Implementation

The new cardiac rehabilitation program is formally implemented. This unique program serves two purposes. First, it provides the therapists with an evidence-based program that can be easily implemented. The information and protocols are clearly outlined and supported by sound research. Second, it demonstrates the facility's commitment to providing quality client care for this population, which may aid in marketing efforts and service reimbursement.

> **BOX 13-4 ■ Example of Program Evaluation**
>
> After the new program has been implemented for several months, it is evaluated by looking at hospital readmission rates, conducting a focus group with therapists on their experiences implementing the program, and surveying clients to determine their satisfaction. Modifications are made as necessary based on these evaluations.

## What Are Grants?

**Grants** are funds commonly provided by charitable foundations, federal agencies, businesses, individuals, or other entities for a distinct purpose. Entities offering grants have the right to specify their grant's purpose and requirements. They may also identify what the money can be used for and what are excluded expenses. For example, some grants may only cover personnel training, whereas others could also be used for supplies. Similarly, some grants may be reserved for research activities, but others may fund quality improvement programming. To receive a grant, you must submit a carefully drafted application or proposal that meets the requirements and be selected from the pool of proposals submitted. Once a grant is received, the funding agency typically requires documentation of grant activities and outcomes. In other words, they want to ensure you have held true to your word and are using the money for its intended purpose. Grants can range from relatively small amounts (for example, $100) to substantial amounts (for example, $1 million or more). Some grants may include a one-time disbursement, whereas others may provide funding over several years. Grants are an excellent funding source for innovative new programs, but you should also consider the program's sustainability once the grant period is over because grant funding is not indefinite. The grant funding process is depicted in Figure 13-2.

## Types of Grants

Grants can be categorized as internal or external. **Internal grants** include funding available *within* an organization that benefits the organization or its members. Examples include an internal grant for quality improvement within a hospital system or funds offered by a local town council for developing new recreational programs for youth in their community. While these grants are generally smaller, they may be more attainable, especially if you are new to grant writing.

**External grants** include funding offered by outside organizations that seek to support individuals, groups, or other institutions with similar missions to their own. Examples of organizations that may offer grant funding are foundations, professional organizations, corporations, or the government. A foundation is a nonprofit "entity that supports charitable activities by making grants to unrelated organizations or institutions or to individuals for scientific, educational, cultural, religious, or other charitable purposes" (Council on Foundations, 2023, *What is a foundation?*). Some well-known examples include the American Heart Association and the Michael J. Fox Foundation. Some professional organizations may provide grant funding to support members' interests and activities. For example, the Foundation for Physical Therapy Research is exclusively dedicated to funding research by physical therapists. Corporations that offer grants may include public or private companies. For example, a tech company may offer science and technology grants, or a home improvement company could provide grants for disaster relief or accessibility projects. Finally, grants are often available through the federal government. For example, a federal grant might support research on COVID-19 or programming to address youth mental health. Grants from external sources are frequently larger in dollar amounts but may require greater time, resources, and skills.

Most grants are awarded to an institution, organization, or a team of people. However, you may find some modest ones, mainly those offered internally, awarded to individuals for small-scale projects or research. Another exception is a fellowship. In healthcare, **fellowships** are training programs for individuals to further develop their clinical skills, research skills, or both. Fellowships are often merit based and may include access to benefits, a

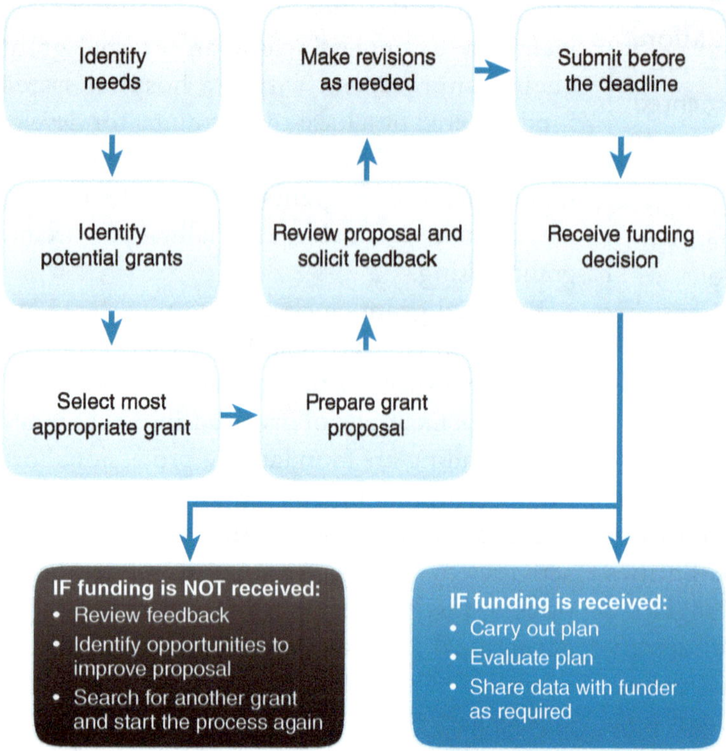


Figure 13-2 Grant funding process.

stipend, and subsidized housing for the duration of the fellowship. Fellowships usually range from several months up to 2 years. For example, the Mayo Foundation for Medical Education and Research (2023) offers fellowships in hand therapy, dysphagia, and neurorehabilitation for occupational therapists. Their website allows you to search for fellowships in your practice area and to learn about the admission requirements and application process.

## Where to Find Grants

The first challenge in grant writing is to locate a grant suitable to your purpose. Table 13-1 includes potential grant sources to begin your search.

## Choosing a Grant

Most grants will include a **Request for Proposal** (RFP), a document describing the funding opportunity, including the purpose, submission guidelines, and the application deadline. This document may also be referred to as a request for application (RFA), notice of funding opportunity (NOFO), or a notice of funding availability (NOFA). You must review this information carefully to determine if your program idea or research aligns with the funder's criteria and aims. An RFP can vary from just one or two pages to more than 50 pages, so it is essential to allow

### TIPS & INSPIRATION

- If you are new to grant writing, consider opportunities in your local community or facility. Contact your facility administration, local religious organizations, town council, community center, rotary club, YMCA, sports clubs, neighborhood associations, schools, or parent-teacher organizations. Many of these entities offer small programming or research grants that align with their missions. Making personal connections can be valuable in getting your ideas funded.
- Sign up for a listserv to receive notifications of new funding opportunities. A listserv is a way for a site (or funder, in this case) to send mass emails to many people simultaneously. Several sites that post funding opportunities have free listservs that you can sign up for by going to their website and submitting your name and email address.

**TABLE 13-1 ■ Potential Grant Sources**

| Source | Information |
|---|---|
| Government database | ■ https://www.grants.gov<br>■ You can sign up to be notified of new grant funding opportunities through their site. |
| Candid database | ■ https://candid.org/?fcref=lr<br>■ Allows you to search for foundation grants. Also allows foundations to search for nonprofits to fund. |
| Corporations | ■ Many corporations offer cause-specific grants, particularly for nonprofit organizations. A couple of examples are provided to get you started.<br>■ https://www.google.org/opportunities<br>They fund innovative programs that address specific problems within communities. You can search their site to see what impact challenges they are currently looking to fund.<br>■ https://corporate.homedepot.com/page/home-depot-foundation<br>They fund community disaster relief efforts, housing for veterans, and training of trade workers. |
| Grantwatch.com | ■ https://www.grantwatch.com<br>■ This is a subscription-based database for searching for various grants, including federal, foundation, nonprofit, small business, and individual grants. |
| Professional organizations or associations | ■ The websites for your professional association or organization may help you locate grants specific to your healthcare discipline. |
| Organizations associated with your target population or community | ■ Consider the target population of your research or program. For example, if your work will benefit clients with dementia or their caregivers, you might search the Alzheimer's Association for possible grant funding.<br>■ If your work targets a specific institution or community, you might explore organizations within the institution or community, for example, the city council, a Rotary Club, or a religious organization. |
| Organizations that funded similar work | ■ Find out if funding was previously secured for similar programs or research. If so, these same organizations may have additional funds for novel projects that build on prior work. |
| Institutional grant office | ■ Some organizations, particularly academic ones, may have an internal grants office. You can share your funding needs, and they may support locating and applying for a grant. |
| Networking | ■ Connect with others interested in your topic, those who might benefit from your work, others who have previously received funding, or individuals responsible for financial decisions within the facility, community, or organization you hope to impact.<br>■ They might be aware of funding opportunities or be able to help you advocate for your needs. |

sufficient time to review this document before applying for the grant. Following are some questions to help you assess the fit of a grant with your program or research ideas. If you answer no to any of these questions, you should consider a different funding opportunity since the grant may not be a good match for your ideas. Table 13-2 also includes some terms and acronyms commonly found in an RFP.

**TABLE 13-2 ■ Common Terms and Acronyms in Grant Writing**

| Term or Acronym | Information |
|---|---|
| **RFP or RFA** | Request for Proposal and Request for Application are documents that describe grant opportunities. |
| **NOFO or NOFA** | Notice of Funding Opportunity and Notice of Funding Availability are other terms for the document that describes the grant opportunity. |
| **Grantor** | The organization providing the grant. |
| **Grantee** | The person, group, or organization applying for/receiving the grant. |
| **PI** | The Primary or Principal Investigator is responsible for directing and coordinating the grant project or research if the grant is received. They are part of the grantee group and are named on the grant application. |
| **Co-investigators** | Other members of the grantee group listed on the grant proposal are responsible for carrying out various activities associated with the program or research if the grant is received. |
| **MOU** | A **Memorandum of Understanding**, while not legally binding, is a written agreement between two parties to collaborate on a grant. For example, perhaps you intend to collaborate with a community organization if grant funding is secured. The MOU submitted with your grant application shows that you have consulted with the community organization, and they are willing to engage in this work with you or your organization. |
| **NoA** | Notice of Award is a document that informs grant recipients that they were selected to receive the grant. This document typically describes the terms and conditions of the funding and any required documentation to support spending. |

1. **Is your program, research, or organization eligible for the grant?** The RFP includes specific eligibility criteria that must be met to be considered. You should explore this first. If you are not eligible, you can avoid spending any more time reviewing the RFP.
2. **Does the funder's purpose align with the aims of your proposed project, program, or research?** Review the RFP carefully to determine if the funder's purpose matches your ideas. A good match can significantly increase your chance of getting funded. You can also scope out the funder's website. Learning about their mission, vision, priorities, and previously funded projects can help you make an informed decision.
3. **Do the parameters of the grant align with your program or project ideas?** Grants usually have specific start and end dates, funding amounts, and spending requirements. Be sure these will work for your program or research ideas. Some grants require matching funds. This means that if you or your organization receive funding, you must match a certain percentage of the award or cover some overhead costs not included in the grant itself. Matching can be accomplished through your organization's budget or donations, but you should ensure you can secure these funds before applying for the grant.
4. **Can you reasonably meet the submission deadline?** Be sure to consider the time required to draft the proposal and the time to secure any additional approvals required from your organization, such as letters of support from key stakeholders.

## Applying for a Grant

You can begin the formal grant writing process after locating a grant that best aligns with your program, project, or research ideas. This process frequently includes a team collaborating to write the proposal and implement the plan if funding is secured. Information commonly contained in a grant proposal is discussed next, but you should always align your proposal with the specific guidelines for your target grant. Without careful attention to the specific details, your proposal could be rejected based on failure to meet the submission guidelines, regardless of the merit of your ideas.

## TIPS & INSPIRATION

- Funders sometimes offer specific training on applying for their grants. If so, this information is usually provided on their website or in the RFP. Taking advantage of the training can improve your grant writing skills, offer the opportunity to ask questions, and allow you to establish connections with individuals at the funding agency.

### Components of a Grant Proposal

Most grant proposals include three primary components—the abstract or summary, the detailed proposal plan, and the budget, summarized in Table 13-3. While the abstract or summary is the first part of the proposal, it is typically written last after the entire grant proposal is finalized. The summary is the first thing funders will read, so it should succinctly summarize the proposal, emphasizing the need for the project, its aims and benefits, and alignment with the grant purpose.

Most of the grant writing time is usually spent crafting the detailed plan. This information is conveyed through narratives and using data to support the need for the project. The organizational background should include relevant details about your site or organization, key individuals involved in the proposed project and their credentials (i.e., the PI and co-investigators), and any experience in the project area. The needs assessment, discussed earlier in this chapter and in Chapter 2, should incorporate data that illustrate the need for the project, who will benefit from it, and how these aspects align with the potential funding source. The RFP may require that specific data be submitted in a particular format so proposals can be compared objectively. You should also consider gathering data from key stakeholders or the community or organization where the project will take place to substantiate the need for the project further.

Next, the plan should outline the goals and steps of project implementation, including who is responsible for each step and the timeline for completion. This should encompass strategies to evaluate project success and the plan for sustaining project outcomes after funding ceases. Funders want to ensure their money is well spent on projects with high chances of success and those that will be maintained long-term. If you have completed similar projects, sharing these outcomes can support the feasibility of your current proposal (Guyer et al., 2021). The detailed plan may include various appendices such as letters of support, memorandums of understanding, resumes and credentials of project personnel, and a reference list of supportive literature. The best practice in grant writing is to submit only relevant materials and those specifically required by the funder; submitting extraneous information or documents could result in immediate rejection.

**TABLE 13-3 ■ Components of a Grant Proposal**

| Summary | Detailed Plan | Budget |
|---|---|---|
| ■ Provides an overview of the proposal<br>■ Highlights need for the project, aims, and benefits<br>■ Asserts commitment to grant purpose | ■ Organizational background<br>■ Needs assessment<br>■ Project goals<br>■ Specific project methods<br>■ How challenges will be addressed<br>■ Project evaluation plan<br>■ Sustainability plan | ■ Detailed breakdown of anticipated costs that funding would cover<br>■ Description of how costs were determined<br>■ Outlines funding provided by your organization |

(Doll, 2010; Karsh & Fox, 2019)

The final component of a grant proposal is the detailed budget. The budget should contain costs associated with supplies and equipment, such as office supplies, program-specific equipment, refreshments, travel expenses, testing supplies, and other resources. Costs may also include funds for staffing. For example, the project may require a dedicated administrative assistant to track spending, order supplies, and manage other grant activities for the duration of the grant. The costs mentioned up to this point are considered **direct costs**—meaning that they are directly associated with completing the project. **Indirect costs** are those not directly tied to the grant, such as costs for utilities in the building, human resources, and library and custodial services, to name a few examples (Karsh & Fox, 2019). The budget should be comprehensive and include all anticipated costs, even if they are small. You might have to consult with other individuals to realistically estimate some of the costs. Additionally, most RFPs specify what the grant funding can be used for. For example, some funders may only support training, education, and costs associated with personnel. If your project requires the purchase of supplies, you must determine whether those costs can be funded through an alternative outlet. Be sure to indicate funding from other sources and explain how you estimated the anticipated costs.

### TIPS & INSPIRATION

- **In your abstract,** clearly articulate why the plan is needed and how it aligns with the funder's aims. Mirror the language of the funder's priorities as you explain your plan. Describe the feasibility of the plan and the expected outcomes or impact. These elements are the primary attention grabbers that will get the reviewers interested in your proposal.
- **Limit the project goals** to no more than three unless the funder specifically asks for more. Keeping your grant proposal sufficiently focused can increase your chance of getting funded.
- **When describing your program or project methods,** address how you will navigate challenges or unexpected obstacles. Rarely does a plan go exactly as planned (and that is okay!). Ensure you have contemplated potential issues and solutions and included these in your proposal (Karsh & Fox, 2019).
- **Enlist help** in constructing your budget. Even the most experienced grant writers may seek assistance to ensure their budget is accurate and realistic. This process often takes some digging to determine accurate cost estimates for supplies, equipment, and salaries, and funders may quickly identify if you have taken shortcuts (Karsh & Fox, 2019).
- **Brevity is a skill.** Aim to be clear and concise in your grant proposal regardless of page or word limits. When you write too much, your message may be lost.

### Partnerships in Grant Writing

While you might be exploring grant writing individually as part of your professional development or academic coursework, most grant writing and subsequent programming or research occurs in teams. This may include a team within one organization—for example, individuals from several healthcare disciplines within a facility collaborating to submit a grant proposal to support an interdisciplinary training program. This could also include partnerships with other organizations or institutions with similar goals and interests. For example, faculty and students from one academic institution could collaborate with several community organizations to submit a grant proposal to support preventive healthcare screenings and activities for individuals in their rural communities. In this scenario, the advantages of partnering with others include sharing resources, impacting a broader audience, and establishing a team with more diverse expertise. Individuals from the academic institution may have more knowledge of current healthcare practices. However, individuals from the community organizations likely have more experience with the targeted beneficiaries of the program, which could help determine where, when, and how the activities will be provided. Each of these advantages could increase your chances of securing funding.

### Grant Writing Tips

Grant writing can take significant time and effort, especially if you are new to the process. Nevertheless, there are several things you can do to hone your skills and improve your chances of securing funding. If you plan to write a grant that supports or builds upon your research study or evidence-based practice project, you already have a good start. You have previously described the problem and gathered literature that justifies your inquiry. If you have completed your inquiry, you have preliminary data that may support the feasibility of continuing or expanding the work. Much of this prior work aligns with the information you must provide in a grant proposal. Here are some other tips:

1. Allow sufficient time to locate a suitable grant and construct the grant proposal. As outlined previously, the process requires gathering data from multiple sources and collaborating with others. Allow at least 50% more time than you think you will need (Boyle, 2020). Create a schedule for meetings, collaborative tasks, and grant writing to keep you on track.
2. Carefully review the guidelines for your target grant with particular attention to formatting and page and word limits. Failure to follow the guidelines is one of the top reasons for grant proposal rejection (GrantNews, 2023).
3. Take time to investigate the funding organization. What is their mission? What kind of projects have they funded previously? This is similar to preparing for a job interview. If you do your homework, you can use the information to draft a proposal that aligns with the funders' priorities.
4. Draft your proposal in language that the reviewers will easily understand. Since reviewers may not have your professional background and expertise, you should avoid professional jargon, acronyms, and abbreviations. Grant proposals are typically written in first or third person; the funder may provide guidelines, or the decision may be yours. Foundations offering smaller grants may respond well to a more casual approach, whereas government grants typically require a more formal style. You can also review and incorporate the suggestions provided in Chapter 14 on becoming a better writer.
5. Ensure your program or research is novel and innovative, as these elements often account for a large percentage of grant-scoring criteria (Doll, 2010; Guyer et al., 2021). Your proposal should be unique and avoid replicating what has already been done. Innovation might include approaching a problem in a new way, combining methods previously shown to be effective in isolation, or exploring completely new methods or ideas. For these innovations, your preliminary inquiry data can support the feasibility of your plan.
6. Avoid overly complex plans or multiple diverse project aims. Having too many aims may require additional funding or more time than the grant allotted. This is a common mistake among new grant proposal writers (Guyer et al., 2021).
7. Find a mentor with experience in grant writing who can provide support and offer feedback (Boyle, 2020). Even experienced grant writers can benefit from mentorship, which can support professional development and funding success.
8. Contact the grant director with questions about the grant requirements or submission process. The grant director is an individual named in the RFP responsible for accepting and processing grant submissions. In most cases, they are open to answering questions ahead of time, saving you time and ensuring your understanding of the funder's aims (Doll, 2010).
9. Establish an organizational system at the beginning of the grant writing process. Consider team collaboration tools and software to draft and store the required documentation to avoid multiple versions of the same document and to ensure all team members have access to the required documents when necessary.
10. Persevere. Approximately 1 in 10 grant proposals are accepted (Professional Grant Writers, 2021, para. 1). Of course, your chances of funding are linked to several factors, including how many submissions are received for the grant, the quality of your proposal, and how well it aligns with the grant opportunity. Submitting more grant proposals may also increase your chances of success (Guyer et al., 2021). The moral of the story is: Do not give up. It is often a matter of finding the right funding opportunity for your ideas.

## Impact of Grant Funding

Now that you have some foundational knowledge about types of grants, where to find them, and the proposal content and process, let us consider their significant role in shaping and influencing healthcare. Grants can fund research that advances evaluation and treatment practices or evidence-based practice initiatives to promote knowledge translation. They can also support the education and training of the healthcare workforce, including current practitioners and students, to enhance the quality of care. Similarly, our healthcare infrastructure and public health programming may be enhanced through grant funding. Many grants address access to healthcare services in underserved communities, health disparities among diverse groups, or global health challenges. Without grant funding, many existing healthcare programs, practices, and research would not be possible. Small internal grants within a community or organization and larger external grants are equally important in bringing innovative programming and research to fruition.

The information in this chapter should inspire you to explore program development and grant funding for your program or research ideas. While grant writing is an advanced skill requiring patience, practice, and collaboration to hone, the impact can be well worth the effort. If you plan to engage in grant writing, collaboration with an experienced grant writer and further exploration of the grant writing process is recommended. More detailed information is beyond the scope of this text, but there are entire books on grant writing that you can consult if additional information is needed. Several options are included at the end of this chapter.

### TIPS & INSPIRATION

- **Identify** a content expert and someone skilled in grant **writing** to review your submission and provide feedback. **Allow** sufficient time to incorporate the feedback before the deadline.
- **If you are applying for a grant,** plan to submit at least **1 to 2 days** before the deadline in case you encounter technical difficulties.
- **Ensure you** provide accurate contact information on **the grant** proposal so that you receive the funders' **decision** promptly. If you receive the funding, you **may be** required to complete additional time-sensitive **paperwork.**
- **If you are** rejected, the funder usually provides feedback. **This** is a learning opportunity; you can use the feedback to improve your next submission. If you have questions about the feedback, most funders are more than willing to provide clarification. Do not be **afraid** to reach out and ask, and most of all, do not **be discouraged** by a rejection. It is the courage to try again that counts!

### CHAPTER SUMMARY

1. Describe the steps of program development.
   - Program development is a four-step process: (1) completing a needs assessment, and (2) planning, (3) implementing, and (4) evaluating a new program or service or improving or expanding an existing one.
     - A needs assessment is a systematic process to uncover existing problems or needs in a situation or setting. Steps include planning the needs assessment, developing the questions and methods of data collection, conducting the needs assessment, and analyzing the data to prioritize future actions.
     - Program planning is a series of tasks to design a quality program and secure funding. Program planning involves exploring supporting literature; selecting a theoretical base; setting measurable program goals; defining programmatic roles and timelines; outlining the program steps, recruitment and marketing strategies, and budgeting; developing a program evaluation plan; and obtaining approvals and funding for the program.
     - Program implementation involves collaborating with individuals with programmatic roles to carry out the program plan.
     - Program evaluation is a continuous process throughout a program to determine if program goals are being achieved.

2. Differentiate types of grants.
   - Grants are funds commonly provided by charitable foundations, federal agencies, businesses, individuals, or other entities for a distinct purpose. Types of grants can include internal grants, external grants, and fellowships.
   - Internal grants include funding available within an organization, which benefits the organization or its members.
   - External grants include funding offered by outside organizations that seek to support individuals, groups, or other institutions with similar missions.
   - Most internal and external grants are awarded to an institution, organization, or team of people. One exception is fellowships, which are training programs for individuals to develop their clinical skills, research skills, or both.
3. Identify potential grant sources.
   - Potential grant sources, outlined in Table 13-1, include databases (government, Candid, grantwatch.com), corporations, professional organizations or affiliations, organizations associated with your target population or community, organizations that have funded similar work in the past, institutional grant offices, or networking with others.
4. Explain how to choose an appropriate grant.
   - The first step in choosing a grant is to thoroughly review the Request for Proposal (RFP), a document describing the purpose, submission guidelines, and deadline for a grant.
   - Table 13-2 includes common terms and acronyms you might find in an RFP.
   - Characteristics of an appropriate grant include the following: (1) The funder's purpose aligns with the aims of your program or research idea, (2) you meet all of the eligibility criteria, (3) the grant start and end dates, funding amounts, and spending requirements work with your program or research idea, and (4) you can meet the submission deadline.
5. Recall the primary components of a grant proposal.
   - Most grant proposals include an abstract or summary, a detailed proposal plan, and a budget, but you should always align your proposal with the specific guidelines of your target grant.
   - The abstract succinctly summarizes the program or research needs, aims and benefits, and how your idea aligns with the grant purpose.
   - The detailed plan is the most significant portion of the proposal. It should include the relevant background of your organization, the needs assessment, the project goals, specific project methods, and the project evaluation and sustainability plans.
   - The budget should include the estimated direct and indirect costs. Direct costs are those directly associated with completing the project, such as office supplies, equipment, refreshments, and personnel. Indirect costs are those not directly tied to the grant, such as facility utilities, human resources, and library services.
6. Explore tips for successful grant writing.
   - Partnerships, including working with a team of people or collaborations with other organizations or institutions that share similar goals and interests, can increase chances of funding. The benefits of partnerships include resource sharing, more diversity in team expertise, and a broader impact.
   - Other tips for grant writing include allowing increased time to prepare the proposal, strictly following the submission guidelines, getting to know the funding entity, and using language the reviewers will easily understand.
   - Ensuring your program or research idea is novel, innovative, yet sufficiently focused can increase your chances of funding.
   - Having a grant writing mentor and contacting the grant director for clarification can support your professional development and funding success.
   - Establish a sound organizational system for collaboration early in the process and do not give up. Success with funding is often a matter of finding the best funding opportunity for your ideas.

## TEST YOUR KNOWLEDGE

1. The parents of children who reside in a rural community are surveyed about potential recreational programming for next summer. Which step of program development is this activity part of?
   a. Program evaluation
   b. Program implementation
   c. Program planning
   d. Needs assessment

2. Which step of program development involves developing an evaluation plan?
   a. Program evaluation
   b. Needs assessment
   c. Program planning
   d. Program implementation
3. A university posts a funding opportunity for faculty and students to develop sustainable on-campus resources to address student mental health. This is an example of what type of grant?
   a. An external grant
   b. A fellowship
   c. An internal grant
   d. A research grant
4. If you are new to grant writing and plan to explore grants related to programming for community-dwelling seniors in your town, which of the following is the BEST place to look for a grant?
   a. Organizations within the community
   b. The American Occupational Therapy Foundation
   c. The grants.gov database
   d. The grant office of your academic institution
5. When reviewing a Request for Proposal (RFP), what is the FIRST item you should confirm?
   a. You should confirm that the funding amount is sufficient for your program.
   b. You should confirm that you can meet the submission deadline.
   c. You should confirm you are eligible for the grant.
   d. You should confirm that the funders' purpose aligns with your aims.
6. Which part of the grant proposal is MOST important for gaining the attention of funders?
   a. The budget
   b. The needs assessment
   c. The project goals
   d. The summary
7. Which of the following is a benefit of partnering with another organization or group on a grant application?
   a. Resources can be shared.
   b. Meetings are more efficient.
   c. The application can be completed faster.
   d. The project will be more sustainable.

Answer key appears at the end of this text.

## NEXT STEPS

1. Outline a needs assessment plan for a specific site or setting. Include the targeted stakeholders, existing information and resources, questions you want to ask, and the chosen data collection methods. Include a justification for each part of your plan. Next, if appropriate, conduct your needs assessment. What is the highest need? What ideas do you have to address this need?
2. Draft a program plan based on an area of need in your setting. Include measurable goals, the chronological steps of program activities (including who is responsible for completing each step), an evaluation plan, and a sustainability plan. Share your plan with a peer, mentor, or advisor for feedback. What elements may require further consideration?
3. Use the information in Table 13-1 to identify two potential grant sources that align with your program or research ideas. Review the RFPs and list the pros and cons of each option. Consider the eligibility requirements, the deadlines, and how well the grant features (purpose, available funds, spending requirements, etc.) align with your ideas. Which one is the best choice and why?
4. If you are applying for a grant, locate and thoroughly review the RFP. Obtain the required application and use the information provided in this chapter to create a working draft of your grant proposal.

## REFERENCES


Boyle, E. M. (2020). Writing a good research grant proposal. *Paediatrics and Child Health, 30*(2), 52-56. https://doi.org/10.1016/j.paed.2019.11.003

Braveman, B. H. (2001). Development of a community-based return to work program for people with AIDS. *Occupational Therapy in Health Care, 13*(3-4), 113-130. https://doi.org/10.1080/j003v13n03_10

Council on Foundations. (2023). *Foundation basics: What is a foundation?* Council on Foundations website. https://cof.org/content/foundation-basics

Doll, J. (2010). *Program development and grant writing in occupational therapy: Making the connection.* Jones and Barlett.

GrantNews. (2023, April 26). *Why are grant proposals rejected?* GrantWatch. https://www.grantwatch.com/grantnews/why-are-grant-proposals-rejected

Grossman, J., & Bortone, J. (1986). Program development. In S. C. Robertson (Ed.), *Strategies, concepts, and opportunities for program development and evaluation* (pp. 91–99). American Occupational Therapy Association.

Guyer, R. A., Schwarze, M. L., Gosain, A., Maggard-Gibbons, M., Keswani, S. G., & Goldstein, A. M. (2021). Top ten strategies to enhance grant-writing success. *Surgery, 170*(6), 1727–1731. https://doi.org/10.1016/j.surg.2021.06.039

Karsh, E., & Fox, A. S. (2019). *The only grant-writing book you'll ever need: Top grant writers and grant givers share their secrets* (5th ed.). Basic Books.

Mayo Foundation for Medical Education and Research. (2023). *Health sciences education: Mayo Clinic School of Health Sciences.* https://college.mayo.edu/academics/health-sciences-education

Professional Grant Writers. (2021, December 14). *What is a good grant writing success rate?* https://www.professionalgrantwriter.org/learn-rejected-grant-proposal

## ADDITIONAL GRANT WRITING RESOURCES

Brooks, M. (2023). *Grant writing: The most up-to-date guide to finding the best funding sources from online databases, writing grant proposals that get noticed, and getting funding for your projects.* Author. https://bukz.co/products/grant-writing-the-most-uptodate-guide-to-finding-the-best-funding-sources-from-online-databases-writing-grant-proposals-that-get-noticed-and-getting-funding-for-your-projects-9798394577413

Gladstone-Highland, M. (2020). *Grant writing: The complete workbook for writing grant proposals that win.* Monkey Publishing.

Karsh, E., & Fox, A. S. (2019). *The only grant-writing book you'll ever need: Top grant writers and grant givers share their secrets* (5th ed.). Basic Books.

Noble, M. (2021). *How to write a grant: Become a grant writing unicorn* (2nd ed.). SenecaWorks.

Rustick, H. (2019). *The beginner's guide to grant writing: Tips, tools, & templates to write winning grants.* Rustick Productions.

# Section 4

# Disseminating Your Outcomes

Section 4 (Chapters 14–16) of this text focuses on ways to share your inquiry outcomes with others. Sharing the methods and results of your inquiry can help others understand, apply, or build on your work, and contribute to your professional development. You might share your outcomes through a formal inquiry report (Chapter 14), a presentation (Chapter 15), or a publication (Chapter 16). Each chapter includes guidance specific to that dissemination method to promote your success. As the designer and conductor of your inquiry, you have so much valuable information to share. Let's begin with the formal inquiry report.

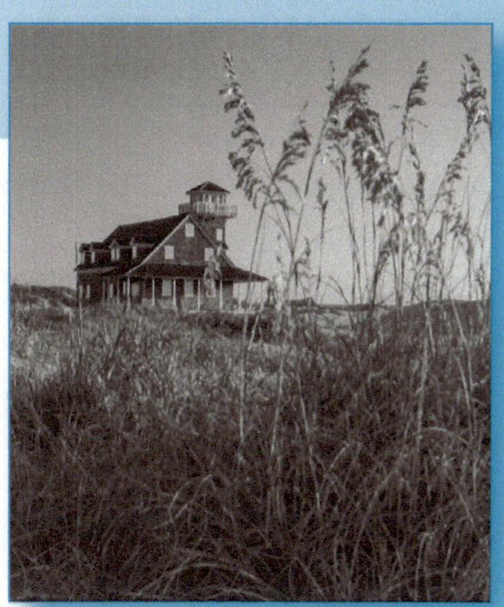

# Chapter 14

# Writing Up Your Inquiry Report

LEARNING OUTCOMES

*The information provided in this chapter will assist you to:*

14.1 Describe the contents of a formal inquiry report.

14.2 State the most effective ways to illustrate data and outcomes.

14.3 Identify the purpose of scientific writing styles.

14.4 Explain tips for becoming a better writer.

14.5 Construct a formal inquiry report.

## Contents of an Inquiry Report

If you are completing an inquiry as part of academic coursework, a grant, or a clinical assignment, you may be required to compile a formal report that summarizes the background, methods, and outcomes of the inquiry. The format and length of the report will likely be dictated by your instructor, funders, supervisor, or institution; in some cases, you may be required to draft a series of chapters that include the key information. In others, a singular paper or manuscript may be necessary. Here, we will focus on the content that is most often required. While the term "inquiry" has been used throughout this text to refer to a research study or an evidence-based practice project, minor variations exist in reporting these two approaches. Whereas the purpose of the research report may be to generalize information gained from scientific inquiry, the function of the evidence-based practice report is to illustrate the application of existing research and evaluate the outcomes to inform future practice or program development.

The distinction will be made when necessary related to report contents. Suggested outlines for a research study and an evidence-based practice project are included in Table 14-1.

### The Abstract

The abstract is a short (no more than 250 words) synopsis of the information contained throughout the inquiry report, including the purpose, methods, primary outcomes, and conclusions of the inquiry. Readers frequently review the abstract to decide if the report warrants further inspection or applies to their purposes. Although the abstract is placed at the beginning of the formal report, it is typically written last after all other sections have been drafted. The abstract should include clear, concise language and avoid technical jargon.

Oregon Inlet Lifesaving Station, Outer Banks, North Carolina.

**TABLE 14-1 ■ Research Versus Evidence-Based Practice Formal Report Outline**

| Research Study Outline | Evidence-Based Practice Project Outline |
|---|---|
| Abstract | Abstract |
| Introduction<br>■ Background of the topic (includes defining key terms and concepts)<br>■ Scope of the study<br>■ Rationale for the study (illustrates gaps in prior literature or work)<br>■ Hypothesis or research question | Introduction<br>■ Background of the topic (includes defining key terms and concepts)<br>■ Detailed setting description<br>■ Description of the problem and rationale for the project (includes results of needs assessment)<br>■ Supports and barriers (including practitioner skills and experience)<br>■ Evidence-based practice question |
| Literature Review<br>■ Methodology of the literature search<br>■ Description of the literature portfolio (may include literature matrix and critical appraisal of individual studies)<br>■ Synthesis of literature portfolio | Literature Review<br>■ Methodology of the literature search<br>■ Description of the literature portfolio (may include literature matrix and critical appraisal of individual studies)<br>■ Synthesis of literature portfolio |
| Methods<br>■ Inquiry design<br>■ Participant recruitment and selection<br>■ Procedures<br>■ Data collection tools | Methods<br>■ Inquiry design<br>■ Participant recruitment and selection<br>  ■ Approach to client-centeredness<br>■ Procedures<br>■ Data collection tools |
| Data Analysis | Data Analysis |
| Results<br>■ Participant description<br>■ Statistical significance of results (if applicable)<br>■ Descriptive or qualitative results (may use tables or figures) | Results<br>■ Participant description<br>■ Descriptive or qualitative results (may use tables or figures) |
| Discussion and Conclusions<br>■ Interpretation of results<br>■ Comparison to existing literature<br>■ Limitations<br>■ Future recommendations | Discussion and Conclusions<br>■ Evaluation of results (including aspects of feasibility)<br>■ Comparison to existing literature<br>■ Limitations (usually site- or population-specific)<br>■ Future recommendations (usually site- or population-specific) |

## Introduction

The introduction helps to "set the stage" for the inquiry and typically includes the content reviewed in Chapter 2 of this text—namely, the inquiry question and the rationale for the inquiry, including the theoretical perspective, if one exists. Key terms or concepts should be clearly defined so their meaning cannot be misinterpreted. Using definitions from dictionaries, textbooks, or topic experts or creating your own definitions is acceptable. In the research report, the introduction orients the reader to the study's scope and explicitly reviews the research hypothesis or question. The need for the research study is illustrated by gaps or shortcomings in prior literature or work.

For the evidence-based practice report, the introduction includes a detailed description of the setting where the project took place. More detail about the setting is included for evidence-based practice because these projects are situated in real-life scenarios, and the details help contextualize the outcomes. The rationale for the project is often substantiated with data from a needs assessment or SWOT (strengths, weaknesses, opportunities, threats) analysis (see Chapters 2 and 13) specific to the setting or organization. Also, when evidence-based practice is used for new program development or quality improvement, a strong rationale can aid in obtaining necessary funding or administrative approval for the project. Finally, while considering supports and barriers is useful in the planning phase of any inquiry, this is particularly important for evidence-based practice initiatives because support from multiple stakeholders may be necessary to fully implement the practice change. This might also include a review of your qualifications for conducting the evidence-based practice project. Be sure to include any applicable education, training, credentials, certifications, and experiences that make you well suited to take on this project. These details are not commonly conveyed in a research study report.

### Literature Review

A literature review is required in formal reporting for both research and evidence-based practice initiatives. Detailed information on the literature search process and constructing a literature review can be revisited in Chapter 3. Your formal report should focus on three key components of the literature review:

1. The methodology of the literature search
2. A description of the literature portfolio
3. Synthesis of literature portfolio content

#### *Methodology of the Literature Search*

The **methodology of the literature search** is an in-depth description of your search process, including the search terms used (including MeSH terms and combinations of search terms, if applicable) and the inclusion and exclusion search criteria for article selection. Reporting on the databases searched and any other search strategies, such as citation tracking, allows the search to be replicated and illustrates the scope of your search. Also, clarify any techniques required to expand or narrow your search. Box 14-1 offers an example of what the search methodology section might look like.

#### BOX 14-1 ■ Methodology of the Literature Search Example

Fifteen articles published between 2017 and 2023 were critically appraised for this inquiry. Search terms included *leadership development, leadership confidence, mentoring, leadership skills, professional development,* and *commitment.* Search terms were used individually and in various combinations, as outlined in the literature matrix. Databases searched include MEDLINE, CINAHL, and Google Scholar. In addition, the reference lists from relevant articles were searched, and the search was determined to be exhaustive when the same articles were found with various combinations of keywords. Studies were included in the portfolio if published within the last 10 years (to provide current practice trends), written in English, and focused on interventions to develop leadership skills in healthcare professionals. Studies were excluded if they did not involve healthcare professionals, if they were published prior to 2017, or if they were not available in English or full text.

#### TIPS & INSPIRATION

- The *Methodology of the Literature Search* section should be fairly easy to write if you did an adequate job tracking your literature search. Revisit Table 3-5 for more information on tracking your literature search.

#### *Description of the Literature Portfolio*

The **description of the literature portfolio** should include a concise picture of your **literature portfolio** (or body of literature you have gathered on your topic). The description is usually a straightforward review of the number of articles, study designs, the time frame of the studies, where the studies took place, and the general topics. It may also be helpful to identify the levels of evidence, especially when applying that evidence through an evidence-based practice project is the aim. Additional information that could be beneficial may include facilities or countries where the studies took place, the populations involved, and other important design features you want to emphasize. For example, did the studies occur in rural communities or involve interprofessional collaboration that you hope to integrate into your inquiry? Box 14-2 contains an example of a portfolio description for an inquiry.

### *Synthesis of Literature Portfolio*

The final section of the literature review is a narrative **synthesis** of the findings from your collective body of literature. Recall that **synthesizing** involves integrating the findings from all the individual studies into an organized literature review that progresses logically to help the reader understand the topic and why your inquiry is necessary. One way to approach this information is by clustering your literature around common **themes**, or central concepts or findings occurring in two or more studies. The aim is to use collective statements that effectively summarize concepts from multiple studies rather than discussing each study singularly. You might also be asked to include your literature matrix or individual article critical appraisals in an appendix to further substantiate your synthesis. An excerpt from a literature review for a study on handwriting interventions with elementary school students is included in Box 14-3

#### BOX 14-2 ■ Example of a Literature Portfolio Description

The final literature portfolio consists of 13 articles published in peer-reviewed journals between 2017 and 2023 that support the proposed inquiry. Eight studies were conducted in the United States, two in Australia, two in France, and one in South Africa. The study designs include two randomized controlled trials (level I), eight pretest-posttest designs (level III), and three qualitative case studies (level IV). The articles demonstrate the effectiveness of sensory-based interventions or environments to improve participation in functional tasks and decrease negative behaviors in clients with dementia. Several articles compare these interventions to alternative interventions such as reminiscence activities, art, or music therapy. Additionally, multiple articles provide background on sensory deficits with dementia, insight into the application of sensory-based interventions with this population, as well as information on potential data collection tools for behavioral outcomes.

#### BOX 14-3 ■ Example of Literature Synthesis

*Those interventions that employ a cognitive approach to handwriting have demonstrated the most effective and successful outcomes for students (Denton, Cope, & Moser, 2006; Howe et al., 2013; Hoy, Egan, & Feder, 2011; Pfeiffer et al., 2015; Zwicker & Hadwin, 2009; Zylstra & Pfeiffer, 2016). A cognitive approach to handwriting intervention is based on learning theories that involve direct handwriting instruction, and that includes repetition, reinforced practice, and feedback to elicit improved performance (Zwicker & Hadwin, 2009). Three studies compared the outcomes related to use of a cognitive approach to handwriting, versus traditional handwriting instruction (Case-Smith et al., 2014; Pfeiffer et al., 2015; Zylstra & Pfeiffer, 2016). In each of these studies, statistically and clinically significant improvements in handwriting legibility were noted in the groups that received the cognitive handwriting support. The control groups which received traditional handwriting instruction support, showed improvement in handwriting legibility but not statistically significant improvements (Pfeiffer et al., 2015; Zylstra & Pfeiffer, 2016). Traditional handwriting instruction often involves a variety of practices depending on the school district's curriculum and grade level to teach and practice handwriting for legibility. Traditional practices include workbooks, visual models, and discussion of the letters to practice that are often taught in alphabetical order (Case-Smith et al., 2014; Pfeiffer et al., 2015; Zylstra & Pfeiffer, 2016). Teaching and practicing handwriting for legibility, is often limited or nonexistent because teachers do not feel adequately prepared to teach handwriting or they devote more effort to other subjects (Applebee & Langer, 2011; Graham, Harris, Bartlett, Popadopoulou, & Santoro, 2016). In light of the evidence which supports a cognitive approach to handwriting deficits, schools should consider instituting a preventive cognitive handwriting program to promote student success in this area (Asher, 2006). (Lee & Lape, 2019, p. 172)* to illustrate good literature synthesis. Notice how summary statements include citations from multiple articles to support those points.

## TIPS & INSPIRATION

- The *Synthesis of the Literature Portfolio* is one of the most labor-intensive sections to write. A common mistake is discussing each study individually rather than sharing collective statements that effectively summarize multiple studies. Your literature matrix (see Table 3-6) will be most helpful in crafting this section.
- For literature on effective interventions, common themes might focus on some of the following:
  - Multiple studies that show positive outcomes after the intervention
  - Multiple studies that show similar approaches (for example, in person, online, in groups, in a particular setting) to providing the intervention
  - Multiple studies that illustrate changes (positive or negative) in the *same* outcome (for example, level of stress, upper extremity strength, handwriting legibility, performance of activities of daily living)
  - Multiple studies that used the *same* or similar outcome measure(s)
  - Multiple studies that used the *same* or similar design features (for example, pretest-posttest design, study duration, timing)

## Methods

The methods section includes the inquiry design, descriptions of the participant recruitment and selection, the inquiry procedures, and the data collection tools. These components should be sufficiently described so that others can fully understand what was done and could replicate the inquiry if needed.

### *Inquiry Design*

The inquiry design specifies whether you are undertaking research or evidence-based practice as well as if you are using a quantitative, qualitative, or mixed methods approach. The specific inquiry design may also be identified and justified related to the inquiry purpose. Lastly, approval for the inquiry via an **Institutional Review Board** (IRB) is noted in the *Inquiry Design* section of a formal report. This conveys to readers that the inquiry plan has been reviewed to ensure the protection of subjects or participants, which further adds to the credibility of the findings. The IRB process is covered in greater detail in Chapter 12.

### *Participant Recruitment and Selection*

For participant recruitment and selection, a list of participant inclusion and exclusion criteria and descriptions of recruitment and sampling methods are included. Your choice of the terms "subjects" or "participants" in this section may be based on your specific discipline, publication or academic requirements, or your preference, as previously discussed. For an evidence-based practice project, this section often clarifies the approach to client-centeredness. The term "client-centered," first coined by Carl Rogers (1959) in relation to the provision of psychotherapy, is widely accepted in all aspects of healthcare today. Being **client-centered** involves allowing the client to become an active member of the clinical team by voicing their concerns and preferences and being a central member of the decision-making process. Recall from Chapter 1 that evidence-based practice involves interweaving three elements—evidence; practitioner skills and knowledge; and client goals, values, and circumstances. Care should be taken to delineate precisely how the procedures will be varied to meet each client's needs in an evidence-based practice project. This section is omitted in a research study that aims to adhere to stricter procedures to generate new information.

### *Procedures*

The procedures refer to the steps taken during the implementation of an inquiry. For inquiries in which interventions are provided, those interventions should be amply described, including when and how they were delivered and by whom. For commercially available interventions (for example, a published handwriting program), a brief description of the program with appropriate citations will usually suffice. Any modifications to the original program should be specified. If you created or designed the intervention, additional details would be necessary to explain the development of the intervention or program.

Additionally, a table (see Table 11-2) or flow diagram (see Figure 14-4) can be effective ways to illustrate the steps of your inquiry. For example, for an inquiry conducted over 8 weeks, a table with one row for each of the 8 weeks might be used to delineate the steps that occurred each week.

For a research study with multiple study groups (for example, an experimental group and a control group), a flow diagram might be used to differentiate the procedures for each group (see Figure 11-3). The procedures for a research study should be rather strict, whereas those for an evidence-based practice project will have some degree of flexibility.

#### *Data Collection Tools*

Finally, the methods section should include an explanation of the data collection tools and methods, including when the tools were administered and by whom. If a standardized assessment is used for data collection, a brief description of the assessment, including the purpose, information on reliability and validity, and prior use with citations, is appropriate. For tools (surveys, interview questions, focus group questions, assessments, observation checklists, etc.) that you develop specifically for your inquiry, additional details should be provided:

- **Purpose of the tool:** Clarify the reason for using this tool. Also include why a standardized tool was not used. For example, perhaps no existing tools effectively assess the construct of interest, or those that exist present other challenges such as being cost-prohibitive, requiring advanced training to administer, or being unavailable in the participants' language.
- **Tool development:** Share details on how the tool was developed and by whom. For example, was it constructed from inception of the idea, or was it based on prior literature, concepts, or existing tools?
- **Reliability and validity information:** While it is unlikely that a tool you created specifically for an inquiry would have undergone advanced testing related to reliability and validity, you should make some effort to promote credibility of the data gathered with this tool. Clarify any strategies used to improve the quality of a tool, such as having an expert on the topic review the tool or piloting it with groups similar to the inquiry participants. If multiple raters will use the tool, some pretesting could also help establish interrater reliability.

For data collection involving observations or record/artifact review, a report of how the site, records, or items were accessed and how the data were extracted is necessary. If equipment was used to gather the data, details about calibration of the equipment and any training completed by the data gatherer should also be included.

### Data Analysis

An explanation of the data analysis procedures is part of the formal report for all inquiries. For quantitative data, you should specify the statistical methods and software used. For qualitative data, more detail is needed to describe the coding and analysis process. Clarify who completed the data analysis and any strategies to confirm the analysis results. For example, did a second person review the quantitative analysis, or did multiple people analyze the qualitative data and compare the resultant themes to reach a consensus?

### Results

The results include a description of the final participant sample and the outcomes of the data analysis.

#### *Participant Description*

The participants should be described numerically; this may include reporting frequencies, percentages, a range, or other measures of central tendency (such as the mean) for the sample's demographic characteristics. This description gives readers a clear picture of the sample as they consider the inquiry outcomes and possible application to other groups of people. The sample description can be in narrative format or supplemented with tables and figures. See Box 14-4 for an example.

#### *Statistically Significant Results*

The results of the data analysis can be discussed in narrative format or displayed in tables and figures. Visual displays of results are discussed later in this chapter. Within the results section, only the results of the inquiry should be presented, with no

> **BOX 14-4 ■ Example of Participant Description**
>
> In Friedman and VanPuymbrouck's (2021) study on the impact of occupational therapy education on students' disability attitudes, they described the participants in a table as well as in the narrative that follows:
>
> *The mean age of participants when they entered their graduate program was 24.79 yr, and it was 27.34 yr after graduation (Table 1). The majority of participants were White, straight, nondisabled, and female. Most participants had at least one significant relationship (e.g., family, partner, friend) with a PWD [person with a disability]. Family socioeconomic status was relatively evenly distributed. The mean political orientation (self-report; measured on a scale from 1 = very liberal to 100 = very conservative) of students when they entered their graduate program was 31.57, and it was 24.64 after graduation. (p. 3)*

interpretation. This factual account of results should include all relevant ones—not just those substantiating your hypothesis or practice needs. For a research study in which inferential statistics were used to analyze the data, each hypothesis should be reviewed and checked against the statistical results; you should report the confidence level (discussed in Chapters 5 and 6) and whether each hypothesis was substantiated. For inquiries in which inferential statistics are not appropriate (descriptive studies, nonexperimental designs, qualitative studies, or evidence-based practice projects), statistical significance cannot be reported. In some cases, reporting clinical significance (discussed in Chapter 6) may be appropriate where the outcomes are deemed clinically meaningful. See Box 5-3 for an example of results with statistical significance.

### *Descriptive or Qualitative Results*

Descriptive quantitative results can be reported similarly to those used to describe the sample, that is, by reporting frequencies, percentages, ranges, central tendencies, or percent change. Presenting these results in narrative or visual form is also appropriate. For a qualitative inquiry, the results are commonly discussed as themes, which are recurrent ideas or patterns within a dataset. These themes should be described, and participant quotes or other narrative data may be used to justify the themes. Sometimes, this information is provided in table format.

Descriptive or qualitative outcomes are most frequently reported for evidence-based practice projects. Inferential statistics are usually inappropriate because these projects tend to be rooted in real-life clinical situations, and participant groups are smaller or restricted to one practice, clinic, or health system. In addition, remember that the goal of evidence-based practice is to apply existing evidence to practice and then evaluate the success of those initiatives. Although standardized measures can be used to gather participant data, the success of the intervention is not based on statistical outcomes but instead on clinical ones. Tables and figures are also commonly used to display data in evidence-based practice projects.

## Discussion and Conclusions

Up until this point, the results should be presented in a straightforward manner, without further interpretation. The discussion and conclusion sections of the formal report reinforce the main results, explain why they are important, and compare them to the existing literature on the topic. For a research study, this involves an interpretation of the results. Ideally, each study contributes to the body of knowledge on a topic, which may further support the efficacy of interventions, reveal relationships between phenomena, or build theory on a particular issue. The results are typically compared with the results of other studies on the topic, and similarities and differences are acknowledged. If you note parallels between your literature review and your study's results, this lends support to prior findings. When dissimilar results are found, it is customary to speculate plausible reasons for the departure. Recognizing confounding results and suggesting plausible reasons for them allows readers to fully understand what happened in your study and may have implications for future studies.

For evidence-based practice projects, the discussion is more of an evaluation of the project's outcomes. Results are compared to the existing literature on the topic but are also considered within the site-specific context and logistics. Many evidence-based practice projects are undertaken as quality improvement projects, so in these instances, the discussion should move beyond superficial consideration of the results. The discussion might focus on aspects of feasibility, including availability of resources, equipment, and staff, safety, alignment with organizational culture and aims, as well as potential benefits of the project for key stakeholders.

### *What If Your Results Do Not Support the Inquiry Question or Hypothesis?*

This brings us to how to handle an inquiry that generates limited data in support of the proposed hypothesis or evidence-based practice question, or one in which the hypotheses are not supported at all. It is important to share the results of such inquiries for these reasons:

- They may put to rest a popular myth that needs to be dispelled. For example, an intervention might be widely accepted as effective when little evidence exists to support it. Sharing that an intervention is ineffective can also promote evidence-based practice.
- They may show that a particular methodology or inquiry design is not a useful way to investigate or approach a particular problem, thus saving others from making the same mistake.
- They may highlight design flaws so others can avoid them in future inquiries.

### *Limitations*

In any inquiry, acknowledging the limitations is respectable and allows readers to decide for themselves if the integrity of the inquiry has been compromised too much to place value on the results. Limitations may be related to an unreliable data collection tool, a small sample, an unforeseen interference in the inquiry, faulty assumptions by the researcher or evidence-based practitioner, or any other form of bias discussed in prior chapters. Limitations for research should focus on challenges in design that may impact the ability to generalize results to the larger population. Limitations in evidence-based practice are likely to be more site-specific and may justify changes in staffing, resources, or other logistics if the project is continued.

## TIPS & INSPIRATION

- It is okay if your results do not align with prior literature or are not what you expected. The discussion is your opportunity to explain why this might be the case. For example, your participants may have differed significantly from what you anticipated, or unforeseen circumstances may have occurred at the inquiry site. You also might have altered the intervention or program to better align with the site requirements or aims.
- Some limitations may be unavoidable. Circumstances beyond your control may have dictated features of the inquiry design or resulted in challenges during the implementation of the inquiry. Just focus on reporting the limitations so that the results can be considered in light of them. An inquiry without limitations is extremely rare!

### *Future Recommendations*

Recommendations for the future are also provided in the formal report and may include suggestions for future research, practice, or healthcare policy; however, recommendations for evidence-based practice are typically specific to the project site or population. Some important questions to consider when writing your discussion and conclusions include the following:

1. What are the main results, and why are they important?
2. Do the results of the inquiry differ from what you expected? If so, what are some plausible reasons for the differences? Why might this information be important?
3. Do your results align with prior literature on the topic? If so, this adds to the body of knowledge on the topic. If not, why might your results have differed?
4. Based on your results, what recommendations do you have for future research or practice improvement? For research projects, you might include suggestions for improvements to the study's design or procedures as well as proposals for new research, if applicable. For evidence-based practice, you might incorporate

ideas for program development, modification, or expansion, as well as changes to healthcare policies or educational opportunities.

5. What are the strengths of the current inquiry? What are the primary limitations of the inquiry?

Thinking critically about your outcomes and the implications for the future can lead to a thought-provoking discussion. Although it is common for readers to skim the more technical sections of an inquiry report, such as the literature review or the data analyses, the discussion and conclusions are usually reviewed in their entirety. This is where the summary of the results and the "take-home message" are clearly delineated.

**TABLE 14-2 ■ Degrees of Elbow Flexion Following Treatment ($N = 50$)**

| Degrees of Elbow Flexion | Frequency of Occurrence |
|---|---|
| **20–40** | 2 |
| **41–60** | 4 |
| **61–80** | 9 |
| **81–100** | 10 |
| **101–120** | 12 |
| **121–140** | 9 |
| **141–160** | 3 |
| **161–180** | 1 |

### TIPS & INSPIRATION

- **Be careful** not to overstate the results of your inquiry. **For example,** a rigorous experimental design is required to show cause-and-effect relationships or the effectiveness of an intervention. In the absence of these designs, results cannot indicate effectiveness or "prove" anything. Instead, consider stating that the results align with prior literature, or that the results *provide support* for the intervention or program in question.

## Visual Displays of Data and Results

Displaying data visually, in tables and figures, allows readers to make sense of larger amounts of data at a glance. As the old saying goes, "A picture is worth a thousand words," or, in this case, a thousand numbers. Tables and figures can eliminate complicated or boring narratives but should be used judiciously; too many can become confusing.

### Tables

**Tables** can be used to present simple lists of frequencies and percentages or to consolidate and present data, such as numbers of pounds squeezed on a dynamometer. For example, if scores are arranged in order from highest to lowest (rank ordering), readers can quickly gain an overview of the responses. They can see the range of scores—the highest, lowest, and middle scores—and compare one person's scores against the others.

Tables are especially useful for condensing large quantities of data so the reader can understand the information more readily. Suppose a study yielded 50 scores of degrees of elbow flexion for a group of patients. Even presenting the 50 scores in order of magnitude would be difficult to digest. In this case, grouping the scores, say into units of 20, would reduce the data and allow the reader to quickly grasp the spread of scores (see Table 14-2). Most patients had flexion in the midrange (60 degrees to 120 degrees), whereas few had flexion at the greater and smaller angles. Even though some detail is lost in this type of grouping, it is generally a useful and efficient representation of data.

Tables can also be used to illustrate findings from descriptive and inferential statistics in less space than would be required by a narrative. It is not necessary to repeat all the table data in the text. The important points should be emphasized in the text, and the reader should be directed to the table for greater detail. Tables 14-3 and 14-4 present results generated from descriptive and inferential statistics.

### Figures

Although tables are invaluable for concisely communicating large sets of numbers, many people find it challenging to get the "big picture" from a table.

**TABLE 14-3 ■ Distribution of Demographic Characteristics of Healthcare Administrators and Clinicians ($N$ = 385)**

| Demographic Characteristics | Administrators ($N$ = 201) | | Clinicians ($N$ = 184) | | Total Group | |
|---|---|---|---|---|---|---|
| | Frequency | Percentage | Frequency | Percentage | Frequency | Percentage |
| Age: | | | | | | |
| 20–25 years | 0 | 0 | 2 | 1 | 2 | 0.5 |
| 26–30 years | 17 | 9 | 46 | 25 | 63 | 16 |
| 31–35 years | 56 | 28 | 52 | 28 | 108 | 28 |
| 36–40 years | 33 | 16 | 26 | 14 | 59 | 15 |
| 41–50 years | 53 | 26 | 40 | 22 | 93 | 24 |
| 51+ years | 42 | 21 | 18 | 10 | 60 | 16 |
| College degree: | | | | | | |
| Associate | 95 | 47 | 113 | 61 | 208 | 57 |
| BA/BS | 13 | 10 | 17 | 9 | 30 | 8 |
| MA/MS | 10 | 6 | 8 | 4 | 18 | 6 |
| Certificate | 21 | 11 | 4 | 2 | 25 | 7 |
| Clinical doctorate | 47 | 25 | 19 | 15 | 66 | 17 |
| Research doctorate | 4 | 2 | 0 | 0 | 4 | 1 |
| Age when took first job: | | | | | | |
| 20–25 years | 178 | 89 | 156 | 85 | 334 | 87 |
| 26–30 years | 14 | 7 | 17 | 8 | 28 | 7 |
| 31–35 years | 4 | 2 | 5 | 3 | 9 | 2 |
| 36–40 years | 2 | 1 | 5 | 3 | 7 | 2 |
| 41+ years | 5 | 2 | 4 | 2 | 9 | 2 |
| Specialty of practice: | | | | | | |
| Psychiatry | 60 | 30 | 49 | 27 | 109 | 29 |
| Pediatrics | 31 | 15 | 59 | 32 | 90 | 24 |
| Physical disabilities | 95 | 47 | 63 | 35 | 158 | 41 |
| Geriatrics | 15 | 8 | 11 | 6 | 26 | 7 |

This is where we turn to figures. **Figures** illustrate visual images of items or events, changes in scores over time, or comparisons of multiple items. Figures can include line graphs, bar graphs, diagrams, flowcharts, pie charts, photographs, schematics, or drawings, to name a few. To further clarify, tables are best for presenting data. In contrast, figures are used to help the reader gain a clearer understanding of the outcomes and to propose relationships among key concepts in the inquiry. Consult Table 14-5 to determine the most appropriate illustration for your goals.

**TABLE 14-4 ■ Differences Between Administrators and Clinicians on Demographic Characteristics ($N = 385$)**

| Role by Characteristic | Pearson Chi-Square | Significance Level |
|---|---|---|
| Role by age | 31.22 | 0.00* |
| Role by degree | 31.22 | 0.00* |
| Role by age entering the field | 2.68 | 0.75 |
| Role by age at taking first job | 2.24 | 0.69 |
| Role by specialty practice | 18.20 | 0.00* |
| Role by mother's education | 3.71 | 0.81 |
| Role by father's education | 7.73 | 0.36 |
| Role by mentor | 6.22 | 0.10 |

*$p < 0.001$.

**TABLE 14-5 ■ Choosing the Most Effective Type of Illustration for a Given Goal**

| To Accomplish This: | Choose One of These: |
|---|---|
| To present exact values, raw data, or data that do not fit into any simple pattern | Table, list |
| To summarize trends, show interactions between two or more variables, relate data to constants, or emphasize an overall pattern rather than specific measurements | Line graph |
| To dramatize differences or draw comparisons | Bar graph |
| To illustrate complex relationships, spatial configurations, pathways, processes, or interactions | Diagram |
| To show sequential processes | Flowchart |
| To classify information | Table, list, pictograph |
| To describe parts or electric circuits | Schematic |
| To describe a process, organization, or model | Pictograph, flowchart, block diagram |
| To compare and contrast | Pictograph, pie chart, bar graph |
| To describe a change of state | Line graph, bar graph |
| To describe proportions | Pie chart, bar graph |
| To describe relationships | Table, line graph, block diagram |
| To describe causation | Flowchart, pictograph |
| To describe an entire object | Schematic, drawing, photograph |
| To show the vertical and horizontal hierarchy within an object, idea, or organization | Flowchart, drawing tree, block diagram |

Matthews, J., & Matthews, R. (2014). *Successful scientific writing: A step-by-step guide for the biological and medical sciences* (4th ed.) Cambridge University Press. Reprinted with permission of Cambridge University Press.

## Line Graphs

Line graphs are used to show changes in a phenomenon over time. Measurements of an attribute are plotted at multiple points during the inquiry, and all points are joined to form a continuous line on the graph. Line graphs can only present continuous data, and more than one line can be included on the same graph to reveal trends among two or more groups or participants. While it is possible to use a line graph with only two data points (for example, a pretest and a posttest), this only illustrates the trend from the first measurement to the second. If the inquiry occurs over a longer period without measurements at set increments, you cannot draw conclusions about trends that may have occurred between the pretest and posttest. A line graph is also inappropriate for comparing multiple groups or participants at a single point in time; in this case, a stacked bar graph, discussed next, is most suitable. An example of a line graph, in which student test scores were plotted for two cohorts of students over an academic year can be found in Figure 14-1. Examination of the graph reveals that scores improved more for Cohort B, possibly because of changes in curriculum design, for example.

## Bar Graphs

Bar graphs are similar, except they are formed by drawing a vertical bar at each frequency gained across the width of the score interval. This offers a strong visual impact and is often effective for comparing scores among all participants or pre- and postscores among individuals or the study groups. See Figure 14-2 for an example of a bar graph. In this example, participants were assessed using the *Agitated Behavior Scale* (Bognar et al., 2000) before and after sensory-based treatments. Because higher numbers on the scale indicate the presence of more behaviors, this graph reveals that behaviors dropped following the treatment sessions.

## Pie Charts

A pie chart is often used to depict a breakdown of some quantity, for example, expenditures for a program or types of inquiry participants, as shown in Figure 14-3. Pie charts may be particularly useful to describe a study sample, but multiple pie charts used to illustrate the distribution of a sample on various

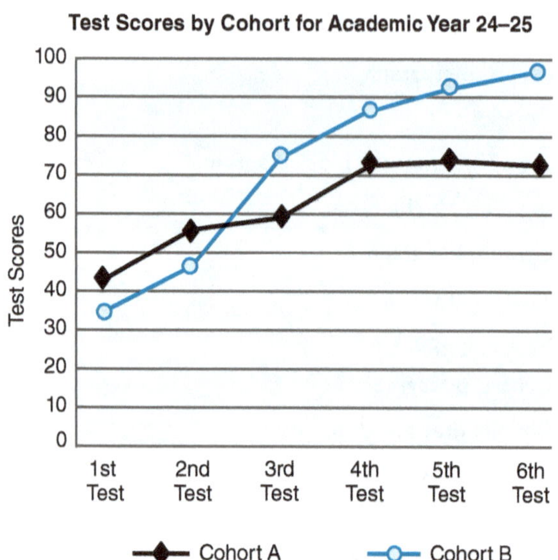


Figure 14-1 Line graph comparing student test scores for two cohorts of students throughout an academic year.

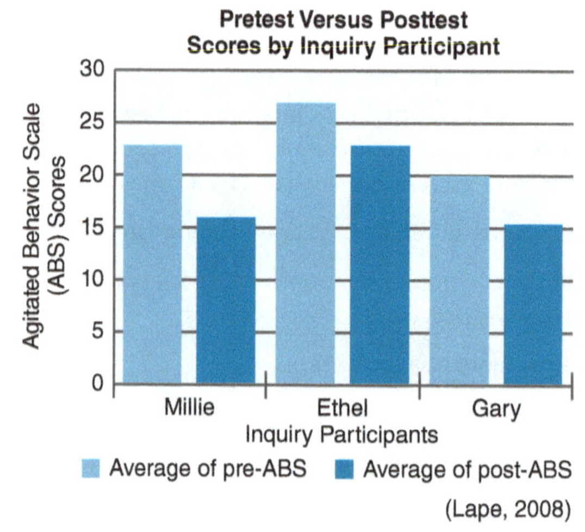


Figure 14-2 Example of a bar graph.

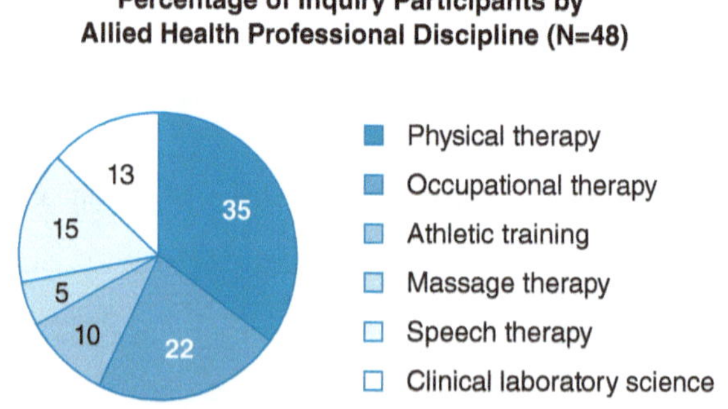


Figure 14-3 Example of a pie chart.

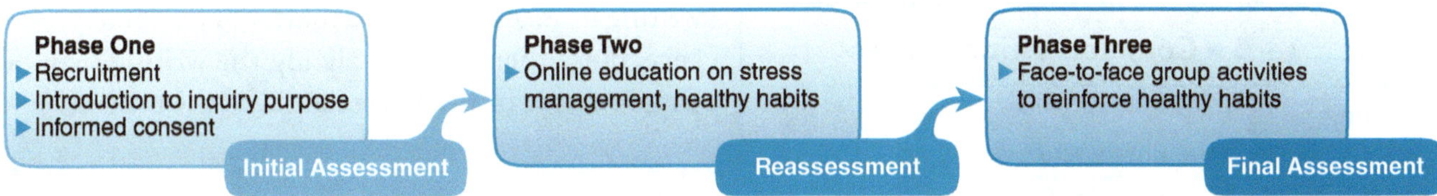


Figure 14-4 Flowchart depicting the phases of a proposed research study.

attributes can be difficult to compare. A single table comprising frequencies of all relevant attributes would be more effective in such a case.

### *Flowcharts and Other Diagrams*

Flowcharts, schematics, drawings, and design trees are all ways of visually explaining processes, systems, or phenomena. In designing these figures, the level of detail should match what is required and understood by the reader. The example in Figure 14-4 depicts the three phases of a proposed research study on the impact of online and group activities in promoting healthy habits in adolescents with obesity. It clearly defines the steps in each phase of the intervention and at what points in the process formal assessments of the participants will occur.

These are just a few of the possibilities for displaying data. For further ideas or descriptions of all types of figures, you may refer *to Successful Scientific Writing: A Step-by-Step Guide for the Biological and Medical Sciences* (Matthews & Matthews, 2014). If you use these visuals for presenting data, be sure to label them correctly—tables are called "tables," whereas graphs, charts, drawings, photographs, and so forth, are called "figures." Include accurate and complete titles, column headings, axes labels, and legends so that tables and figures can be understood on their own, without text. In addition, always refer to each table and figure within the body of the formal report. Tell readers what to look for and point out salient features.

#### TIPS & INSPIRATION

- Share your planned tables and figures with others for feedback. This can help you determine if you have selected the best way to illustrate your data and outcomes.
- Review features in Microsoft Excel for the creation of graphs. If your data are in an Excel spreadsheet, you can select the desired graph, label the axes, and make a legend or key. Once completed, the graph can be copied into your inquiry report.
- Use the SmartArt feature (from the Insert menu in Microsoft Word) or the Diagram feature (from the Insert menu in Google Docs) to create other diagrams that illustrate processes, hierarchies, or relationships. Other word processing programs include similar features.

## Scientific Writing Styles

Now that we have addressed the content for each section of the report, let us turn to the topic of writing style, which is commonly dictated by the setting and purpose of the report. In academic settings, the instructor or discipline usually sets forth the accepted writing style, whereas clinical settings lack specific requirements. If you plan to publish, the writing style is specified in the author guidelines for your target journal, and publication of your work is discussed in greater detail in Chapter 16. Various writing styles exist; Table 14-6 includes some of the most popular style manuals applicable to the allied health professions.

Each style manual outlines specific methods for formatting headings, in-text citations, and reference lists, as well as for organizing the various sections of the report. The manuals also address plagiarism, grammar, and syntax. Although many online resources are available for each style, having a hard copy of the appropriate style manual at your disposal will prove invaluable. Reviewing the manual before the start of writing allows you to become familiar with the overall content and know where to find the

**TABLE 14-6 ■ Common Writing Styles**

| Writing Style | Manual Reference |
|---|---|
| APA | American Psychological Association. (2020). *Publication manual of the American Psychological Association: The official guide to APA style* (7th ed.). Author. |
| MLA | Modern Language Association. (2021). *MLA handbook* (9th ed.). Author. |
| AMA | AMA Manual of Style Committee. (2020). *AMA manual of style: A guide for authors and editors* (11th ed.). Oxford University Press. https://doi.org/10.1093/jama/9780190246556.001.0001 |
| *The Chicago Manual of Style* | University of Chicago Press. (2017). *The Chicago manual of style* (17th ed.). Author. |

information when needed. A well-worn highlighted manual with dog-eared pages is a sign of a meticulous writer.

## Becoming a Better Writer

Although basic writing skills are necessary in the allied health professions for documenting patient progress, recording program outcomes, or taking notes in education or meetings, many of us do not view ourselves as professional writers. However, with the emphasis on research and evidence-based practice, there is a push to disseminate information from these inquiries. Whether your report is submitted to a facility administrator, course instructor, or a professional organization, you must clearly and concisely articulate the main points of your inquiry. Some additional tips for the writing process are reviewed here.

### Using an Outline

Basic outlines for a research study or an evidence-based practice project have been provided in Table 14-1. These outlines provide a good starting point where additional details individualized to your inquiry can be inserted. Many writers prefer to begin with a detailed outline and progress to a draft of the formal report, whereas others do better starting the writing immediately. It is a matter of personal preference, but either way, visualizing the writing plan on paper or in your head is essential to the process.

**TIPS & INSPIRATION**

- Congratulate yourself when you write something! A paragraph can sometimes take an entire day, whereas you will write many pages on other days. Writing that requires citations and referencing also takes longer than passages of text where you are summarizing information that you already know or have experienced. Planning for more writing time than you think you might need can help you avoid late-night cramming and make you feel accomplished if you finish ahead of schedule.

### Grammar and Organization

The grammatical style and organization of the information sets the tone for the report and ensures that the reader can understand the information provided. Care should also be taken to ensure that the level of writing is appropriate for the target audience. These strategies can be helpful:

1. **Organization:** Present information in a logical order, building on each point to develop the next one. Begin each paragraph with a compelling topic sentence and then elaborate on those points as you progress through the paragraph. Go back and compare your topic sentence to the information in the corresponding paragraph. Did you include extraneous information not connected to the topic sentence? If so, remove it.
2. **Concise language:** Use clear and concise language, choosing words wisely. Avoid inserting extra words that do not add to the content. In scientific writing, more is not always better. Brevity is a skill that requires diligent effort to achieve.
3. **Comprehension:** Limit the use of technical jargon, acronyms, and abbreviations to aid in comprehension. Consider your audience and be sure the writing is geared to that group. Using layperson's terms and writing out most words allows your work to be understood by a broader audience.
4. **Verb tense:** Writing in the past tense is customary because the inquiry has already been completed. Although you may have written some

sections in future or present tenses when the inquiry was in development, going back and revising everything into past tense at the end places your work in the appropriate context.

5. **Grammatical person:** There is much debate regarding use of first-person versus third-person writing in scientific endeavors. For most academic programs and publications, the general rule of thumb is to use first person sparingly or only when it is absolutely necessary. Third-person professional writing is generally preferred for formal reports and peer-reviewed publications. First-person writing may be acceptable in clinic-based settings or when recording outcomes of evidence-based practice projects, as these situations warrant more personal connections with participants, and procedures are not as strict.
6. **Grammatical voice:** Grammatical voice refers to the placement of nouns and verbs in a sentence, and two types are active and passive voice. With active voice, the noun performs the action indicated by the verb, whereas with passive voice, the noun is acted upon *passively* by the verb. See the following example:

   **Active:** The researcher conducted the study.
   **Passive:** The study was conducted by the researcher.

   Active voice is generally preferred because it is more direct and easier to understand.
7. **Use of direct quotations:** Reserve use of direct quotes for situations when you are unable to paraphrase the material effectively (i.e., when technical phrases or terms are used that cannot be stated another way or when the original authors stated the information in such a unique way that meaning would be lost with paraphrasing). Using too many direct quotes in one section or paragraph limits the flow of the writing and does not show that you understand the material and can effectively integrate it. A general rule of thumb is to limit direct quoting to no more than one quote per several pages of your own words. When using direct quotes, always follow the guidelines outlined in the style manual for proper formatting and citation. Remember that failure to cite appropriately can be considered plagiarism.

### TIPS & INSPIRATION

- Avoid contractions in professional writing.
- Never end a paragraph with a direct quote. Summing up the paragraph in your own words creates ownership of the content you are sharing.
- Steer clear of absolutes in your writing. Using words such as *always* or *never* can create inaccuracies in your conclusions.

### Use of Software Features

Consider using features within your word processing program to increase the quality of your writing and eliminate errors. These features include spelling and grammar checks, readability formulas, a thesaurus, document statistics, translators, and support for automating creation of reference lists and a table of contents. Although it might take some extra time to figure out how to activate these features, the benefits outweigh the initial effort. Each of these features is discussed here:

1. **Spelling and grammar checks:** This feature can be activated to check the document as you write or the entire document after you have finished. Most programs also provide suggestions as to how to correct the identified errors.
2. **Readability formulas:** Readability formulas are used to analyze the average sentence and word length used in the document to determine the level of writing. Two of the most common tests are the Flesch Reading Ease Test and the Flesch-Kincaid Grade Level Test. The Flesch Reading Ease Test rates reading ease on a 100-point scale (with a score of 90 to 100 easily understood by a fifth grader, 60 to 70 easily understood by eighth or ninth graders, and a score of 0 to 30 understood by college graduates; Flesch, 1948; Kincaid et al., 1975). Writing at 60 to 70 is appropriate for most purposes; however, one might expect levels to be closer to 30 for doctoral-level projects or education. The Flesch-Kincaid Grade Level Test transfers the readability score into a U.S. school grade level. So, if the Flesch-Kincaid Grade Level score

is 10.8, we expect students in 10th to 11th grade to be able to understand it. These two tests are inversely proportional. As the readability score increases (meaning it gets easier to understand), the grade level score gets lower (meaning those in a lower grade can understand it). Although these are just one measure of the level of writing, these tests provide a quick way for you to screen your writing to see if it is at the appropriate level. Most word processing programs will perform these calculations automatically, or various calculators are available online (ReadabilityFormulas.com, n.d.). For example, in Microsoft Word, this option can be activated by selecting "Options" from the File Menu, then clicking "Proofing" and then ensuring that "Show readability statistics" is checked. Results are shown once the entire document has been checked.

3. **Thesaurus:** Most word processing programs have a built-in thesaurus that allows you to select any word within the document to check for alternative word choices. This is especially useful when you struggle with a word choice or use the same word repetitively. Using the thesaurus can add variety to your writing and may even help you choose a stronger word than what initially came to mind.
4. **Document statistics:** Most word processing software is equipped with features to calculate your document statistics automatically, including the number of pages, words, characters, and lines. This can be useful if you are striving to adhere to the word limits outlined in the author's guidelines for a particular publication or trying to be clear and concise in a particular passage (for example, trying to limit your abstract to 250 words). Additionally, this feature can be used to verify the length of directly quoted material for proper citation. For instance, in American Psychological Association (APA) style, direct quotes that are 40 or more words in length require special formatting (APA, 2020).
5. **Translators:** Translators can convert text from one language to another. Although opponents of these features argue that accuracy is somewhat limited, it is a viable option. It can be helpful if your literature search turns up a quality piece of evidence in another language. Using the translation feature in your word processing software or one of the many programs found online may allow you to integrate this applicable information into your report.
6. **Automatic reference lists and table of contents:** Creating these items manually is an option, but utilizing your word processing software's automated features can help ease the burden. Most programs allow you to create a database of references used within the body of the formal report. This is accomplished by selecting the writing style, say APA style, and then manually entering vital information, such as the authors, article title, journal name, volume, issue, and page numbers for each reference used. Once references are added to the database, they can be inserted within parenthetical citations, in footnotes, or in a master reference list as needed. The table of contents feature works similarly. Headings are formatted according to the selected style guide via an automated heading feature in the software program. After the formal report is finished, this feature allows you to insert the entire table of contents with only a few keystrokes.

## TIPS & INSPIRATION

- When writing your formal report, take the time to automate your table of contents and reference list. The extra time now will save much time later!
- Consider using a writing assistant program to improve your writing further. Examples of these programs include Grammarly, ProWritingAid, and WordTune, to name a few. Most charge a fee to enable full functionality across your devices. For example, Grammarly extends to your web browser and computer applications to assess your writing, including grammar, plagiarism, style, and tone, and makes suggestions for improvements in addition to suggestions made by your word processing software.

- Enlist the help of at least three proofreaders to review your writing. Select one person who is familiar with your topic and can review the content, one outside your content area so that you will know if you are writing for a broader audience or if your content can be easily understood by those outside your discipline, and one who is skilled in grammar, writing, and formatting.

## CHAPTER SUMMARY

1. Describe the contents of a formal inquiry report.
   - A formal inquiry report summarizes an inquiry's background, methods, and outcomes. Your instructor, funders, or institution will likely dictate the format.
   - Sections of a formal inquiry report include the abstract, introduction, literature review, methods, data analysis, results, discussion, and conclusions.
   - Differences in a formal report for a research study and for an evidence-based practice project are outlined in Table 14-1.
2. State the most effective ways to illustrate data and outcomes.
   - Data and outcomes can be displayed visually in tables and figures. Table 14-5 can help you choose the best illustration for your goal.
   - Tables can be used to consolidate and present larger quantities of data so that the reader can understand the information more readily.
   - Figures, including line graphs, bar graphs, diagrams, flowcharts, pie charts, photographs, or other schematics, illustrate outcomes, relationships, and changes in scores over time or compare multiple scores.
     - Line graphs are used to show changes over time. They can only be used with continuous data, and more than one line can be included on the same graph to reveal trends among two or more groups or participants.
     - Bar graphs include a vertical bar at each frequency across a width of the score interval and are effective for comparing scores among all participants or when comparing pre- and post-scores among individuals or study groups.
     - Pie charts are useful to examine distributions of some variable—for example, a sample of some attribute such as years since diagnosis or spending by category.
     - Flowcharts or other diagrams can be useful for illustrating processes or systems.
3. Identify the purpose of scientific writing styles.
   - Common scientific writing styles include APA, MLA, AMA, and *The Chicago Manual of Style* (see Table 14-6). The instructor or discipline usually sets forth the required writing style for a formal report.
   - Each writing style outlines specific methods for formatting, referencing and citations, organization of the report, and grammar.
4. Explain tips for becoming a better writer.
   - Using an outline can be an effective method to organize your thoughts before you begin writing.
   - Tips for organization and grammar include presenting information logically; using clear and concise language; avoiding technical jargon and excessive acronyms and abbreviations; writing in past tense, third person, and active voice; and limiting direct quoting.
   - Word processing software features that can be helpful include spelling and grammar checks, readability formulas, a thesaurus, document statistics, translators, and automatic reference list and table of contents generation features.
5. Construct a formal inquiry report.
   - The information and strategies offered in this chapter should allow you to construct a quality formal inquiry report should you be required to do so.

## TEST YOUR KNOWLEDGE

1. Formal reports for research studies and evidence-based practice projects include the same content. True or false?
2. Which section of a formal inquiry report is typically written last?
   a. Conclusion
   b. Abstract
   c. Results
   d. Limitations
3. Which of the following BEST describes the content of a quality literature review?
   a. A summary of search methods and portfolio synthesis
   b. A synthesis of literature portfolio themes
   c. A summary of the search process, terms, and strategies
   d. A synopsis of how the literature will be applied

4. What should be included in the description of a new data collection tool that you created specifically for an inquiry?
   a. A description of how the tool was normed
   b. An explanation of the tool's development
   c. The names of similar standardized tools
   d. Citations supporting the tool's validity and reliability
5. Which of the following should be reported in the *Results* section of a formal inquiry report?
   a. Comparison of the results to existing literature
   b. Outcomes of statistical tests without interpretation
   c. Limitations of the inquiry and how those impact results
   d. Recommendations for future research, practice, or healthcare policy
6. Identify the appropriate visual display (bar graph, flowchart, line graph, pie chart, table) for each presentation aim.
   a. Share large quantities of data
   b. Illustrate changes over time
   c. Demonstrate the distribution of a phenomenon
   d. Explain a sequential process
   e. Compare pretest and posttest scores
7. Which of the following is recommended in formal scientific writing?
   a. Use abbreviations to condense the writing when possible.
   b. Write in present or future tense to improve clarity.
   c. Use third-person perspective for greater objectivity.
   d. Use passive voice to limit the risk of writing bias.
8. Using one direct quote per page of text is generally acceptable. True or false?
9. Which feature in your word processing software can help you determine if your writing is appropriate for your target audience?
   a. Flesch Reading Ease Test
   b. Thesaurus
   c. Document statistics
   d. Automatic table of contents

Answer key appears at the end of this text.

## NEXT STEPS

1. Rate your professional writing skills on a scale of 1 (being poor or with significant errors in writing style, grammar, and organization) to 10 (being excellent or at the level of a peer-reviewed journal article). Be honest with yourself and know that it takes much practice to become a skilled writer. Most students and allied health professionals fall somewhere in the midrange unless professional writing is part of their everyday tasks (such as those working in academia). Explore the strategies for improving your writing provided in this chapter. Which strategies will you use and why? What additional supports might be necessary for you to improve your writing?
2. If you need to draft a formal inquiry report, begin with the appropriate outline from Table 14-1. Then, bullet specific information you need to include under each topic or subsection. This should provide a solid outline to guide your writing.
3. Review a published inquiry, paying particular attention to the visual displays of data and results. How do the illustrations contribute to your understanding of the content? Were the most appropriate illustrations chosen, or do you have suggestions for alternative illustrations that would have increased your understanding? Be sure to justify your response.

## REFERENCES

American Psychological Association. (2020). *Publication manual of the American Psychological Association: The official guide to APA style* (7th ed.). Author.

Bognar, J., Corrigan, J., Bode, R., & Heinemann, A. (2000). Rating scale analysis of the agitated behavior scale. *Journal of Head Trauma Rehabilitation, 15*(1), 656-669. https://doi.org/10.1097/00001199-200002000-00005

Flesch, R. (1948). A new readability yardstick. *Journal of Applied Psychology, 32*(3), 221-233. https://doi.org/10.1037/h0057532

Friedman, C., & VanPuymbrouck, L. (2021). Impact of occupational therapy education on students' disability attitudes: A longitudinal study. *American Journal of Occupational Therapy, 75*(4), 7504180090. https://doi.org/10.5014/ajot.2021.047423

Kincaid, J. P., Fishburne, R. P., Rogers, R. L., & Chissom, B. S. (1975). *Derivation of new readability formulas (Automated Readability Index, Fog Count, and Flesch Reading Ease Formula) for Navy enlisted personnel. Research Branch Report 8-75.* Chief of Naval Technical Training: Naval Air Station Memphis.

Lape, J. (2008). Use of a multisensory environment to decrease negative behaviors in dementia patients. *Unpublished manuscript.* Chatham University.

Lee, A., & Lape, J. E. (2019). A cognitive, self-monitoring intervention for handwriting with second-grade students. *Journal of Occupational Therapy, Schools, & Early Intervention, 13*(2), 170–185. https://doi.org/10.1080/19411243.2019.1672604

Matthews, J., & Matthews, R. (2014). *Successful scientific writing: A step-by-step guide for the biological and medical sciences* (4th ed.). Cambridge University Press.

ReadabilityFormulas.com. (n.d.). *Readability formulas.* https://readabilityformulas.com

Rogers, C. (1959). A theory of therapy, personality, and interpersonal relationships as developed in the client-centered framework. In S. Koch (Ed.), *Psychology: A study of a science. Formulations of the person and the social context.* (Vol. 3, pp. 184–256). McGraw-Hill.

## ADDITIONAL WRITING RESOURCES

Belcher, W. L. (2019). *Writing your journal article in twelve weeks: A guide to academic publishing success* (2nd ed.). University of Chicago Press.

Glasman-Deal, H. (2021). *Science research writing for native and non-native speakers of English* (2nd ed.). World Scientific Publishing.

Hofmann, A. H. (2020). *Scientific writing and communication: Papers, proposals, and presentations* (4th ed.). Oxford University Press.

Hopper, V. F., Gale, C., Foote, R. C., & Griffith, B. W. (2010). *Essentials of English: A practical handbook covering all the rules of English grammar and writing style* (6th ed.). Barron's Educational Services.

Lindsay, D. (2020). *Scientific writing = Thinking in words* (2nd ed.). CSIRO Publishing.

Matthews, J., & Matthews, R. (2014). *Successful scientific writing: A step-by-step guide for the biological and medical sciences* (4th ed.). Cambridge University Press.

Mewburn, I., Firth, K., & Lehmann, S. (2019). *How to fix your academic writing trouble: A practical guide.* Open University Press.

Sternad, D., & Power, H. (2023). *The thesis writing survival guide: Research and write an academic thesis or dissertation with less stress.* Econcise.

Strunk, W., Jr., & White, E. B. (2022). *The elements of style* (4th ed.). Pearson.

Whitney, R. V., & Davis, C. A. (Eds.). (2013). *A writer's toolkit for occupational therapy and health care professionals: An insider's guide to writing, communicating, and getting published.* AOTA Press.

Chapter 15

# Presenting Your Inquiry

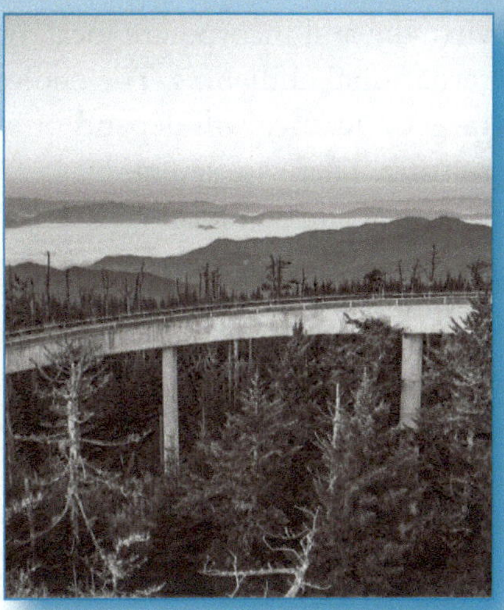

**LEARNING OUTCOMES**

*The information provided in this chapter will assist you to:*

15.1 Explain the scope of a presentation.
15.2 Outline reasons for formally presenting your inquiry.
15.3 Differentiate synchronous and asynchronous presentations.
15.4 Describe features of oral presentations and recommendations for presentation slide design.
15.5 Describe features of poster presentations and recommendations for poster design.
15.6 Identify key tasks to prepare for a presentation.
15.7 Conduct a professional presentation using appropriate etiquette.

## Scope of a Presentation

A **presentation** refers to a method of verbally communicating specific information to an audience to educate, inspire, persuade, or call others to action. This sharing of information is purposeful and tailored to the targeted audience. A presentation could be a lecture or a speech with little interaction from the audience. Conversely, a presentation might be very interactive, offering hands-on experiences for the attendees or the opportunity to engage in lively discussions or question-and-answer periods. Greater audience participation may be more common in presentations that are part of short courses, workshops, demonstrations, or formal coursework with laboratory experiences. While all presentations use the spoken word to share information, many include visual aids, electronic media, or other equipment to enhance the experience for the audience further. This could include visual slides (for example, a PowerPoint presentation or a poster), virtual media (for example, videos, virtual polls, audio recordings, games, or other media), or other equipment (for example, therapeutic tools, art supplies, or materials specific to the topic). Reasons for presenting and several presentation options are discussed in this chapter.

## Why Present?

Presenting your research study or evidence-based practice project is an effective way to disseminate your inquiry methods and outcomes. Some places where you could share your work include an academic setting, a clinical site, a professional conference, a continuing education venue, or a community location. Your presentation could occur in person or

Kuwohi (formerly Clingman's Dome), Great Smoky Mountain National Park, Tennessee.

virtually and incorporate local, national, or even international audiences. The choice of venue and the target audience will depend on your goals for presenting. There are several reasons for presenting the methods and results of your inquiry:

- Helping others to understand your work
- Sharing your work with those not easily reached by other methods
- Networking and collaborating with other professionals who are interested in your topic
- Expanding your professional skills

First, presentations are used to translate the information in your detailed inquiry report so that others can easily understand it. Your audience may have little interest or skills for reading and understanding a lengthy report, but they might benefit from a tailored presentation with relevant information. In academic settings, presentations in formal coursework may allow students to succinctly summarize their work for other students, faculty within the discipline, or individuals within the university community and beyond. Conducting a master's or doctoral thesis can take months or even years, yet a successful presentation recaps the entire inquiry in significantly less time. Clinical presentations can be used to distribute inquiry results applicable to practice. These presentations might include an in-service, where treatment ideas are presented, discussed, and practiced. In addition, clinical presentations can address program development, with the aim of gaining support from supervisors and administrators for practice changes.

The second reason for presenting is to reach audiences that may otherwise be unavailable. Depending on the venue, these audiences could include fellow researchers, students, policymakers, administrators, or the general public. For example, if you conducted a research study on the effectiveness of massage on joint pain in geriatric clients, you would be unlikely to reach potential clients themselves by presenting at a national conference or publishing in a professional journal. Although there are definite benefits to each of these actions, they are not appropriate if your goal is to convey the information to geriatric clients. In this case, a presentation at a local senior center, hospital, or gym might be more fitting. Getting the word out about your inquiry can allow others to use the information in practice (where applicable) or to design and conduct future inquiries.

Third, presentations at professional conferences or continuing education venues allow you to share your knowledge with other professionals interested in your topic. This is an excellent way to network, collaborate, and advance the science of your discipline. The professional exchanges that occur at professional or discipline-specific conferences can lead to increased knowledge for you as well as your attendees. These professional connections can lead to other collaborative projects, publications, and friendships!

Finally, for some, presentations can be used to hone public speaking skills, to accrue required continuing education units for licensure or certification, or to develop a professional profile worthy of promotion. Being able to clearly articulate details about your inquiry and field questions from various audiences are worthy skills for any allied health professional. Moreover, adding multiple presentations to your resume emphasizes your commitment to your professional development and the advancement of your profession. Let us begin by discussing two broad categories of presentations—synchronous and asynchronous.

### TIPS & INSPIRATION

- At this point, if you are not an experienced presenter, you may get nervous at even the thought of being in front of an audience presenting. Some degree of public speaking jitters is quite normal. Take a few deep breaths, maintain your composure, and remember that you are an expert on your topic.
- Beginning with an informal presentation to a small group of individuals and progressing to more formal or larger scale settings is the perfect way to hone your public speaking skills and promote expansion of your topic and your professional growth.

## Synchronous Versus Asynchronous Presentations

A **synchronous presentation** is one in which the presenter and attendees are online or in the same physical location at the *same time*. An **asynchronous**

**presentation** refers to a presentation that is recorded and made available virtually so that attendees can access it whenever it is convenient for them. Synchronous presentations allow for greater collaboration between attendees and the presenter; questions can be answered immediately, and attendees may be more committed to the learning experience. However, synchronous presentations may be less convenient and pose challenges to accessibility. Asynchronous presentations, which offer great flexibility for presenters and attendees, tend to be highly focused on topic content with little emphasis on collaboration or support, so attendees must be self-disciplined. Therefore, synchronous presentations are most appropriate for sharing complex topics, networking, and collaboration, whereas asynchronous sessions are better suited for straightforward material when few questions are anticipated. The advantages and disadvantages of each are further delineated in Table 15-1.

Presentations can also occur in person (synchronous) or virtually (synchronous or asynchronous). The advantages of virtual presentations include being cost-effective (i.e., no travel expenses for the presenter or attendees) and convenient (i.e., ability to present or access information from most geographic locations and electronic devices), and the ability to reach larger, more diverse audiences. However, technological

**TABLE 15-1 ■ Synchronous Versus Asynchronous Presentations**

| | Synchronous Presentations | Asynchronous Presentations |
|---|---|---|
| **Advantages** | ■ Generally, a more immersive experience.<br>■ May involve hands-on learning.<br>■ Direct contact between presenter and attendees to clarify concepts and answer questions.<br>■ Presenter can gauge attendees' understanding and adjust the presentation as needed. | ■ Flexibility in scheduling—attendees can view the presentation at their convenience.<br>■ Attendees can control the pace. Increased time to reflect on the content before asking questions.<br>■ Increased accessibility—attendees could view the content repeatedly if needed. More accessibility features may be available for recorded virtual presentations.<br>■ The presenter has multiple opportunities to practice and record the content.<br>■ No travel is required for the presenter or attendees. |
| **Disadvantages** | ■ No flexibility in scheduling—attendees may not be available when the presentation is scheduled.<br>■ Accessibility challenges (for example, attendees may not be able to access the presentation after it occurs, or it may be difficult to enable closed-captioning for a live presentation).<br>■ May require travel for the presenter or attendees.<br>■ Requires greater planning and spontaneous decision-making of the presenter to keep the presentation on track.<br>■ For virtual presentations: Requires strong internet connection for attendees and the presenter, and the presenter must have strong skills in managing the virtual platform. | ■ Generally, a less immersive experience.<br>■ Lack of hands-on learning opportunities.<br>■ Limited connection between attendees and the presenter. The presenter cannot adjust the content to meet the needs of attendees.<br>■ Limited opportunities for attendees to ask questions.<br>■ Requires attendees to be self-motivated, disciplined, and manage distractions. |

malfunctions or difficulty navigating the technology may pose challenges for the presenter and attendees.

Presentation formats can include an oral presentation supplemented with visual media (such as a Prezi presentation) or a poster presentation. Both oral and poster presentations can occur synchronously or asynchronously, as well as in person or virtually. Because these two presentation formats (oral and poster) require distinctly different skills, they are discussed separately in this chapter.

## Oral Presentations

An **oral presentation** can follow a lecture format but may also include demonstrations of techniques or equipment, individual or group learning activities, role-playing, question-and-answer periods, interactive discussions or brainstorming, case studies, hands-on learning experiences, or any combination of these strategies. **Lectures** are formal oral presentations with little to no interaction between the presenter and the attendees. Although this one-way communication may limit comprehension of the material, lectures are commonly used with larger audiences when increased interaction is impractical, when the goal is to share straightforward information for which limited questions are anticipated, or when the presentation occurs asynchronously. Oral presentations may include short courses, workshops, or training sessions.

While presentations without interactive elements have their place, using interactive strategies within a presentation is preferred to promote understanding of the material being presented. Interactive strategies, such as demonstrations, discussions, or hands-on learning experiences, are most common in synchronous presentations. Interactive presentations tend to be less formal, and audiences are smaller and more engaged. Disadvantages of interactive presentations include more preparation time. Presenters must be prepared to field questions, give additional clarification when needed, and keep the presentation on track. With more interaction from the audience, a discussion or activity can quickly derail the presentation if the presenter is not skilled in adjusting or guiding the audience appropriately. Gauging the time for a presentation with interactive elements requires much more planning and practice.

### TIPS & INSPIRATION

- In addition to the interactive strategies mentioned here, consider using storytelling, case studies, or personal and real-life examples to bring life and passion to your presentation. These elements often help gain your audience's attention and establish a connection between you and the attendees.

### Visual Support for Oral Presentations

Handouts, presentation slides, or other visual or virtual media often accompany oral presentations. These visual elements should support or enhance the spoken word but should not take its place. Nothing is worse than a presentation in which the presenter reads directly from the handouts or slide presentation. **Handouts** may be provided to the audience for ease of note-taking or when you wish to reference detailed or complex elements that would be difficult to see on a slide or screen. Handouts, which are often shared electronically, are also an effective method for sharing your references and contact information, should attendees wish to learn more about the topic or have questions later.

During the presentation, you can share visuals that were developed ahead of time (such as presentation slides and other visual media), as well as those created as the presentation progresses (such as brainstorming ideas, responses to a poll, etc.). For in-person presentations, your computer screen is projected onto a large screen; for virtual presentations, you can use the screen share function in the video conferencing software (for example, Zoom or Microsoft Teams). Flip charts, chalkboards, whiteboards, or Smart boards are other options for generating lists, figures, and other clarifying visuals during the presentation. Additionally, virtual mediums such as podcasts, blogs, videos, gamification, and other immersive software and applications are increasingly used to improve learner engagement, inclusion, and knowledge acquisition (Haleem et al., 2022). These types of technology may be especially useful when explaining complex concepts or when increased interaction is deemed beneficial. In each case, you should carefully select the most appropriate technology for

**The Problem**

- Projected increase in elderly population through 2050 (US Census Bureau, 2008)
- An estimated 10 million baby boomers expected to develop dementia (Alzheimer's Association, 2008)
- Around 47% of nursing home residents have some form of dementia (US Department of Health & Human Services, 2009)
- Among the most common symptoms are mood and behavior changes (agitation, lethargy, wandering, etc.)
- Cost of managing behaviors is $183 billion per year, with increase to $1.1 trillion projected by 2050 (Alzheimer's Association, 2011)
- Typical management includes restraints, medications, behavior modification techniques
- Lack of awareness of the role of the sensory system in dementia patients

Figure 15-1 Presentation slide tailored to the presenter with too much text.

the aims of your presentation. If the visual media or technology is cumbersome, it may hinder your presentation instead of supporting it.

### Presentation Slide Design

Oral presentations supplemented with visual slides are the most common, with Microsoft PowerPoint ranking as the most popular presentation software since it is widely available and easy to use (Velarde, 2023). Although the purpose of any presentation software is to enhance the presentation, without effective slide construction, the presentation becomes boring, and the intended message may not be successfully conveyed to the audience. The slides should *supplement* what you have to say; however, many presenters make the mistake of trying to include everything they want to say on the slides (see Figure 15-1), but this creates a presentation devoid of spontaneity and interest. You should develop the slides with your audience in mind, and then create a separate set of notes for yourself to use as a guide during the actual presentation. See Figures 15-1 and 15-2 for a comparison of two presentation slides. The first slide (Figure 15-1) is constructed based on the presenter's needs and includes a significant amount of text. The second slide (Figure 15-2) is simplified and includes only guiding points that the presenter will expand upon during the presentation; this is the preferred layout.

**The Problem**

- Rise in elderly population
- Increased incidence of dementia
- Behavioral symptoms of dementia
- Costs associated with behavior management
- How behaviors are typically managed
- Limited awareness of the sensory system's role

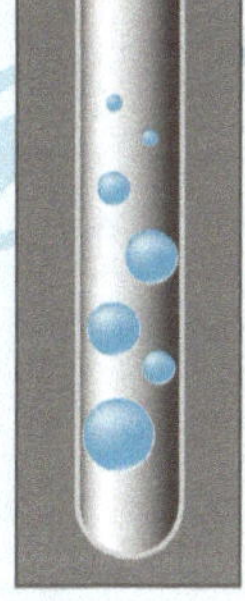

Figure 15-2 Presentation slide tailored to the audience with guiding points.

As these two examples show, content and design are important considerations. Regarding content, the prevailing belief is "Less is more." The presentation should not replicate your formal inquiry report; it should summarize only your inquiry's most relevant details and outcomes. Your time with the audience is limited, so it is critical to use the time efficiently. When considering whether to include a particular detail in the presentation, it is often effective to ask yourself, "So what?" If you cannot come up with a strong reason for including the information, then leave it out. Although some details are important to you, they may have no bearing on the audience's understanding of the inquiry. After you have decided on the slide content, the focus turns to slide design. Table 15-2 includes recommendations for designing your presentation slides.

**TABLE 15-2 ■ Recommendations for Presentation Slide Design**

| Feature | Recommendations |
|---|---|
| **Organization** | ■ Use a consistent theme and simple font (for example, Arial). Frequent changes can distract the audience.<br>■ Arrange slides in chronological order, beginning with a title slide and objectives, and then progress through the stages of your inquiry.<br>■ Present only one topic or idea per slide. |
| **Accessibility** | ■ Follow accessibility guidelines to ensure everyone can access the content. Use the software accessibility checker to assess your slides during development.<br>■ For example, enable closed captioning for video; use slide designs that ensure that fonts, colors, and images are accessible and function with screen readers and other accessibility tools; use alternative text for images. |
| **Visual appeal** | ■ Ensure the display is visually appealing and uncluttered.<br>■ Dark text on a lighter background is generally preferred. Very bright white or other vivid colors can be harsh on the eyes. |
| **Language** | ■ Know your audience; avoid technical jargon, terminology, and abbreviations unless your audience will understand them. |
| **Text** | ■ Use a minimum of 14- to 28-point font.<br>■ Headings should be at least 2 points larger than general content.<br>■ Avoid using all capitalized letters.<br>■ Reserve bold and italics for points that really need emphasis.<br>■ Use short phrases to summarize points rather than whole sentences. A general rule: no more than six words per line and six lines per slide.<br>■ Use graphics, photos, and figures in place of text when possible. If you include everything you intend to say on the slides, there is no need for the presentation. |
| **Tables** | ■ Limit use of tables as they may present accessibility challenges.<br>■ Simplify tables from your inquiry report if you plan to include them. A table with too many numbers will be difficult to read.<br>■ If you need to share a table in its original form, distribute it in your handouts and skip putting it into the presentation slides. |
| **Figures** | ■ Include a title and key (if needed).<br>■ Label all components and axes.<br>■ Choose colors wisely so that attendees can easily discern differences in the components and will understand the relationships or outcomes being illustrated.<br>■ Check the scale to eliminate distortion; the height-to-length ratio is usually 1:2. |
| **Images** | ■ Resolution should generally be set at 1024 × 768 pixels for good quality when the image is portrayed on a larger screen. Often images will look adequate on your computer screen but will be very grainy when enlarged. Testing your presentation on a larger screen ahead of time or zooming in on your computer screen to 200% to view each image are ways to ensure the images are of adequate quality. |
| **Visual effects and media** | ■ Limit use of animations. A good rule is to use no more than two types of animations in a presentation and avoid use on every slide. Animations should be used for a distinct purpose only (for example, to unveil the steps of your inquiry).<br>■ Insert only relevant video or audio clips of short duration (no greater than a few minutes). Disable autoplay so you can start the media when you are ready. |
| **References** | ■ Always include citations for information, tables, and figures in your presentation, where applicable. Include the author's name and the year; using a smaller font for this information is acceptable.<br>■ Include full references in your handout rather than on the presentation slides. |

### TIPS & INSPIRATION

- Constructing your slides is just one aspect of preparing for your presentation. Once you start rehearsing what you will say in the presentation, it may be necessary to modify your slides. This could include adding, removing, or reordering the content.
- Use the Rule of Three when considering what content to include in an oral presentation. People can easily remember three things, and as the number of items increases beyond that, the ability to remember decreases. Consider what three take-home messages you want the audience to get from your presentation. Designing your presentation and supporting visuals around these three points will increase your chances of success.
- While PowerPoint is the most popular presentation software, do not be afraid to experiment with some alternatives. These might include Google Slides, Prezi, Canva, Keynote, or Microsoft Sway, to name a few.

## Poster Presentations

**Poster presentations** involve the creation of an eye-catching vertical display, which typically includes a combination of text and figures or graphics portraying the methods and results of your inquiry. Synchronous poster presentations often occur at professional conferences and meetings, where many posters are displayed together in one location for a set period of time, and the poster authors are physically present to discuss their work. A poster session may also be conducted virtually, with presenters dispersed among breakout rooms within a video conferencing platform. This setup allows attendees to move in and out of the breakout rooms to interact with the presenters. A final option is an asynchronous poster session for which presenters make video recordings of their digital posters with brief audio narrations describing the inquiries; the recordings are then distributed to attendees to view at their leisure.

Poster presentations are an effective method for informing others about your inquiry, eliciting feedback before expanding your inquiry or seeking publication, networking with others interested in your topic, and promoting your own professional development (Plunkett, n.d.). In contrast to oral presentations, poster presentations allow you to connect with many attendees from more diverse backgrounds and interest areas individually. If you are a novice presenter, a poster presentation provides an excellent opportunity because the format is less formal and intimidating than an oral presentation.

### Poster Design

Many of the presentation slide design recommendations shared previously also apply to poster design. In fact, most professional posters are created using just one presentation slide, which is scaled appropriately for the finished size of the poster. A template (36" × 56") is included in the supplemental materials of this book, and some additional online poster templates you can customize to suit your needs are referenced at the end of this chapter.

Although using a single slide for poster construction is most common, another option is to create individual presentation slides for each section of the poster (for example, methods, results, discussion, and so on), which are then assembled on a larger board for an in-person presentation. The presentation venue most often dictates the style and size of your poster, and checking the specifications beforehand will avoid last-minute revisions to the poster's formatting or a stressful situation when you arrive at the presentation site.

The poster is commonly organized into multiple sections that summarize different phases of your inquiry. For research studies, sections should consist of the introduction, literature review, methods, results, limitations, and implications of results. For evidence-based practice projects, sections include the background with details about the setting, the literature review, project design, results, and implications of the results, including the project's significance to the profession or practice area. Each section can be customized to suit your needs and any requirements of the presentation venue. The key elements of a professional poster and the recommended content are summarized in Table 15-3.

**TABLE 15-3 ■ Key Elements of a Professional Poster**

| Key Element | Recommended Content |
|---|---|
| Title | ■ Concise inquiry title.<br>■ Author(s) names with credentials and affiliation (school or place of employment). |
| Introduction | ■ Brief problem description that led to the inquiry.<br>■ Rationale for the inquiry—may include statistics or visuals that illustrate the need for the inquiry.<br>■ Description of the inquiry setting (for evidence-based practice projects).<br>■ Relevant literature reviewed (for research studies). |
| Literature review | ■ Summary of existing literature on the topic.<br>■ It is common to review the number of studies and to describe the portfolio in terms of levels of evidence and common themes (evidence-based practice only). |
| Methods or project design | ■ Summary of the inquiry steps; may be outlined in a numbered list, a table, or a figure.<br>■ For research, this section is titled *Methods*. For evidence-based practice projects, it is more commonly titled *Project Design*. |
| Results | ■ Primary findings of the inquiry.<br>■ Frequently includes tables, graphs, or other figures to illustrate the results. |
| Limitations | ■ Brief review of limitations that may have impacted results.<br>■ Limitations may include those related to inquiry design, data collection tools, subjects/participants, or the researcher or evidence-based practitioner.<br>■ This section is often omitted for evidence-based practice projects. |
| Implications of results | ■ Compares the inquiry results to existing literature.<br>■ Outlines implications of the results for future practice or research.<br>■ The significance of the inquiry to the profession or area of practice is often incorporated for evidence-based practice projects. |

After selecting a poster template and determining the key elements and content to be included, attention must be given to the visual layout and design. Your poster should be a striking visual representation of your inquiry rather than a duplication of your inquiry report. "Many people find it helpful to view the poster-writing process not as trying to condense a paper but rather as expanding and enriching the abstract" (Matthews & Matthews, 2014, p. 232).

A quality poster includes a balance of text and graphics, a visually pleasing layout and color scheme, and adequate information about the inquiry, such that it can be understood, even if the author is not present. Consolidating text and using photographs, tables, and figures in place of text, where possible, can add visual interest and attract more viewers. Moreover, a three-column format works best, and the material should flow from top to bottom and left to right. Attendees will be most interested in the results and implications of them, so avoid excessive detail about the background, literature, and methods. Table 15-4 provides additional recommendations for poster design, and Figure 15-3 shows an example of a professional poster.

## TIPS & INSPIRATION

- Drafting your professional poster can be a welcome, creative task after completing large amounts of professional writing required for your formal inquiry report or publication. Downloading a poster template and experimenting with colors and design is a great first step.

## TABLE 15-4 ■ Recommendations for Professional Poster Design

| Feature | Recommendations |
|---|---|
| Visual appeal | ■ Use a consistent theme and font.<br>■ Information should flow from top to bottom and left to right.<br>■ Avoid photographs as background. Instead, use photographs on the poster to illustrate a point or to add visual interest.<br>■ Format section headings to emphasize them and guide attendees from one section to the next in a logical progression. Use thin borders around each section heading and a light-colored background to highlight the different sections or to group sections together if necessary.<br>■ Balance text and graphics. Placing all the graphics on one side of the poster will create visual imbalance.<br>■ Strive for an uncluttered poster with sufficient white space to improve flow and balance. Some suggest as much as 50% blank space (Matthews & Matthews, 2014, p. 233).<br>■ Limit text. Use short phrases to summarize points rather than whole sentences. Use graphics, photos, and figures in place of text when possible. |
| Text | ■ Use a minimum of 28- to 36-point font for all content; 48-point font for section headings, author(s) names, and affiliations; and 72-point font for the title.<br>■ Dark text on a lighter background is preferred. Very bright white or other vivid colors can be harsh on the eyes.<br>■ Content should be readable from 4 feet away (if presenting in person).<br>■ Choose a simple font (e.g., Arial), as more complex fonts are difficult to read from a distance.<br>■ Avoid use of all capital letters.<br>■ Reserve bold and italics for points that really need emphasis.<br>■ Keep headings centered; keep content text justified. |
| Tables | ■ Simplify tables from your inquiry report if you plan to include them on the poster. A table with too many numbers will be difficult to read.<br>■ Use a minimum of 28-point font for all tables. |
| Graphs and figures | ■ Include a title and key; label all components and axes.<br>■ Choose colors wisely so that attendees can easily discern differences in the components, or understand the relationships or outcomes being illustrated.<br>■ Check the scale to eliminate distortion; the height-to-length ratio is usually 1:2.<br>■ Use a minimum of 28-point font for all graphs. |
| Images | ■ Resolution should generally be set at 1024 × 768 pixels for good quality when the image is enlarged. Often, images will look adequate on your computer screen but will be very grainy when enlarged. Viewing your poster on a large screen or zooming in on your computer screen to 200% to view each image are ways to ensure images are of adequate quality.<br>■ Be aware that images copied and pasted from the internet are usually of poor quality when enlarged.<br>■ Use photos you have taken yourself or ones in the public domain to avoid copyright infringement.<br>■ Obtain informed consent if you use photos of subjects or participants. |
| References | ■ Always include references, where applicable. Include the author's name and the year; using a smaller font for this information is acceptable.<br>■ Include full references on a handout. |
| Handouts | Craft a one-page handout on your inquiry that can be offered to interested attendees. Many venues now require you to upload your handout to a central repository to make it electronically available to attendees. Handout options include the following:<br>■ A miniature reproduction of your poster on one page, and your key references or other relevant information on the reverse side.<br>■ The abstract on one page, and key references or other relevant information on the reverse side.<br>■ A handout with bullet points highlighting key elements of your inquiry. You may also want to include a graph or chart depicting the results.<br>■ Regardless of what format you choose, be sure to include your name and contact information. |

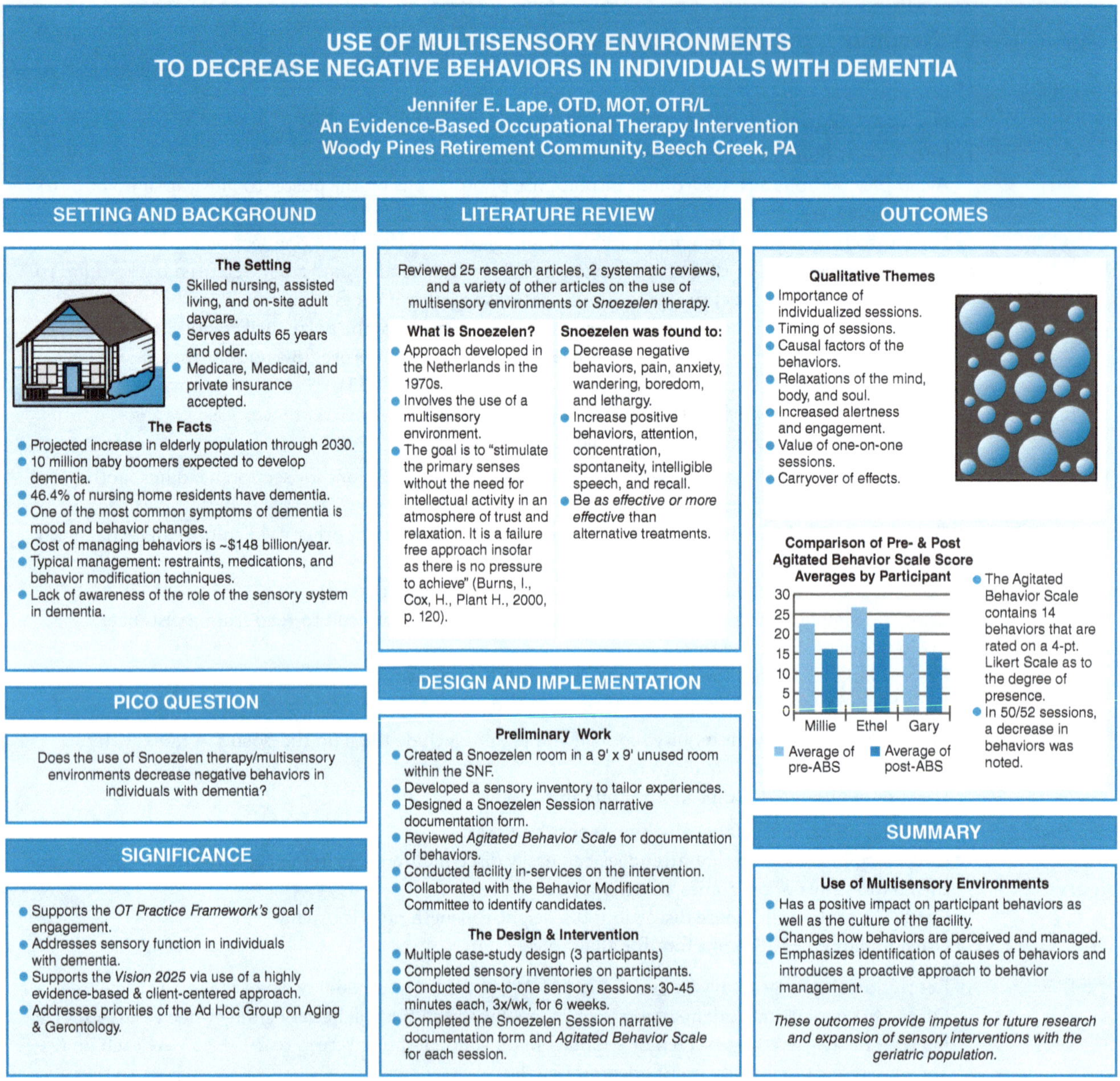

# USE OF MULTISENSORY ENVIRONMENTS TO DECREASE NEGATIVE BEHAVIORS IN INDIVIDUALS WITH DEMENTIA

Jennifer E. Lape, OTD, MOT, OTR/L
An Evidence-Based Occupational Therapy Intervention
Woody Pines Retirement Community, Beech Creek, PA

## SETTING AND BACKGROUND

**The Setting**

- Skilled nursing, assisted living, and on-site adult daycare.
- Serves adults 65 years and older.
- Medicare, Medicaid, and private insurance accepted.

**The Facts**

- Projected increase in elderly population through 2030.
- 10 million baby boomers expected to develop dementia.
- 46.4% of nursing home residents have dementia.
- One of the most common symptoms of dementia is mood and behavior changes.
- Cost of managing behaviors is ~$148 billion/year.
- Typical management: restraints, medications, and behavior modification techniques.
- Lack of awareness of the role of the sensory system in dementia.

## PICO QUESTION

Does the use of Snoezelen therapy/multisensory environments decrease negative behaviors in individuals with dementia?

## SIGNIFICANCE

- Supports the *OT Practice Framework's* goal of engagement.
- Addresses sensory function in individuals with dementia.
- Supports the *Vision 2025* via use of a highly evidence-based & client-centered approach.
- Addresses priorities of the Ad Hoc Group on Aging & Gerontology.

## LITERATURE REVIEW

Reviewed 25 research articles, 2 systematic reviews, and a variety of other articles on the use of multisensory environments or *Snoezelen* therapy.

**What is Snoezelen?**

- Approach developed in the Netherlands in the 1970s.
- Involves the use of a multisensory environment.
- The goal is to "stimulate the primary senses without the need for intellectual activity in an atmosphere of trust and relaxation. It is a failure free approach insofar as there is no pressure to achieve" (Burns, I., Cox, H., Plant H., 2000, p. 120).

**Snoezelen was found to:**

- Decrease negative behaviors, pain, anxiety, wandering, boredom, and lethargy.
- Increase positive behaviors, attention, concentration, spontaneity, intelligible speech, and recall.
- Be *as effective or more effective* than alternative treatments.

## DESIGN AND IMPLEMENTATION

**Preliminary Work**

- Created a Snoezelen room in a 9' x 9' unused room within the SNF.
- Developed a sensory inventory to tailor experiences.
- Designed a Snoezelen Session narrative documentation form.
- Reviewed *Agitated Behavior Scale* for documentation of behaviors.
- Conducted facility in-services on the intervention.
- Collaborated with the Behavior Modification Committee to identify candidates.

**The Design & Intervention**

- Multiple case-study design (3 participants)
- Completed sensory inventories on participants.
- Conducted one-to-one sensory sessions: 30-45 minutes each, 3x/wk, for 6 weeks.
- Completed the Snoezelen Session narrative documentation form and *Agitated Behavior Scale* for each session.

## OUTCOMES

**Qualitative Themes**

- Importance of individualized sessions.
- Timing of sessions.
- Causal factors of the behaviors.
- Relaxations of the mind, body, and soul.
- Increased alertness and engagement.
- Value of one-on-one sessions.
- Carryover of effects.

**Comparison of Pre- & Post Agitated Behavior Scale Score Averages by Participant**

30 25 20 15 10 5 0
Millie Ethel Gary
Average of pre-ABS Average of post-ABS

- The Agitated Behavior Scale contains 14 behaviors that are rated on a 4-pt. Likert Scale as to the degree of presence.
- In 50/52 sessions, a decrease in behaviors was noted.

## SUMMARY

**Use of Multisensory Environments**

- Has a positive impact on participant behaviors as well as the culture of the facility.
- Changes how behaviors are perceived and managed.
- Emphasizes identification of causes of behaviors and introduces a proactive approach to behavior management.

*These outcomes provide impetus for future research and expansion of sensory interventions with the geriatric population.*

Figure 15-3 Example of a professional poster.

## Printing and Transporting the Poster

If your poster presentation will occur synchronously at a professional conference or another in-person venue, printing and transporting your poster are usually necessary. Because of their size, posters require a specialized printer. Many local print shops or office stores can print them, as can various online sites. The advantage of online sites is that you can upload your poster from home, and they can usually e-mail you a proof of the poster before they print it. Posters can be printed on an array of paper or fabrics with varying quality and finishes, depending on personal preference or the specifications of your institution or conference. Scoping out printing options in advance will allow you to determine the best choice for your needs and ensure adequate turnaround time.

There are various ways to transport your poster to the presentation site. Posters printed on paper are usually rolled up and transported in a carrying case, ranging from more expensive options with shoulder straps to less expensive cardboard tubes. If traveling by air, you must check with the airline to determine if you can take the poster as a carry-on item. From experience, some airlines will permit this free of charge, whereas others charge additional fees. If you must pay a fee, consider coordinating poster transport with others in your area presenting posters at the same venue. Multiple posters can be placed in one carrying case, and presenters can share the expense. Another popular and convenient option is to have your poster printed on fabric, eliminating the need for a poster tube since you can easily fold the poster and place it in your carry-on or suitcase. Still other options include shipping your poster to the hotel ahead of time or arranging to have it printed near the conference site.

## Presentation Preparation

In addition to designing your visual aids, preparation for a presentation includes choosing a presentation venue and format, submitting your presentation proposal (if applicable), and practicing what you will say. Each of these tasks is discussed in further detail.

### Choosing a Presentation Venue and Format

If your presentation is required for formal coursework or a clinical affiliation, your course instructor or site supervisor will likely dictate the presentation venue and format. For example, you may be required to complete a poster presentation at a campus-wide research symposium. In other instances, you may be free to choose the presentation venue and format. Asking yourself these questions can help you select the best presentation option for your goals and skills:

1. **What are your goals for presenting?** For example, if you aim to connect with others in your discipline who are interested in future collaborations on your topic, a professional discipline-specific conference would likely be the best choice.
2. **Who is your target audience?** Ensure the chosen venue and presentation format are conducive to your target audience. For example, if your inquiry investigated the effectiveness of strategies to promote developmental milestones in young children, and you want to share this information with parents of young children, you might consider presenting in person at a local day-care center and using demonstration and hands-on activities to ensure parents' ability to apply the information. Know your audience and their unique needs so you can select the presentation format, visual supports, and accessibility features necessary to effectively share your information.
3. **What content do you want to share?** The most appropriate venue and format can vary based on the content you intend to share. Content at professional venues tends to be focused on inquiry methods and results or on improving the clinical skills of other professionals. Content at clinical or community-based sites may be less formal and presented at a level appropriate for comprehension by the public or those outside your discipline. Also, the volume of content should align with the presentation duration.
4. **What presentation options are available to you?** Different venues may include different presentation options. For example, one venue may only permit poster presentations, whereas another may have options for short courses, half- or full-day workshops, and poster presentations. The choice of in-person versus virtual presentations may be based on your geographic location and budget. Some venues also require submission and acceptance of a presentation proposal, which is discussed later in this chapter. Fully understanding your options is a foundational step in making an informed decision.
5. **Do you have prior experience with this topic and prior presentation experience?** If you have prior experience with the topic and/or presenting, an oral presentation such as a short course or a workshop may be an excellent choice to build on that prior experience. These presentation formats require greater skill and are generally longer presentations, which would allow you to share your depth of knowledge on the topic. Conversely, if you are a novice presenter or are new to your topic, a poster presentation permits one-on-one interaction with attendees and can be less intimidating than speaking to a large audience; this could build your confidence and skills for more advanced presentation options in the future.

TIPS & INSPIRATION

- If you have lots of content, a longer presentation, such as a conference course or a workshop, may be a good choice. A shorter session or a poster might be best if you have less content.

### Submitting a Presentation Proposal

As noted previously, most professional conferences require you to submit a proposal for your presentation to the conference committee or a group of blinded proposal reviewers. The conference committee typically puts out a call for proposals that includes specific guidelines for required content and the deadline for submission. You should check the submission guidelines for any conference you are considering and follow them explicitly; failure to submit the required information or not adhering to page or word limits could result in immediate rejection. Information typically requested includes the presentation title, chosen format from the available options (for example, short course, poster presentation), a presentation abstract, key references, and your professional affiliation and biography. Proposals are usually peer-reviewed and scored based on the quality, relevance, and innovation of the topic and alignment with the purpose of the conference. Top-scoring proposals are accepted for presentation, and lower-scoring presentations are rejected.

TIPS & INSPIRATION

- Each conference has limited presentation slots, so if you are unsuccessful initially, do not be afraid to try again. Many conferences provide feedback for rejected proposals, which you can use to strengthen your submission the next time.
- Poster presentations and shorter presentations (those 15–30 minutes long) are great choices if you are new to presenting at a professional conference.
- If you are a novice presenter, consider presenting *with* a colleague or faculty mentor who has more experience in the topic or presenting.

### Practicing

Regardless of the presentation venue or format, practicing allows you to become familiar with the content, prepare your notes, gauge how much time it will take to get through the material, and make any modifications that might be necessary. You want to be familiar enough with the content so that you do not need to read from your slides or notes, but not so familiar that it sounds like a memorized speech. You should be confident presenting your topic—after all, you know it better than anyone else! Practice can help to decrease nervousness, but some level of public speaking jitters is normal. During your practice sessions, you can fine-tune your notes to best support your presentation delivery.

A good oral presentation includes some level of spontaneity and entertainment; your skills in using these elements can be honed through practice. Spontaneity allows you to adjust the presentation as you go by offering additional examples or clarification as needed. In a synchronous presentation, watching your audience will let you know if they are engaged (and perhaps you should elaborate more on a point they are interested in) or if they are bored (in which case you may need to do something to gain their attention again). While you will not be able to read your audience in an asynchronous presentation, you can still infuse your presentation with examples, personal stories, or other media to enhance the more routine content. Finally, adding some element of entertainment to the presentation can help sustain the audience's attention; these elements can be effective in both synchronous and asynchronous presentations. Starting with a personal story, interactive activity, or another attention-getting technique, such as the use of an audience poll or a short video clip, can really enhance the presentation. Giving examples or adding humor (when appropriate) can further increase your connection with the audience and contribute to their understanding of the content.

For oral presentations, practicing can help you gauge how long it will take to cover your planned material. Without sufficient practice, you may run out of time to cover everything you prepared; as the presenter, you may appear rushed toward the end or need to skip important information to stay within the time limit. The opposite can also occur; you could finish the presentation too early, creating an awkward feeling about what to do with the excess time. Practicing your presentation several times allows you to judge when you need to add more content or remove some.

For synchronous poster presentations, attendees usually spend a few minutes scanning your poster before asking for a general verbal summary of your inquiry. This is your invitation to give them your brief elevator speech—usually no more than a few minutes' summary of your inquiry from start to finish. Brevity is a skill, and practicing this ahead of time will help you identify the most important points you want to share. This same information is recorded for asynchronous poster presentations, and you might need several takes until you are satisfied with your recording.

### TIPS & INSPIRATION

- A good rule of thumb is to practice your oral presentation no more than five times. This is usually sufficient practice to become familiar with the content and make any necessary adjustments to the presentation and your notes. More practice than this can lead to delivering a memorized speech devoid of spontaneity, which can disengage your audience.
- Audio or video record yourself presenting, or practice in front of a mirror to help you identify errors in speaking, posture, and hand gestures. Another alternative is to practice your presentation with friends or colleagues. Ask them to be brutally honest with you regarding the quality of the presentation and be willing to accept constructive criticism.

## Presentation Etiquette

You should be familiar with some basic etiquette for conducting effective presentations. For synchronous presentations, ensure you dress appropriately for the venue, and arrive at the presentation location or log in to the video conferencing platform early. Arriving early allows sufficient time to check technical components, such as your presentation slides or supporting videos, microphone, and speakers, and to address any issues proactively. This is also a good time to connect with the presentation moderator if one is provided. Many conferences use moderators, often volunteers, who are present during the presentations to assist with technology issues, monitor the time, introduce and thank the presenter, facilitate question-and-answer sessions, and record attendance for attendees. For in-person presentations, moderators might also help prepare the session room by ensuring the lighting, temperature, and seating arrangement are adequate.

For synchronous poster presentations, ensure you have an adequate number of handouts or upload your handouts to the conference's electronic platform. You should stand close to your poster (for in-person poster presentations—see Figure 15-4) or remain in the virtual presentation space (for virtual poster presentations) throughout the presentation session. Greet attendees professionally and give them time to view the poster on their own prior to offering your elevator speech on your inquiry. Then, be prepared to field additional questions on your inquiry. However, if you do not know the answer to a question, it is reasonable to share that you are unsure or have not explored the topic under discussion, rather than attempting to offer an answer that may be inaccurate. One of the purposes of presenting your poster is to network with others interested or experienced in your topic, and it is quite possible that you will

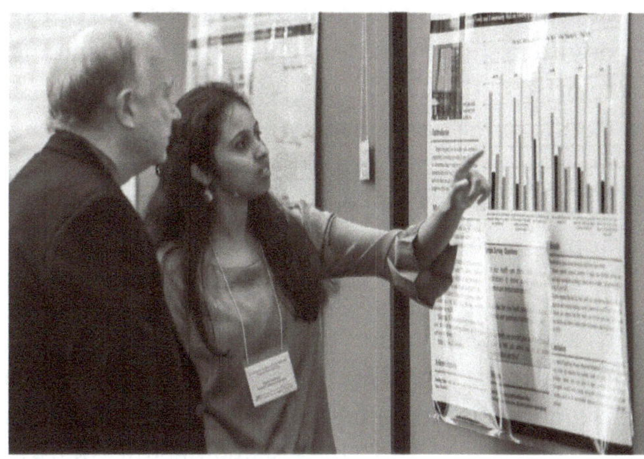

Figure 15-4 Example of a synchronous in-person poster presentation. *From The University of Texas Health Science Center at San Antonio, Texas.*

make valuable connections and learn something new in the process. After answering questions, it may be helpful to ask attendees if they understand or need more detail. Remember not to spend too much time with one attendee if others are waiting; connecting with all interested attendees is the goal, and socializing with friends or colleagues should be reserved for after-conference hours.

Additional etiquette for virtual presentations includes the following:

- Knowing how to operate the virtual platform (such as Zoom), including muting/unmuting yourself and others, turning your video on/off, enabling polls or setting up breakout rooms (if necessary), monitoring the chat feature, raising/lowering of attendees' hands, and sharing your screen.
- Muting yourself unless you are speaking and turning your camera off if you need to step away (for example, during a break in the presentation).
- Looking directly at your camera and speaking clearly.
- Minimizing distractions. Ensure you are in a quiet space. Do not have other tabs open on your computer or attempt to multitask, and silence all notifications on all electronic devices.
- Ensuring your background is professional and free of clutter. A blank wall behind you is preferred to a virtual or blurred background. Virtual or blurred backgrounds can result in distortions or glitches in your video, which can be distracting to others.
- Confirming your screen name reflects how you want to be addressed professionally. Include your credentials and preferred pronouns as appropriate.

Regardless of the presentation venue or format, with adequate attention to design, content, delivery, and adherence to proper etiquette, you can expect to make professional connections, advance your skills and knowledge, and share valuable information about your inquiry. Some additional resources for creating effective presentations are included in the reference list for this chapter.

## TIPS & INSPIRATION

- If you experience technical issues during a synchronous presentation, do not spend more than 5 to 10 minutes trying to resolve them. Doing so will decrease your ability to cover the planned content. In case of technical difficulties, be sure you have a backup plan in mind.
- Begin your presentation by telling your audience what you will tell them (review the objectives for the presentation); then tell them (give the presentation); then end by reminding them what you just told them (recap and summarize the presentation). Follow these three steps, regardless of whether the presentation is formal or informal, synchronous or asynchronous, or in person or virtual.
- For synchronous presentations, always allow time for questions and answers.
- For all presentations, be sure to provide attendees with your contact information should they have questions later.
- Presenting your work is an excellent way to inspire others to explore your topic through future research or evidence-based practice, or to make positive changes to their clinical practice. Just imagine the impact YOU could have!

## CHAPTER SUMMARY

1. Explain the scope of a presentation.
   - A presentation is a method of verbally communicating information to an audience to educate, inspire, persuade, or call others to action. This could include sharing information with little to no interaction with the audience or various interactive experiences and visual aids or other media.
2. Outline reasons for formally presenting your inquiry.
   - Reasons for presenting the methods and outcomes of your inquiry include helping others to understand your work, sharing your work with others who may not be reached via other methods, networking and collaborating with professionals interested in your topic, and expanding your professional skills.

3. Differentiate synchronous versus asynchronous presentations.
   - Synchronous presentations involve the presenter and attendees being online or in the same physical location at the *same time.*
   - Asynchronous presentations refer to presentations that are recorded and made available virtually so that attendees can access them whenever convenient.
   - Table 15-1 summarizes the advantages and disadvantages of synchronous versus asynchronous presentations.
4. Describe features of oral presentation and recommendations for presentation slide design.
   - Oral presentations can follow a lecture format or involve more interactive strategies and visual support, including presentation slides. Oral presentations often take the form of short courses, workshops, or training sessions. Handouts are often provided for oral presentations for ease of note-taking, or when you want to reference more detailed figures or concepts.
   - Presentation slides should serve as a guide for the presentation with only the most relevant details included. Slides should be visually appealing, uncluttered, and tailored to your audience. Table 15-2 lists additional recommendations for presentation slide design.
5. Describe features of poster presentations and recommendations for poster design.
   - Poster presentations involve an eye-catching, balanced display of text and graphics to portray the methods and results of an inquiry. Typically, a poster is available for viewing while the author is present so that attendees can ask questions. A poster presentation is less formal than an oral presentation and provides an excellent opportunity to network with others.
   - A poster consists of multiple sections summarizing phases of an inquiry, including the introduction, literature review, methods/project design, results, limitations, and implications of the results. Sections may vary depending on the venue and whether a research study or evidence-based project is the presentation's focus. Table 15-3 provides additional guidance regarding poster content.
   - Recommendations for poster design include using a three-column format, arranging content from top to bottom and left to right, and using clear, concise text and simplified high-quality graphics. Table 15-4 provides additional guidance regarding professional poster design.
6. Identify key tasks to prepare for a presentation.
   - The first task is choosing a presentation venue and format. Important considerations in making these decisions include your goals for presenting, your target audience, the content you wish to share, the options available, and your prior experience with your topic and with presenting.
   - The second task is submitting a presentation proposal, if applicable. This involves carefully examining the submission guidelines for your chosen venue and constructing a relevant quality proposal that aligns with the conference's purpose by the deadline. Proposals are peer-reviewed, with top-scoring proposals being accepted for presentation.
   - The final task is practicing your presentation, which allows you to become familiar with the content, prepare your notes, gauge how much time it will take to get through the material, and make any modifications that might be necessary.
7. Conduct a professional presentation using appropriate etiquette.
   - Basic presentation etiquette includes dressing appropriately and arriving at the venue or logging into the presentation early to make final preparations and check technical components and equipment.
   - Etiquette for poster presentations includes staying with your poster for the duration of the session, having a sufficient supply of handouts or uploading your handout to a digital platform ahead of time, and being prepared to provide a brief elevator speech about your inquiry and field questions.
   - Additional etiquette for virtual presentations includes knowing how to operate the virtual platform, minimizing distractions, and presenting from a quiet, professional, uncluttered space.

## TEST YOUR KNOWLEDGE

1. Identify whether each advantage is related to a synchronous or an asynchronous presentation.
   a. More immersive experience
   b. Direct contact between attendees and presenter
   c. Attendees can control the pace of the presentation
   d. No travel required for attendees and presenter
   e. Can include hands-on learning
   f. Flexibility in scheduling

2. Presentation slides should contain all relevant information that will be shared during a presentation. True or false?
3. Which of the following is recommended when designing presentation slides?
   a. Remove citations to decrease visual clutter.
   b. Use animations on each slide to add visual interest.
   c. Use very bright colors to make your figures stand out.
   d. Present only one idea per slide.
4. Which of the following is recommended for poster design?
   a. Use images from the internet to ensure sufficient quality.
   b. Organize information from top to bottom and left to right.
   c. Use a minimum of 12-point font for content.
   d. Use darker backgrounds and lighter text for contrast.
5. The aim of your presentation is to share your inquiry methods and results with other professionals within your discipline. As part of the presentation, you intend to have attendees practice the inquiry intervention for later application in their practice. Which of the following would be the BEST presentation format?
   a. A synchronous poster presentation at a discipline-specific conference
   b. A synchronous oral presentation at an interdisciplinary conference
   c. An asynchronous presentation at a virtual healthcare conference
   d. A synchronous oral presentation at a discipline-specific conference
6. Practicing your presentation can help you become familiar with your content and prepare your speaking notes. True or false?
7. In a scholarly presentation, what is the MOST IMPORTANT consideration for effectively communicating with your targeted audience?
   a. Tailoring the content to the audience's knowledge and expertise
   b. Highlighting the results of the inquiry with limited methodological details
   c. Avoiding the use of visual aids to limit distractions
   d. Using informal language and humor to keep the audience engaged

Answer key appears at the end of this text.

## NEXT STEPS

1. Consider your inquiry topic, methods, and results. Outline the three main points you want your attendees to take away from your presentation and why they are most important. Consider how this information might impact your presentation venue and format.
2. Identify your target audience for your presentation, and then consider your presentation from their perspective. What would they most want to know? What presentation format aligns best with their needs? What presentation strategies and visual aids would help them most to understand the content?
3. Most presentation proposal submission guidelines require you to share your presentation title and an abbreviated abstract, typically not more than two or three sentences, that can be included in a conference program to advertise your presentation to attendees. Using a highly descriptive, catchy title and a succinct abstract increases the likelihood of getting your proposal accepted and may increase the number of people interested in your topic. Brainstorm some possible titles for your presentation and write a two- or three-sentence abstract. Share these with others for feedback.
4. Visual aids can enhance the delivery of a presentation. Use the recommendations from Table 15-2 (presentation slides) or Table 15-4 (poster) to create a rough draft of a visual aid for a presentation on your inquiry.

## REFERENCES

Haleem, A., Jacaid, M., Qadri, M. A., & Suman, R. (2022). Understanding the role of digital technologies in education: A review. *Sustainable Operations and Computers, 3*, 275–285. https://doi.org/10.1016/j.susoc.2022.05.004

Matthews, J., & Matthews, R. (2014). *Successful scientific writing: A step-by-step guide for the biological and medical sciences* (4th ed.). Cambridge University Press.

Plunkett, S. W. (n.d.). *Tips on poster presentations at professional conference.* Retrieved June 26, 2023, from https://www5.iasnr.org/wp-content/uploads/2022/10/Poster_Presentations_Tips.pdf

Velarde, O. (2023, May 18). *15 best presentation software for 2023 (full comparison guide).* Visme. https://visme.co/blog/best-presentation-software/#powerpoint

## ADDITIONAL RESOURCES

### Poster Templates

Various other templates are available online that you can customize to suit your needs; the links are included here and in the supplemental materials.

1. https://www.posterpresentations.com/free-poster-templates.html
2. https://www.posternerd.com/sciposters-templates
3. https://www.canva.com/posters/templates/research

### Resources for Creating Presentation Slides

Atkinson, C. (2018). *Beyond bullet points: Using PowerPoint to tell a persuasive story that gets results* (4th ed.). Pearson Education.

La Counte, S. (2019). *Getting started with Google slides: A practical guide to cloud-based presentations*. Self-published.

Laguna, I. (2023). *Declutter your slides: Creating clear and effective technical presentations*. Laguna Peralta Publishing.

Matthews, J., & Matthews, R. (2014). *Successful scientific writing: A step-by-step guide for the biological and medical sciences* (4th ed.). Cambridge University Press.

Thakur, A. J. (2023). *Tapping the power of PowerPoint for medical posters and presentations*. Springer.

### Resources for Creating Poster Presentations

Carter, M. (2021). *Designing science presentations: A visual guide to figures, papers, slides, posters, and more* (2nd ed.). Elsevier.

Erren, T. C., & Bourne, P. E. (2007). Ten simple rules for a good poster presentation. *PLoS Computational Biology, 3*(5), e102. https://doi.org/10.1371/journal.pcbi.0030102

Faulkes, Z. (2021). *Better posters: Plan, design, and present an academic poster*. Pelagic Publishing.

Zaumanis, M. (2022). *Scientific presentation skills: How to design effective research posters and deliver powerful academic presentations* (Book 3). Self-published.

### Resources for Creating Virtual Presentations

Allen, S. J., & Young, M. S. (2020). *Captovation: Online presentations by design*. Self-published.

Clay, C. (2019). *Great webinars: Interactive learning that is captivating, informative, and fun* (revised and updated ed.). Punchy Publishing.

### Presentation Resources

Hofmann, A. H. (2020). *Scientific writing and communication: Papers, proposals, and presentations* (4th ed.). Oxford University Press.

Reynolds, G. (2020). *Presentation Zen: Simple ideas on presentation design and delivery* (3rd ed.). Pearson Education.

Schreim, S. (2023). *Storytelling with charts—The full story: The ultimate playbook to master the art and science of captivating audiences by telling stories with data and framework charts*. SCAS.

# Chapter 16

# Publishing Your Inquiry

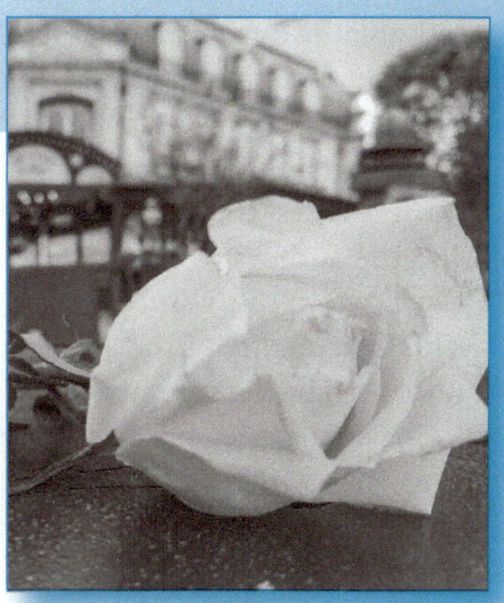

LEARNING OUTCOMES

*The information provided in this chapter will assist you to:*

16.1 Outline reasons for formally publishing your inquiry.

16.2 Differentiate peer-reviewed and non–peer-reviewed publications, and open-access and closed-access journals.

16.3 Describe factors in choosing an appropriate target publication.

16.4 Use formatting guidelines to draft an article for your chosen target publication.

16.5 Explain potential responses to your article submission and how to respond to them.

## Why Publish?

Publishing can be time-consuming and even daunting, especially if you have not done it before. As such, this is often the point at which researchers and evidence-based practitioners lose momentum. However, sharing your inquiry findings in a written publication increases the long-term accessibility of your work to those who are interested in your topic. It is customary to present your work first, which allows you to gain feedback from colleagues interested in the topic, which you can incorporate into your publication. Additional benefits to publishing may include the following:

- Sharing knowledge gained to allow informed decision-making by professionals and consumers
- Inspiring fellow researchers or practitioners to build on your work
- Enabling others to avoid pitfalls noted in your inquiry in their future endeavors
- Networking and collaborating with others in your discipline or those interested in your topic
- Expanding your professional research and writing skills
- Building your resume for future employment or funding opportunities
- Contributing to the body of literature in your discipline or topic area

## Peer-Reviewed Versus Non–Peer-Reviewed Publications

Generally, the two publication options for your inquiry are peer-reviewed and non–peer-reviewed publications. These are described in more detail in the next sections.

### Peer-Reviewed Publications

**Peer-reviewed publications** (sometimes called scholarly or refereed publications) are articles

France Pavilion, Orlando, Florida.

authored by one or more experts in a field or topic area and reviewed by other experts in the field or topic area to confirm each article's quality before acceptance for publication. To minimize biased reviews of the articles, the reviewers are usually unaware of who the authors of an article are when they are reviewing it. In this way, the reviewers must assess the value and quality of the article itself without being influenced by the reputation of the authors.

The publication process for peer-reviewed journals is rigorous, with multiple revisions required over long periods of time. Most peer-reviewed journals aim to disseminate quality research or evidence-based practice. Peer-reviewed journals are usually inappropriate for informational-type articles or articles geared toward the general public. Some features of peer-reviewed articles are as follows:

- Evidence of completion of a research study or formal evidence-based practice project. Keep in mind that some journals may only publish research, while others will consider high-quality evidence-based practice projects.
- Approval or exemption by an Institutional Review Board (IRB) for the inquiry being published. See Chapter 12 for additional information on the IRB process.
- Possible use of complex statistical methods, graphs, or tables to support outcomes.
- Highly structured format, with required sections specified in the publication's author guidelines.
- Inclusion of multiple references from other scientific or professional journals to support the work.
- Use of complex professional language and terms that may not be easily understood by those outside the profession or unfamiliar with the topic.

Peer-reviewed journals typically appear very plain, with black-and-white photos or illustrations and little or no advertisements; many peer-reviewed journals publish exclusively online. Publication in these journals is highly respected among academicians, who are often required to publish for continued employment. Others may seek publication in peer-reviewed journals to gain professional respect and recognition for future employment or funding opportunities.

Some examples of peer-reviewed journals are *The International Journal of Telerehabilitation, The British Journal of Occupational Therapy, The American Journal of Physical Medicine & Rehabilitation,* the *Journal of Clinical Nursing,* and the *Journal of Public Health,* to name a few. Most professional organizations publish discipline-specific peer-reviewed journals, and there are many interdisciplinary or subject-specific journals that you might consider. A list of some common health-related journals is included in Appendix D to get you started.

### Closed-Access Versus Open-Access Journals

If you pursue a peer-reviewed publication, an additional consideration is whether you will target a closed- or open-access journal. A **closed-access journal** is a traditional subscription-based journal, meaning that individual readers or institutions must pay a subscription fee to access articles within the journal. Some examples of closed-access journals are *The American Journal of Occupational Therapy, PTJ: Physical Therapy & Rehabilitation Journal,* and the *Journal of Allied Health.* Fees can range from an annual membership that provides full access to the journal to an individual fee to access a single article. If you are affiliated with a medical or academic institution, you likely have access to many subscription-based journals through the institution's library. Similarly, if you belong to a professional discipline-specific organization, your membership likely affords you access to the organization's publications. While closed-access journals are solid choices for publication, it is important to consider that only individuals who have access to the journal will have access to your article.

A viable alternative is an **open-access journal**, which means the publication and all the articles within it are freely available to readers, institutions, and the public. The benefits of publishing in an open-access journal include a wider audience since readers do not need a subscription, and the potential for greater impact since this model allows access to current evidence in a timely manner; this can be especially important to practitioners with limited financial resources. At this point, you might think open-access publishing sounds like a great choice. However, since the reader does not pay a subscription, the publication costs are covered in other ways, including author publication fees, grants, or institutional or association budgets. Open-access journals are also sometimes referred to as **pay-to-publish journals**, but there is no guarantee of publication, and articles submitted still undergo rigorous review. Authors submitting to pay-to-publish journals may have to pay review costs as well as per-page or per-article charges if the article is accepted. You should scope out the fees before deciding on an open-access journal and avoid submission if you disagree with the terms. Some examples of open-access journals are the *Journal of Athletic Training, The Internet Journal of Allied Health Sciences and Practice,* and *The Open Journal of Occupational Therapy.*

#### TIPS & INSPIRATION

- Discuss peer-reviewed publication options with others in your discipline or those who are knowledgeable about your topic. If you can connect with someone who has personal experience with a journal (perhaps they have reviewed articles for the journal or published in the journal themselves), they can provide valuable insight into the process and whether the journal might be a suitable choice for you.
- If you aim to publish in an open-access journal, many viable options do not charge author publication fees (they subsidize their costs in other ways) or charge nominal fees of $300 or less. Avoid options that charge significantly more, as this may signify predatory journals that place profits above the quality of their review process and information published (Memon, 2019).

### Non-Peer-Reviewed Publications

**Non-peer-reviewed publications** include magazines, books, pamphlets, or other works that publish articles intended to provide more general information. Authors are usually professionals with some advanced experience in the subject area; however, conducting research or evidence-based practice in the subject area is usually not required. In contrast to peer-reviewed articles, non-peer-reviewed articles are typically reviewed only by the editor(s) of the publication, who are not necessarily experts in the field or subject area. Non-peer-reviewed articles must be appraised by the individual readers to determine the quality and applicability of the information contained within them.

The publication process for non-peer-reviewed publications is less demanding than that of peer-reviewed ones, although some revisions are usually necessary. Non-peer-reviewed articles are less scientific, intended for general audiences, and aim to publicize information on a focused topic. Other features of non-peer-reviewed articles are as follows:

- Less structured organization, with sections designed and arranged by the authors
- Provision of news or other general information to the public or other professionals
- Possible use of anecdotal evidence, photographs, simplified charts and figures, or personal or procedural narratives to illustrate the main points of the article
- Limited to no inclusion of references from other sources to support the work
- Use of layperson's terminology that is easily understood by those outside the profession or unfamiliar with the topic

While non-peer-reviewed publications have distinct benefits, peer-reviewed ones usually require more time and skill and are often the aim when a formal inquiry has taken place. For this reason, this chapter focuses primarily on peer-reviewed publications, though some content may also apply to non-peer-reviewed publications.

## Choosing a Target Publication

Once you have decided to pursue publication, the next step is choosing your target journal or other publication. Many factors weigh into this decision:

- What publication opportunities exist related to your topic?
- What are your publishing goals? Do you have publication experience?
- Who is your target audience?
- What is your key argument?
- Are the target publication's aims and author guidelines congruent with your topic?

Although each factor is discussed separately here, you must consider them collectively. It is reasonable to rank your top two to three publication options so that you have a backup plan if your first choice does not accept your article. Also, know that it is unethical to submit your article to more than one journal simultaneously. You can submit your article to your first-choice journal, and if the article is rejected, then, and only then, is it permissible to submit it to another publication.

## Publication Opportunities

There are usually multiple publication opportunities within a single inquiry. Boxes 16-1 and 16-2 show examples of a research study and an evidence-based practice project, respectively, with some potential publication avenues for each. Although these examples are not exhaustive, they illustrate the variety of opportunities. As illustrated in these examples, publishing multiple articles related to your inquiry is possible, though each article should have a distinct

### BOX 16-1 ■ Example Research Study and Potential Publication Opportunities

A research study was conducted by three physical therapy students and their faculty advisor to explore the impact of a balance training program on the incidence of falls within one senior retirement community. Seventy-six participants were randomized into two study groups: an experimental group that participated in the balance training program three times per week for 2 months and a control group that did not participate in the balance training program in the initial phase of the study. Results indicate that the experimental group had significantly fewer falls than the control group during the study. Publication opportunities might include the following:

- Publishing in a professional peer-reviewed physical therapy journal to share the study's outcomes with others in the field who might want to expand on this research or apply the results to their practice
- Writing an article for a discipline-specific magazine on the steps involved in setting up a balance training program similar to that used by the researchers
- Composing a piece for a senior citizens' newsletter on the risk factors for falls, how physical therapy can help, and how to get more information or find a physical therapist in the area

### BOX 16-2 ■ Example Evidence-Based Practice Project and Potential Publication Opportunities

A school-based occupational therapist interested in the effectiveness of sensory-based activities to improve attention and emotional regulation in 5-year-olds with sensory-processing difficulties gathered and appraised 13 research articles on the use of this intervention with similar populations. Then, he designed and implemented an evidence-based program that incorporated findings from the research; his prior knowledge and experiences with sensory-based treatments; and the goals, values, and circumstances of the 5-year-olds on his caseload. He collected data during the treatments to determine changes in the children's attention and emotional regulation after participating in this new program and whether his outcomes matched the literature he reviewed. Publication opportunities might include the following:

- Publishing in a discipline-specific journal or magazine (peer-reviewed or non–peer-reviewed) to share his experiences or the procedures he used in conducting the evidence-based project as well as the outcomes from the project
- Writing an article for a parenting magazine on how to recognize signs of sensory-processing difficulties, tips for managing behaviors, and where to locate additional resources if needed
- Publishing in an education journal or magazine focusing on collaboration between teachers and other professionals to address sensory-processing difficulties with children

purpose and content. As noted previously, submitting the same article to multiple publications simultaneously is never appropriate.

## Defining Your Publishing Goals

Your personal and professional goals and publishing experience can impact your publication decisions. For faculty in academic institutions or those intending to pursue an academic career, peer-reviewed publications are often the best choice because these are typically required for promotion and tenure. This is also a suitable option to build your expertise in the topic and connect with other experts. For clinicians wanting to share information about their services with consumers, non-peer-reviewed publications, which are less formal and more readily accessible to those outside the field, are a great alternative. Likewise, if you aim to share direct clinical application of your inquiry with practitioners (such as how to set up a similar program or challenges to consider in using an intervention), a non-peer-reviewed, discipline-specific publication that uses layperson's descriptions might best accomplish this goal.

If you are a student or new to publishing, you might consider publishing with one or more experienced coauthors. Authorship may be attributed to those involved in the inquiry design, implementation, data analysis, and/or actual article writing (American Psychological Association [APA], 2022). It is important to credit those who have contributed significantly to the work in some way; this might include faculty advisors, individuals at the inquiry site, colleagues, peers, or others. Sharing authorship can strengthen the quality of your article and may lead to future collaborative inquiries and professional development. The order of authorship is customarily determined by the level of contribution to the work, with authors ordered from the greatest to the least contribution.

### TIPS & INSPIRATION

- Write down your reasons for publishing. If you are in a situation in which you are required to pursue publication, consider the benefits if the article gets published. Identifying your motivation or the benefits can help you define your publishing goals and ensure your decisions align with your goals.
- Discuss coauthorship early in the publication process. Identify each person's role, negotiate the authorship order as necessary, and establish collaboration methods. Using shared documents is a common way to allow multiple contributors and avoids the confusion resulting from multiple versions of a manuscript emailed back and forth. Also, if roles shift, the authorship order may need to be renegotiated.

## Identifying Your Audience

Identifying your potential audience can help you choose an appropriate publication and will usually dictate the approach and style of writing. For example, if you hope to reach consumers of your service, publishing in a discipline-specific, peer-reviewed journal is unlikely to be effective. Similarly, the general public may not easily understand the writing style and professional language of an article geared toward other professionals. Some publications are discipline-specific; others span multiple disciplines. If you choose an interdisciplinary publication, it will be important that the message and language appeal to those beyond your own discipline. Still other publications target specific groups of people, for example, those over the age of 65 or those caring for a child with disabilities. Identifying your audience is a key factor in choosing a publication.

## Outlining Your Key Argument

The **key argument** is the primary idea, supported with evidence, that you want to convey in your article (Belcher, 2019). Clarifying your key argument is an essential step before choosing a target publication. The key argument is often confused with the article's topic or the primary results, but a good key argument goes a step further to interpret those findings. In other words, why do the results matter? See Box 16-3 for an example comparing these differing elements.

Reducing your message to a single persuasive idea can be challenging, but this step is foundational in selecting a publication and organizing your first draft. You likely have a good argument if you can answer yes to the questions in Box 16-4.

**BOX 16-3 ■ Example Comparing a Topic, Primary Results, and Key Argument**

**Topic:** Use of multisensory environments with clients with dementia

**Primary results:** Negative behaviors were reduced in 96% of the participants who were clients with dementia after use of a multisensory environment.

**Key argument:** The use of multisensory environments for clients with dementia may be an effective nonpharmacological intervention to manage their negative behaviors and promote engagement in meaningful life activities.

*Note:* The argument should be directly stated within an article and substantiated by the inquiry results and prior research. For example, research on the benefits of nonpharmacological interventions (such as decreased healthcare costs, drug dependency, and side effects) and engagement in meaningful life tasks (such as the role in quality of life) can be discussed in conjunction with the inquiry's results. So, it is not just that negative behaviors decreased; instead, it is about why these results matter.

**TIPS & INSPIRATION**

- Drafting a concise, quality argument can take multiple attempts, so do not be discouraged. Writing down your argument and asking yourself, "So what?" can help you separate the meaningful from the unimportant.

**BOX 16-4 ■ Questions to Assess Your Argument**

- **Can someone disagree with your argument?** With a proper argument, individuals can rest on one side or the other of an issue; if you present a fact, disagreement is unlikely. In the example in Box 16-3, it would be difficult to argue with the primary findings (negative behaviors were reduced in 96% of the subjects) if the data support them. However, one could argue that using multisensory environments is not the most appropriate way to manage negative behaviors or promote engagement in meaningful tasks.
- **Does your data support your argument?** In other words, does your data logically lead to your interpretation of the findings? If it is too much of a stretch, your argument may be flawed and quickly refuted by readers. For example, if the primary results were a reduction in negative behaviors for only 10% of subjects, the key argument is not well substantiated.
- **Does your argument address a gap in the literature or a clinical problem (or both)?** Consider that readers will be most interested in your work if it significantly contributes to the literature on the topic. This means it should add some *new* information that was not previously known or understood; if your inquiry does not provide new information, no one will be interested in publishing or reading it.

## Publication's Aims and Author Guidelines

A **publication's aim** describes its purpose, including a summary of the topics covered, the types of articles published (for example, some journals only publish original research, while others also publish applied research or evidence-based practice projects), publishing options (such as open- or closed-access), and the peer review policy (if applicable as in the case of peer-reviewed publications). This information is typically found on a journal's website. Conducting a preliminary review of these details can help you determine if you should consider a journal further. Consider if your work aligns with the journal's purpose and is relevant to the journal's target audience. For example, if your goal is to publish an evidence-based practice project and a journal only accepts original research, this journal should be rejected. Likewise, if your inquiry is very specific to your discipline without application to other allied health professions, an interdisciplinary journal is likely inappropriate.

### TIPS & INSPIRATION

- Consider exploring journals in which articles from your literature review were published. This is an indication of interest in the topic and alignment with the journal's aims. However, be sure your work contributes something new or novel compared to prior articles. If you cannot make this distinction, there may be little interest in your article.
- Review some recently published articles from a journal you are considering to help you determine if it is a good fit for your work.

In addition to a publication's aims, **author guidelines**, also provided on the journal's website, outline the specific requirements for submitting your work. Author guidelines can include information about the writing style used by the publication (for example, APA style), page or word limits, and any requirements for photographs, tables, figures, and so forth. Some publications have distinct guidelines for different types of articles, meaning that the requirements vary depending on whether you are submitting a case study, an editorial, or original research, for example. Submission requirements, including the need to provide additional items such as a cover letter, author biography, conflict of interest declarations, copyright forms, or any associated publication or review fees, are also specified in the author guidelines.

It is essential to strictly adhere to the guidelines set forth by the chosen publication. Your work may be rejected simply because of improper formatting or failure to provide the necessary forms and information, regardless of the topic or quality of your work. Do not rely on past articles in a journal related to formatting or other requirements since author guidelines are frequently updated. Table 16-1 can help you evaluate if a journal's features align with your topic and publication goals. Identify the journal's details in the middle column and make your evaluation in the far right column.

**TABLE 16-1 ■ Journal Evaluation Tool**

***Journal Name:***

***Journal Website:***

| Journal Feature | Journal Details | Evaluation* |
|---|---|---|
| **Aim** | **State the journal's aim:** | **Aim aligns with your topic:**<br>☐ Yes ☐ No |
| **Audience**<br>*Check all that apply* | ☐ Discipline-specific ***within*** your discipline<br>☐ Discipline-specific ***outside*** your discipline<br>☐ Interdisciplinary<br>☐ General public<br>☐ Other specific population: ____________<br>☐ Local ☐ National ☐ International | **Journal audience aligns with your target audience:**<br>☐ Yes ☐ No |
| **Review process** | ☐ Peer-reviewed<br>☐ Non-peer-reviewed | **Review process aligns with your publication goals:**<br>☐ Yes ☐ No |
| **Access**<br>*Check all that apply* | ☐ Closed-access options<br>☐ Open-access options | **Access options align with your publication goals:**<br>☐ Yes ☐ No |

*Continued*

**TABLE 16-1 ■ Journal Evaluation Tool—cont'd**

***Journal Name:***

***Journal Website:***

| Journal Feature | Journal Details | Evaluation* |
|---|---|---|
| **Author fees** | ☐ None<br>☐ Membership to the organization sponsoring the journal (indicate fee if not already a member: ______)<br>☐ Pay-to-publish (indicate fees: ______________________) | **You have adequate funds for associated fees:**<br>☐ Yes ☐ No<br>☐ N/A (no fees) |
| **Writing style** | ☐ APA ☐ MLA ☐ AMA<br>☐ *Chicago Manual of Style*<br>☐ Other: ________________ | **You are familiar with the required writing style:**<br>☐ Yes ☐ No<br>☐ N/A (no required style) |
| **Page/word limits** | Describe any page or word limits: | **Page/word limits are reasonable given the scope of your work and publishing experience:**<br>☐ Yes ☐ No<br>☐ N/A (no limits) |
| **Impact factor** | ☐ >1<br>☐ 1.0 to 0.50<br>☐ <0.5 | **Impact factor is acceptable:**<br>☐ Yes ☐ No<br>☐ N/A (none available) |
| **Reputation**<br>*Check all that apply* | ☐ Publication >5 years<br>☐ Widely accepted in the discipline<br>☐ Published by a reputable organization or institution<br>☐ Reputable editorial board members<br>☐ Prior publication of quality inquiries<br>☐ Rigorous peer review process<br>☐ Specific quality reporting guidelines | **Reputation is acceptable:**<br>☐ Yes ☐ No |
| **Acceptance rate** | ☐ ≥20% ☐ <20% ☐ Unknown<br>☐ N/A | **Acceptance rate is acceptable:**<br>☐ Yes ☐ No<br>☐ N/A (unknown or N/A) |
| **Other favorable features** | List any other favorable features of journal (such as special issues, features, connections to editorial board, or incentives): | **Special features align your topic and aims:**<br>☐ Yes ☐ No<br>☐ N/A (No features) |

*Caution should be exercised in choosing a publication with 50% or greater No responses in the evaluation column. Additional caution is warranted if you are unable to confirm multiple journal details.

AMA, American Medical Association; APA, American Psychological Association; MLA, Modern Language Association.

### *Additional Journal Features*

Some additional journal features, included in Table 16-1, that bear consideration when selecting a publication are the impact factor, reputation, and acceptance rate. The **impact factor**, which cannot be computed for journals with less than 3 years of publication, represents the average frequency of citations of each article published in a journal over the past 2 years (Paulus et al., 2018; Sharma et al., 2014). The greater the average number of citations a journal receives for its published articles, the higher the impact factor. An impact factor of 3 or greater is considered high, though the average impact factor for most journals is 1 or less. The impact factor is most useful for comparing journals within the same field.

Journals with higher impact factors are often considered more prestigious; however, the impact factor does not reflect the quality of individual articles and is often based on very high citation rates for a small number of articles within a journal (Mech et al., 2020; Paulus et al., 2018). Despite these concerns, some academic institutions still use publication in high-impact journals as a benchmark for promotion and tenure; for all others, the impact factor of a journal may be less of a deciding factor.

Other measures of a journal's **reputation** include the journal's publishing history and established credibility in the field. Newer journals with a short publication history may not yet be widely accepted within the discipline. Other signs of a solid reputation include prior publication of scientifically rigorous inquiries (you might identify these from your earlier article appraisals), a well-established peer-review process, and specific quality reporting guidelines that authors must adhere to (Suiter & Sarli, 2019). Journals published by professional organizations or well-known healthcare institutions, and those whose editorial board members include respected experts in the discipline are also solid choices (Suiter & Sarli, 2019). You might consider a journal's reputation acceptable if you can identify two or more details listed in Table 16-1 (see Reputation section), but your assessment may vary based on your professional goals.

The **acceptance rate**, or the number of articles accepted by a journal divided by the total number of submissions, is another metric to consider when selecting a journal. However, it is important to understand some challenges with using acceptance rates as a deciding factor. First, acceptance rates are calculated in varying ways by journals. Some journals use the total number of submissions in the calculation, whereas others use the total number of submissions sent to reviewers, thereby omitting submissions initially rejected by the editor.

Second, the aim and scope of a journal can impact the acceptance rate. Some journals may have higher acceptance rates if they publish on specialized topics that they get very few submissions on (i.e., if they get fewer submissions, they may accept more of them). Conversely, interdisciplinary journals, by nature of their broad focus, receive more submissions and may have lower acceptance rates. Acceptance rates also tend to be lower for older, larger, and higher-impact journals, but a lower acceptance rate does not necessarily equate with higher quality (Herbert, 2020). For this reason, the acceptance rate should be considered along with the other journal features in Table 16-1.

The other challenge is finding the journal's acceptance rate. Some journals share this information on their website along with other metrics, such as the impact factor. In other cases, you might obtain the acceptance rate by directly contacting the journal's editor or referencing a library database, though some journals may not share this information at all. Acceptance rates vary but average around 32% (Herbert, 2020, p. 3). If you are a new author, you may want to avoid submissions to journals with acceptance rates lower than 20% to increase your odds of acceptance.

A final consideration in choosing a target publication is other favorable features that align with your goals and topic. For example, some journals have special features such as editorials, brief reports, book reviews, or practice innovations. Others also publish special issues from time to time that are dedicated to a particular topic or focused on a specific population. For example, *The Open Journal of Occupational Therapy* has called for papers for dedicated issues on topics ranging from the use of technology in practice

(Grajo & Boisselle, 2018) to global occupational therapy practice (Wagenfeld & Martin, 2019). If you are fortunate enough to find a journal with an upcoming special issue or feature that fits your aims, this might be a solid choice. Other favorable features may include connections to the editorial board, outreach from the journal with interest in your topic (this could stem from a prior presentation of your work), or honorariums or other incentives to publish there. Completing Table 16-1 for any journal you are considering and comparing this information with your publication goals and inquiry content can help you choose the most appropriate journal. Use caution in selecting a publication that you cannot answer "yes" (in the rightmost column) to at least half of the items in Table 16-1.

### TIPS & INSPIRATION

- After you have chosen a publication, retrieve one or two recent (within the last 2 years) articles from that journal that will serve as model articles when you are drafting yours. You might choose articles that represent the required formatting, are on a similar topic, or represent a similar design to your inquiry (for example, a pilot study, a feasibility study, or applied research). While you will still need to align your article with all aspects of the author guidelines, having a recently published article can be helpful.

## Writing Your Article

The format and amount of detail for an article will vary based on the intended audience, topic, chosen publication, and author guidelines. The biggest mistake new authors make is copying and pasting content from their formal inquiry report or chapters into a publication. This is usually ineffective since the purpose and level of detail are distinctly different. Formal inquiry reports or chapters are generally academic or institutional requirements, so they may have greater detail and redundancy to justify your decision-making and illustrate your understanding of the topic. For a publication, the aim is to convey the most relevant details clearly and concisely to your audience. To accomplish this goal, you will refer to your formal inquiry report or chapters, but in most cases, you must start the writing afresh to align with the publication's requirements, avoid extraneous details, and ensure continuity of the content.

### Peer-Reviewed Article Format

A peer-reviewed journal article should be formatted according to the publication's author guidelines, which specify the style, length, headings, and other requirements. A sample outline with sections typically included in a peer-reviewed article is provided in Table 16-2. This can help you get organized, but you should always follow the publication's author guidelines once you have chosen your target publication.

**TABLE 16-2 ■ Sample Peer-Reviewed Article Outline**

| Common Sections | Section Content |
|---|---|
| Abstract | ■ Include a concise summary of the inquiry purpose, methods, primary outcomes, and conclusions.<br>■ Journals often require specific headings within an abstract and limit word or character counts. |
| Introduction/ literature review | ■ Include a brief background on the topic, including definitions of key terms and concepts.<br>■ Discuss the existing literature, but do not include an exhaustive historical review. This section will require the most condensing, given the amount of material you have amassed and the journal's space constraints.<br>■ Point out gaps in the existing literature or results of a needs assessment to justify the inquiry.<br>■ State your inquiry's purpose, question, and hypotheses. |

*Continued*

**TABLE 16-2 ■ Sample Peer-Reviewed Article Outline—cont'd**

| Common Sections | Section Content |
|---|---|
| **Methods** | *The method section is usually subdivided:*<br>Inquiry design:<br>■ Identify whether you completed research or evidence-based practice, and note the specific quantitative, qualitative, or mixed methods approach used and why it was chosen.<br>■ Clarify any Institutional Review Board (IRB) approval or exemption.<br>Participants:<br>■ Describe inclusion and exclusion criteria, and recruitment and sampling methods.<br>■ State the sample size (including if participants were lost to attrition) and relevant demographics.<br>■ If participants were assigned to groups, clarify the method of assignment and number in each group.<br>Procedures:<br>■ Describe what was actually done in the inquiry.<br>■ If any intervention or treatment was provided, give a detailed description, including duration and frequency, how and where it was provided, under what conditions, and by whom.<br>■ If applicable, include details on how the intervention was developed and by whom; for commercially available interventions/programs, provide citations.<br>Outcome measures:<br>■ Identify all data collection tools, including a brief description, the purpose, and information on the reliability and validity of the tools, who administered the tools, and when.<br>■ Cite standardized measures or those from other sources.<br>■ For tools you created, describe the purpose, why you did not use an existing tool, development, and any strategies used to improve the quality of the tool. Include a copy of the tool if appropriate.<br>Data analysis:<br>■ For quantitative data, specify the statistical methods and software used.<br>■ For qualitative data, describe the coding and analysis process and strategies used to confirm results (multiple analyzers, member checking, triangulation, etc.). |
| **Results** | ■ Summarize the main findings (do not include interpretation of findings in this section).<br>■ Use figures and tables, if necessary, to illustrate results.<br>■ When reporting the findings from inferential statistics such as *t* tests or chi-squares, include information about the significance level and the degrees of freedom. Style manuals give information on how to type statistical results. |
| **Discussion** | ■ Reinforce the main results and why they are important/meaningful.<br>■ State whether the hypotheses were supported.<br>■ Compare your inquiry results to the literature. Highlight results that are unique or differ from the literature. Speculate plausible reasons for these results.<br>■ Discuss the implications of the results to practice.<br>*The discussion may be further subdivided:*<br>Limitations:<br>■ Review limitations related to the inquiry procedures or site that may have impacted results.<br>Future recommendations:<br>■ Review recommendations for future research or evidence-based practice.<br>■ Provide a brief conclusion. |
| **References** | ■ Include only those references used in the article (in the style specified in the author guidelines). Omit references from your formal inquiry report that do not appear in the article. |

### Non–Peer-Reviewed Article Format

In contrast to the structured format for peer-reviewed articles, the format of a non–peer-reviewed article is generally less formal, with the information tailored to a specific audience and organized as deemed appropriate by the author. The publication may still provide guidance on the length of submissions or other technical requirements, such as the resolution for photographs or accepted file formats. From the sample study in Box 16-1, a possible non–peer-reviewed publication opportunity is composing a piece for a senior citizens' newsletter on the risk factors for falls and the associated benefits of physical therapy. Box 16-5 includes an outline for this article to illustrate how the organization of a non–peer-reviewed article contrasts with that of the peer-reviewed article outline included in Table 16-2. In this example, the sections of the article are unique and logically organized. The goals of the article are to grab the senior citizens' attention about falls, provide them with background information on fall risks in a language they can understand, enable them to assess their fall risk via a short questionnaire, and explain that help is available for them if they need it.

#### BOX 16-5 ■ Sample Non–Peer-Reviewed Article Outline

**Introduction**

- Attention-getting statistics on falls

**What Are the Risk Factors for Falls?**

- Intrinsic factors: decreased strength, vision, reflexes, cognitive changes, disease-related changes (dementia, cardiovascular disorders, osteoporosis), fear of falling
- Extrinsic factors: environment, medication, time of day, staff and caregivers

**Am I at Risk for Falls?**

- Plan to include a short 10-item self-questionnaire that readers can use to identify their risk for falls as minimal, moderate, or maximum

**What Physical Therapy Can Do If You Are at Risk for Falls**

- Environmental modifications
- Strengthening and coordination activities
- Balance retraining
- Set up a home program

**How to Get More Information**

- Consult your doctor
- How to find a physical therapist near you
- How to learn more about falls

#### TIPS & INSPIRATION

- Take some time to contemplate the title for your publication as this often "sells" your article initially. For peer-reviewed articles, consider a concise title that clearly articulates the population, intervention, and outcome. Consider a creative or catchy title for a non–peer-reviewed article.
- Use well-designed figures, graphs, and tables as appropriate to support the written word. Be sure to label all elements, include clear titles, and follow the additional recommendations provided in Chapter 14 regarding visual displays of data and results.

### Submitting Your Article

Once you have chosen a target publication and written your article, you are ready to submit it. The author guidelines typically outline the submission procedure, with most publications requiring electronic submission. Some also have a submission checklist to ensure you provide all required items. The author guidelines may specify the review process so that you know how many people will review your article and the expected turnaround time. If the expected review period has passed and you have not heard from the editor, it is permissible to send a professional inquiry about the status of the review. There have been instances of delayed processing, and a gentle nudge can allow the editor to prompt reviewers or further investigate the delay.

## Responses to Your Submission

After your article submission is reviewed by the journal reviewers as outlined in their procedures, you will receive one of three responses—a request for revisions, a rejection, or an acceptance. Each is discussed here, with guidance provided for your next steps. Decisions are based on whether the topic is relevant to the readership, if the topic has been adequately covered, and if the inquiry is of good quality as well as the alignment with the author guidelines. The length of time your article is under review can vary, with some journals responding within a few weeks and others taking several months. The expected turnaround time is sometimes provided on the journal's website, but it is also reasonable to politely inquire about the status of your submission after a couple of months if you have not received an update.

### Requests for Revisions

Requests for revisions could be of two types—a request for revisions and then reconsideration of the article by the reviewers (or editor in the case of non-peer-reviewed articles) or an acceptance with revisions. With the first option, the reviewers see potential in your work, but they want to examine your revisions before making a final decision. With the second option, they have accepted the work but request that revisions be made before publication. In either case, this is great news! Revisions may be requested to clarify confusing points, adjust the focus, fix grammatical errors, or reorganize the content to better align with the publication's aims or current research. It is important to respond promptly to an editor's request for revisions.

First, remember that the purpose of the feedback and the request for revisions is to strengthen your work. Reading the comments through the first time can often be discouraging, particularly if there are many or you perceive them to be overly critical or negative. Taking a few days to process the feedback often leads to the realization that at least some of the points are valid and require your attention. Eventually, you will need to respond to each comment or request for revisions, even if you disagree. In cases of disagreement, you should respond professionally and explain to the reviewer why you did not make the requested revisions. For example, perhaps their suggestion is based on conflicting, confusing, or missing information in the article; clarifying these points can justify why the requested revision is inappropriate. When responding to reviewer comments, a revised version of the article and a cover letter that explains the edits are usually submitted. The cover letter can take several forms, though a table format, illustrated in Table 16-3, is recommended so that the reviewers can easily compare their comments to your revisions and responses. Responding clearly, concisely, and promptly can effectively expedite the review process.

Do not be surprised if your article goes back and forth between you and the editor a few times before it is acceptable. Above all, do not become so discouraged that you stop revising and resubmitting. If the editor considers the material suitable for publication, it is merely a matter of time before you have it in publishable form.

### Rejection

If your article is rejected for publication, you will usually be given the reason for rejection. Some common reasons for rejection are as follows:

1. **Failure to adhere to the author guidelines.** Examples can include using the incorrect writing style, submitting the wrong file format, or failing to format your article with the required headings, line numbers, or other requirements. Rejections of this nature usually come quickly and may prevent your work from being considered, even if you are willing to correct the issues.
2. **Your topic is outside the scope of the publication.** If your topic does not align with the aims and audience of the chosen publication, your work could be rejected. A thorough review of the publication's website and some currently published articles can help you determine if it is a good match before submission.
3. **Lack of a sufficient key argument.** Although you could discuss many aspects of your inquiry, you must identify a single persuasive idea and say why it is important. To gain focus, try writing your key argument in no more than two sentences. Review the information earlier in this chapter on developing a key argument to ensure your article is not rejected for this reason.
4. **Poor writing.** It is quite possible to have a quality inquiry and a solid key argument but have your work rejected based solely on the quality of the writing. Always review your article for proper

**TABLE 16-3 ■ Example Cover Letter to Respond to Reviewer Comments**

July 26, 2023

To: Reviewer #2

*Internet Journal of Allied Health Sciences and Practice*

Thank you for reviewing our article, "Use of the Kawa Model for Teambuilding with Rehabilitative Professionals: An Exploratory Study." We have reviewed your comments and made revisions accordingly. Please find your specific comments and our responses below. We appreciate your time in reviewing our manuscript and look forward to hearing from you.

| Reviewer Comments | Author Revisions/Comments |
|---|---|
| My biggest concern has to do with the quality of the research. I understand that the authors are considering this a pilot study. | The purposeful selection of an exploratory study design is further clarified in the Study Design section of the manuscript. An exploratory design aims to generate new ideas without definitive conclusions. Since there is limited research on the model, the exploratory design aligns well with our intended purpose of generating possible ways to use the model for teambuilding. |
| Methods: Were the focus groups audio recorded and transcribed? Also, if that is not the case, please provide more information about notetaking during the focus groups. Explain how the researchers can ensure that the comments collected were the participants' and not sentiments that the researchers reframed during the notetaking process. | Focus groups were not audio recorded. The rationale for this and the process of notetaking was clarified in the Procedures section of the manuscript.<br>The trainings occurred during regularly scheduled staff meetings, which are not typically recorded. We believed deviation from the typical meeting norms might impact the team's willingness to participate and share. We also used structured forms, described in this section, to take notes. Each training session was conducted by the team manager, with a manager from a different team observing and taking notes. Member checking was also used to confirm participant responses. |
| Data Analysis: How much time elapsed between focus groups? | The focus groups were one week apart; this is now clarified in the Procedures section. |
| Results: Under theme two, the authors state that both groups "proposed" that the Kawa model was an effective tool. Based on the stated research questions, were the participants guided at all to come to this conclusion? | The term "proposed" was purposefully chosen by the authors since team members generated this concept without prompting. The questions asked in the focus groups did not deviate from the questions outlined in Table 2 of the article. |
| In qualitative research, quotes are often presented in the results section. The lack of quotes here may make a reader suspicious about the quality of the investigation. | Quotes were not included since the sessions were not audio recorded; the lack of audio recording has been addressed in the Limitations section of the manuscript. |

Excerpts from responses to reviewer comments for later published manuscript: Lape and Scaife (2017).

grammar and spelling before submission; a variety of software features (discussed in Chapter 14) are readily available to polish your writing further. Also, avoid verbosity and technical jargon that might confuse readers.

5. **Poor organization.** Your article should flow logically, with later points building on the prior ones. Poor organization is common when information is copied and pasted from a formal inquiry report. To avoid this problem, do not

copy and paste information directly from your report. Also, having someone unfamiliar with your inquiry review your article is often helpful to see if it makes sense. They can help you identify confusing points, allowing you to reorganize the information before submission.

6. **Methodological concerns.** Your article could be rejected due to concerns with your methodology—for example, a small sample size, lack of a control group, other forms of bias, or flaws in the procedures or data collection. If there are methodological concerns related to your inquiry, it is best to acknowledge them in your article. Be careful not to overstate the implications of your findings and consider how the limitations in your inquiry can inform future ones. In the end, some journals have strict requirements regarding certain methodological features, such as minimum sample sizes, which could result in a rejection. Other journals may still be willing to accept your article if you have been forthcoming regarding the limitations and how these impact your results. Even if things did not go as planned in your inquiry, you likely still have valuable information to share, so it is really a matter of finding a fitting publication outlet. An additional option is to reframe the focus of the article; this might include writing a scoping review on the topic, highlighting the positive outcomes via a case study, or drafting an article focused on the feasibility of the intervention or program in question.

### TIPS & INSPIRATION

- **If your work** is rejected, do not be discouraged. Even **experienced** authors can experience rejection. You **have valuable** information to share with others—it **is just** a matter of finding the right publication and **approach.** With a little hard work, your publication **goals** are achievable.
- **Be open** to shifting the focus of your article, trying **another** target publication (perhaps your second, **third,** or even fourth choice!), and getting help from **others.** Imagine the satisfaction you will feel when you are successful.

### Acceptance

Once your article has been accepted, it will be copy-edited to clarify any uncertainties, polish the writing and flow of the article, and finalize the layout. This process may involve multiple revisions and collaboration with the editor. Your editor may require you to review proofs of the article, submit additional forms (such as those related to copyright or conflict of interest), or remit publication fees if applicable. You should respond promptly so as not to delay your publication or risk rejection due to failure to respond. The editor can let you know the anticipated publication date of your article. Some journals publish a set number of issues at specific times during the year, whereas others, particularly those that publish exclusively online, may publish on a rolling basis. During this waiting time, it is perfectly acceptable to list this publication on your resume, noting that it is "in press."

### TIPS & INSPIRATION

- **If you are** a new author, some publications include **shorter** features, often called brief reports of research **or evidence**-based practice. While it may be challenging **to condense** the volume of information you have, if you **can identify** a solid key argument, these shorter articles **are an excellent** way to get started with publishing.
- **Be prepared** to receive constructive feedback throughout the publication process—from choosing a target **journal,** to revising drafts of the article, to submission **and the** journal's response. Those who are successful **are open** to feedback, do not take it personally, and do **not give** up.
- **Experience** is the best teacher related to publishing. **The more** you attempt it, the better you become at it.

### CHAPTER SUMMARY

1. Outline reasons for formally publishing your inquiry.
   - Reasons for publishing your inquiry include sharing knowledge with others so they can build on your work, avoid challenges you encountered, and make informed decisions; networking and collaborating

*Continued*

with others; expanding your professional skills and resume; and contributing to the literature in your discipline or topic.

2. Differentiate peer-reviewed and non–peer-reviewed publications, and open-access and closed-access journals.
   - Peer-reviewed publications disseminate research and evidence-based practice articles authored by experts in the field or topic, which other experts blindly review to confirm quality before publication. Peer-reviewed articles are highly structured and include references to professional literature. They may include inquiries that were IRB-approved and used complex statistical or qualitative analysis methods to support the outcomes.
     - Closed-access journals are traditional, subscription-based journals that require a subscription fee to access articles within the journal.
     - Open-access journals are freely available without a subscription and, for this reason, have the potential to reach a wider audience. Publication costs are covered by author publication fees, grants, or institutional or association budgets.
   - Non–peer-reviewed publications include less scientific magazines, books, pamphlets, and other works intended to provide more general information, often to the public. Non–peer-reviewed articles are less structured, may have limited or no references to professional literature, and use layperson's terminology.
3. Describe factors in choosing an appropriate target publication.
   - Factors in choosing a target publication include the publication opportunities, publishing goals and experience, target audience, key argument, and the target publication's aims and author guidelines.
     - There are usually multiple publication opportunities within a single inquiry, including peer-reviewed and non–peer-reviewed options.
     - If you aim to pursue an academic career or connect with other experts on your topic, a peer-reviewed publication is the best choice. You might consider coauthorship if you are new to publishing. If you aim to share your information with fellow clinicians or consumers, a non–peer-reviewed publication may be the best choice.
     - Authorship may be attributed to those involved in the inquiry design, implementation, data analysis, and/or actual article writing.
   - The target audience of your chosen publication should align with your target audience.
   - You should determine your key argument before choosing a target publication. The key argument is the primary idea, supported with evidence, that you want to convey.
   - A publication's aim describes its purpose, topics covered, types of articles published, publishing options, and review process, and these should align with your topic and goals.
   - Author guidelines are provided on a journal's website and include requirements related to writing style, page or word limits, and tables and figures. Table 16-1 can be used to evaluate a journal you are considering.
     - The impact factor (usually 1 or less for most journals) is the average number of citations per article in a journal over the past 2 years and is most useful for comparing journals in the same field.
     - A journal's reputation is related to its affiliations, publishing history, established credibility in the field, peer-review process, the rigor of previously published articles, and the presence of quality reporting guidelines.
     - The acceptance rate is the number of accepted journal articles divided by the number of submissions. Journals with a broad scope, and those that are older, larger, and higher-impact tend to have lower acceptance rates, so this must be considered along with the journal's other features.
     - Special features or issues, connections to the editorial board, or other incentives may provide support for choosing a target publication.
4. Use formatting guidelines to draft an article for your chosen target publication.
   - An article's format and level of detail vary based on the intended audience, topic, chosen publication, and author guidelines.
   - Table 16-2 provides a sample outline for a peer-reviewed journal article, though you should always follow the author guidelines once you have chosen a publication.
   - Box 16-5 provides an example of the flexible structure of a non–peer-reviewed article.

5. Explain potential responses to your article submission and how to respond to them.
   - Responses to your article submission may include a request for revisions, a rejection, or an acceptance.
   - A request for revisions could be of two types—a request for revisions and then reconsideration, or an acceptance with revisions. Either request is good news and aimed at strengthening your work.
     - Take time to process the feedback and promptly respond to each reviewer's comment. Table 16-3 provides an example of a cover letter to respond to reviewer comments.
   - Rejections can occur for various reasons: failure to adhere to author guidelines, misalignment of your topic with the publication's scope, a poor key argument, poor writing, poor organization, or methodological concerns. Proactively address these elements before submission, and if you are still rejected, you may need to revise your article or find a more fitting target publication.
   - If your article is accepted, you may still need to respond to requests from the editor, review proofs, or submit additional forms or fees. Respond promptly so as not to delay your publication.

## TEST YOUR KNOWLEDGE

1. Identify whether each item is related to a peer-reviewed or non–peer-reviewed publication.
   a. Rigorous review process
   b. Format frequently decided by the author
   c. Required with most academic appointments
   d. Structured format
   e. Limited to no references included
   f. May be more appropriate for the general public
2. Which of the following is TRUE of open-access journals?
   a. They are freely accessible to everyone.
   b. They all charge authors to publish.
   c. Articles submitted do not undergo rigorous review.
   d. Publishing costs do not exceed $300 per article.
3. You could publish a peer-reviewed article and a non–peer-reviewed article on the same topic or inquiry. True or false?
4. You can submit an article to multiple journals simultaneously for consideration. True or false?
5. A coauthor is anyone who has significantly contributed to the work in some way. True or false?
6. Which of the following is a good key argument?
   a. Aging in place increases psychological well-being and quality of life.
   b. The impact of tailored education on aging in place to promote well-being.
   c. Tailored aging in place education is effective in increasing psychological well-being, which can contribute to quality of life. This finding supports future development of preventive community-based programming for the aging population.
   d. Individuals who participated in tailored education on aging in place showed increased psychological well-being as measured by the Psychological General Well-being Index.
7. The impact factor represents the quality of individual articles within a publication. True or false?
8. Which of the following BEST describes features of a reputable journal?
   a. Longevity of the publication, a rigorous review process, and acceptance within a discipline
   b. Longevity of the publication, APA writing style, and acceptance within a discipline
   c. High rejection rates, a rigorous review process, and a reputable editorial board
   d. A rigorous review process, higher publication fees, and an international audience
9. Which journal is likely to have the highest acceptance rate?
   a. A new journal
   b. A journal with an impact factor of 10
   c. A journal that has existed since 1940
   d. A large interdisciplinary journal
10. You must respond to each comment from a journal reviewer, even if you disagree. True or false?
11. For which of the following reasons may a journal reject an article for publication?
    a. The submission strictly adheres to the author's guidelines.
    b. The journal lacks sufficient skilled reviewers on the topic.
    c. A thorough review reveals significant methodological concerns.
    d. The sample size for the inquiry was too large to draw meaningful conclusions.

Answer key appears at the end of this text.

## NEXT STEPS

1. Consider that multiple publication opportunities exist within a single inquiry (as illustrated in Boxes 16-1 and 16-2). Brainstorm and list at least five publication opportunities for your inquiry.
2. Try writing your key argument in no more than two sentences. Compare it to the example in Box 16-3 and assess it using the questions in Box 16-4. Make modifications as necessary and share with others for feedback.
3. Complete Table 16-1 for a publication you are considering. Is this publication a good choice? Why or why not?
4. Use the author guidelines for your chosen publication to create a template with the required headings and formatting. Once you have this in place, outline the content for each section related to your topic or inquiry. If you plan to write a peer-reviewed article, use Table 16-2 to ensure you do not omit vital information. This will help you organize your thoughts before beginning the writing process.

## REFERENCES


American Psychological Association. (2022). *Publication practices and responsible authorship.* https://www.apa.org/research/responsible/publication

Belcher, W. L. (2019). *Writing your journal article in twelve weeks: A guide to academic publishing success* (2nd ed.). University of Chicago Press.

Grajo, L. C., & Boisselle, A. (2018). Technology in occupational therapy and occupational science: Evidence, education, and impact [Special issue]. *The Open Journal of Occupational Therapy, 6*(3). https://scholarworks.wmich.edu/ojot/vol6/iss3

Herbert, R. (2020). *Accept me, accept me not: What do journal acceptance rates really mean?* International Center for the Study of Research. https://doi.org/10.2139/ssrn.3526365

Lape, J. E., & Scaife, B. D. (2017). Use of the KAWA model for teambuilding with rehabilitative professionals: An exploratory study. *The Internet Journal of Allied Health Sciences and Practice, 15*(1), Article 10, 1–8. https://doi.org/10.46743/1540-580X/2017.1647

Mech, E., Ahmed, M. M., Tamale, E., Holek, M., Li, G., & Thabane, L. (2020). Evaluating journal impact factor: A systematic survey of the pros and cons, and overview of alternative measures. *Journal of Venomous Animals and Toxins including Tropical Disease, 26,* e20190082. https://doi.org/10.1590/1678-9199-JVATITD-2019-0082

Memon, A. R. (2019). Revisiting the term predatory open access publishing. *Journal of Korean Medical Science, 34*(13), e99. https://doi.org/10.3346/jkms.2019.34.e99

Paulus, F. M., Cruz, N., & Krach, S. (2018). The impact factor fallacy. *Frontiers in Psychology, 9,* Article 1487. https://doi.org/10.3389/fpsyg.2018.01487

Sharma, M., Sarin, A., Gupta, P., Sachdeva, S., & Desai, A. V. (2014). Journal impact factor: Its use, significance and limitations. *World Journal of Nuclear Medicine, 13*(2), 146. http://doi.org/10.4103/1450-1147.139151

Suiter, A. M., & Sarli, C. C. (2019). Selecting a journal for publication: Criteria to consider. *Missouri Medicine, 116*(6), 461–465. https://www.ncbi.nlm.nih.gov/pmc/articles/PMC6913840

Wagenfeld, A., & Martin, S. (2019). Global perspectives on occupational therapy practice and education [Special issue]. *The Open Journal of Occupational Therapy, 7*(3), 1–4. https://doi.org/10.15453/2168-6408.1654

# Test Your Knowledge Answer Key

The following are the answers to the chapter Test Your Knowledge questions.

## Chapter 1

1. a
2. b
3. c
4. b
5. a. evidence-based practice project; b. research study; c. research study; d. evidence-based practice project

## Chapter 2

1. b
2. d
3. c
4. d
5. a
6. c
7. c
8. a

## Chapter 3

1. a
2. b
3. b
4. c
5. b
6. True
7. a

## Chapter 4

1. b
2. a
3. c
4. c
5. d
6. a

## Chapter 5

1. c
2. a
3. False
4. b
5. d
6. a. nominal; b. interval; c. ordinal; d. ratio
7. c
8. a. descriptive; b. inferential; c. inferential; d. descriptive

## Chapter 6

1. a
2. d
3. d
4. a
5. c
6. c
7. a
8. c

## Chapter 7

1. c
2. b
3. b
4. a
5. d

## Chapter 8

1. c
2. False
3. d
4. False
5. b
6. a
7. c
8. a. thematic analysis; b. content analysis; c. content analysis; d. thematic analysis

## Chapter 9

1. d
2. c
3. a
4. c
5. b

## Chapter 10

1. d
2. c
3. c
4. False
5. a
6. c
7. c

## Chapter 11

1. a
2. c
3. c
4. d
5. b
6. b
7. c
8. d

## Chapter 12

1. True
2. b
3. d
4. d
5. b
6. c
7. b
8. a. confidentiality; b. privacy; c. anonymity

## Chapter 13

1. d
2. c
3. c
4. a
5. c
6. d
7. a

## Chapter 14

1. False
2. b
3. a
4. b
5. b
6. a. table; b. line graph; c. pie chart; d. flowchart; e. bar graph
7. c
8. False
9. a

## Chapter 15

1. a. synchronous; b. synchronous; c. asynchronous; d. asynchronous; e. synchronous; f. asynchronous
2. False
3. d
4. b
5. d
6. True
7. a

## Chapter 16

1. a. peer-reviewed; b. non-peer-reviewed; c. peer-reviewed; d. peer-reviewed; e. non-peer-reviewed; f. non-peer-reviewed
2. a
3. True
4. False
5. True
6. c
7. False
8. a
9. a
10. True
11. c

# Appendix A

# Evidence-Based Practice Resources by Healthcare Discipline

The following resources, grouped by healthcare discipline, can further support you in engaging in the evidence-based practice process. An internet search of the resource titles will guide you in obtaining these resources.

## GENERAL HEALTHCARE


Cullen, L., Hanrahan, K., Farrington, M. M., Tucker, S. J., & Edmonds, S. (2022). *Evidence-based practice in action* (2nd ed.). Sigma Theta Tau International.

Hall, H. R., & Roussel, L. A. (2020). *Evidence-based practice: An integrative guide to research, administration, and practice* (3rd ed.). Jones & Bartlett Learning.

Hoffman, T., Benett, S., & Del Mar, C. (2023). *Evidence-based practice across the health professions* (4th ed.). Elsevier.

Melnyk, B. M., Gallagher-Ford, L., & Fineout-Overholt, E. (2019). *Implementing the evidence-based practice (EBP) competencies in healthcare: A practical guide for improving quality, safety, & outcomes.* Sigma Theta Tau International.

Rubin, A., & Bellamy, J. (2022). *Practitioner's guide to using research for evidence-informed practice* (3rd ed.). John Wiley & Sons.


## ATHLETIC TRAINING AND EXERCISE SCIENCE


Amonette, W. E., English, K. L., & Kraemer, W. J. (2016). *Evidence based practice in exercise science: The six-step approach.* Human Kinetics.

Arnold, B. L., & Schilling, B. K. (2016). *Evidence-based practice in sport and exercise: A guide to using research.* F.A. Davis.

Frenn, M., & Whitehead, D. K. (2021). *Health promotion: Translating evidence to practice.* F.A. Davis.

Prentice, W. E. (2020). *Principles of athletic training: A guide to evidence-based clinical practice* (17th ed.). McGraw-Hill Education.


## LABORATORY SCIENCE


Casler, K. S., & Gawlik, K. S. (Eds.). (2022). *Laboratory screening and diagnostic evaluation: An evidence-based approach.* Springer.


## MASSAGE THERAPY


Andrade, C. (2013). *Outcome-based massage: Putting evidence into practice* (3rd ed.). Lippincott Williams & Wilkins.

Lebert, R. (2021). *Massage therapy: An evidence-based guide for clinical practice.* Lulu.com.


## NURSING


Christenbery, T. L. (Ed.). (2017). *Evidence-based practice in nursing: Foundations, skills, and roles.* Springer.

Dang, D., Dearholt, S. L., Bissett, K., Ascenzi, J., & Whalen, M. (2021). *Johns Hopkins evidence-based practice for nurses and healthcare professionals: Model & guidelines* (4th ed.). Sigma Theta Tau International.

Melnyk, B. M., & Fineout-Overholt, E. (2023). *Evidence-based practice in nursing & healthcare: A guide to best practice* (5th ed.). Lippincott Williams & Wilkins.

Nowak, E. W., & Colsch, R. (2023). *Brown's evidence-based nursing: The research-practice connection* (5th ed.). Jones & Bartlett Learning.

Schmidt, N. A., & Brown, J. M. (2024). *Evidence-based practice for nurses: Appraisal and application research.* Jones & Bartlett Learning.


## OCCUPATIONAL THERAPY


Taylor, R. R. (2023). *Kielhofner's research in occupational therapy: Methods of inquiry for enhancing practice* (3rd ed.). F.A. Davis.

Law, M., & MacDermid, J. (Eds.). (2014). *Evidence-based rehabilitation: A guide to practice* (3rd ed.). Slack.

Brown, C. (2023). *The evidence-based practitioner: Applying research to meet client needs* (2nd ed.). F.A. Davis.


## PHYSICAL THERAPY


Fetters, L., & Tilson, J. (2018). *Evidence based physical therapy* (2nd ed.). F.A. Davis.

Jewell, D. V. (2022). *Guide to evidence-based physical therapist practice* (5th ed.). Jones & Bartlett Learning.


## PHYSICIAN ASSISTANT


Kathirvel, S., Singh, A., & Chockalingam, A. (Eds.). (2023). *Principles and application of evidence-based public health practice.* Academic Press.

Pines, J. M., Bellolio, F., Carpenter, C. R., & Raja, A. S. (Eds.). (2023). *Evidence-based emergency care: Diagnostic testing and clinical decision rules* (3rd ed.). Wiley-Blackwell.

Straus, S. E., Glasziou, P., Richardson, W. S., & Haynes, R. B. (2018). *Evidence-based medicine: How to practice and teach EBM* (5th ed.). Elsevier.

## RADIOLOGIC SCIENCE

Kelly, A., Cronin, P., Puig, S., & Applegate, K. E. (Eds.). (2018). *Evidence-based emergency imaging: Optimizing diagnostic imaging of patients in the emergency care setting.* Springer.

Medina, L. S., Sanelli, P. C., & Jarvik, J. G. (Eds.). (2013). *Evidence-based neuroimaging diagnosis and treatment: Improving the quality of neuroimaging in patient care.* Springer.

Otero, H. J., Kaplan, S. L., Medina, L. S., Blackmore, C. C., & Applegate, K. E. (Eds). (2024). *Evidence-based imaging in pediatrics: Clinical decision support for optimized imaging in pediatric care* (2nd ed.). Springer.

## SOCIAL WORK

Grinnell, R. M., Jr., & Unrau, Y. A. (2018). *Social work research and evaluation: Foundations of evidence-based practice* (11th ed.). Oxford University Press.

Thyer, B. A., Dulmus, C. N., & Sowers, K. M. (Eds.). (2013). *Developing evidence-based generalist practice skills.* John Wiley & Sons.

Appendix B

# Literature Search Tracking Log

Using a spreadsheet is helpful for tracking your literature search. You can use the following blank Search Tracking Log to help track your own literature search. For more details on performing a literature search, see Chapter 3.

## Literature Search Tracking Log

*PIO or PICO Question:*

| Database Searched | Date | Search Terms Used | Limiters or Additional Criteria Set | No. of Results | Notes/Comments | No. of Articles Selected | Citations for Selected Articles |
|---|---|---|---|---|---|---|---|
| | | | | | | | |
| | | | | | | | |
| | | | | | | | |
| | | | | | | | |
| | | | | | | | |
| | | | | | | | |
| | | | | | | | |
| | | | | | | | |
| | | | | | | | |
| | | | | | | | |
| | | | | | | | |
| | | | | | | | |
| | | | | | | | |
| | | | | | | | |
| | | | | | | | |
| | | | | | | | |
| | | | | | | | |
| | | | | | | | |
| | | | | | | | |
| | | | | | | | |
| | | | | | | | |
| | | | | | | | |

# Appendix C

# Critically Appraised Paper Template

A critically appraised paper (CAP) is a short analysis of an individual research study. The following template can be used to analyze individual research studies of varying designs. The first annotated version describes the information you might add as you complete your appraisal. The second version of the template is blank so you can populate each section with information specific to an individual research study. For more details on appraisal of quantitative, qualitative, and mixed methods designs, and levels of evidence, see Chapters 6, 9, and 10.

**Critically Appraised Paper Template**

| Study Components | Appraisal |
|---|---|
| Study Reference | Insert reference for the study being appraised. |
| Purpose | State the study's purpose in layperson's terms. |
| Setting | Describe the setting type (inpatient rehab unit, skilled nursing facility, public school, etc.) and geographic location (e.g., United States, Australia, rural/urban). For systematic reviews, summarize the types of settings of reviewed studies. |
| Sampling and Recruitment | State the number of participants, how they were recruited (via flyers, social media, phone, etc.) and sampled (random, convenience, purposive, etc.), and any relevant demographics. For systematic reviews, include the number of studies reviewed, their designs, and a general description of the study participants. |
| Study Design/ Procedures | ▪ State the specific quantitative, qualitative, or mixed methods research design (randomized controlled trial, phenomenology, etc.).<br>▪ Summarize the procedures (i.e., what did the researchers do?). |
| Level of Evidence | **Quantitative Level of Evidence:**<br>☐ I ☐ II ☐ III ☐ IV ☐ V ☐ N/A<br>**Qualitative Level of Evidence:**<br>☐ I ☐ II ☐ III ☐ IV ☐ N/A |
| Data Collection Tools/ Methods | ▪ List the data collection tools/method(s) used. THIS IS NOT THE STATISTICS USED—THESE ARE THE TOOLS/MEASURES.<br>▪ State if the tools are valid and reliable. If the authors created the tools, were they reviewed by experts and piloted? You may need to look beyond the article to find this information.<br>▪ For a systematic review, describe how the studies were assessed for quality. |

*Continued*

| Critically Appraised Paper Template—cont'd | |
|---|---|
| Study Components | Appraisal |
| Results/<br>Main Findings | ■ State the results in layperson's terms. (Do not copy statistics from the study.)<br>■ Were results statistically significant and/or clinically significant? If so, what does this mean? |
| Limitations | List any limitations in the study that need consideration when evaluating results. Look beyond limitations noted in the article, where applicable. |
| How is this study useful for your purposes? Check all that apply. | Indicate SPECIFIC application of study information related to each item checked on the left:* |
| ☐ Provides background information (justifies a need, defines key terms, establishes theoretical background) | |
| ☐ Shows the effectiveness or support for a proposed intervention (shows effectiveness of the intervention for desired/similar outcome) | |
| ☐ Supports methodology (supports procedures, data collection methods or tools, data analysis) | |
| ☐ Other | |

* Use bullet points to concisely and *specifically* explain how the study is useful for your purposes. Remember that you can glean valuable information from *all* studies regardless of whether the results are favorable. For example, imagine you are interested in fall prevention strategies and believe using appropriate footwear can decrease the risk of falls. Then, you locate a study that reports this is false. It would *still* be important to include this study—remember that "best" evidence combines the research with your skills/knowledge and the needs of your client/population. You must also consider how applicable this study is to what you are proposing.

| Critically Appraised Paper Template | |
|---|---|
| Study Components | Appraisal |
| Study Reference | |
| Purpose | |
| Setting | |
| Sampling and Recruitment | |
| Study Design/<br>Procedures | |
| Level of Evidence | **Quantitative Level of Evidence:**<br>☐ I ☐ II ☐ III ☐ IV ☐ V ☐ N/A<br>**Qualitative Level of Evidence:**<br>☐ I ☐ II ☐ III ☐ IV ☐ N/A |
| Data Collection Tools/Methods | |
| Results/<br>Main Findings | |
| Limitations | |

| Critically Appraised Paper Template—cont'd | |
|---|---|
| How is this study useful for your purposes? Check all that apply. | Indicate SPECIFIC application of study information related to each item checked on the left: |
| ☐ Provides background information (justifies a need, defines key terms, establishes theoretical background) | |
| ☐ Shows the effectiveness or support for a proposed intervention (shows effectiveness of the intervention for desired/similar outcome) | |
| ☐ Supports methodology (supports procedures, data collection methods or tools, data analysis) | |
| ☐ Other | |

# Appendix D

# Critically Appraised Topic Template

A critically appraised topic (CAT) is a summary appraisal of multiple studies on a single topic or intervention, which results in a clinical "bottom line" or summary recommendations. The following template can be used to complete a CAT in an area of interest. The first annotated version describes the information you might add as you complete your appraisal of your topic. The second version of the template is blank so you can populate each section with information specific to your topic. For more details on appraisal of quantitative, qualitative, and mixed methods designs, and levels of evidence, see Chapters 6, 9, and 10.

| Critically Appraised Topic Template | |
|---|---|
| **Topic Identification** | |
| Inquiry Question | Insert your inquiry question in the PIO or PICO format. |
| Clinical Scenario | Describe the clinical situation or problem motivating this investigation of the literature. What is your rationale for pursuing this topic? |
| **Search Methods and Review Process** | |
| Databases Searched | State all databases and websites searched. |
| Search Terms by PICO Element | Include applicable search terms for each category:<br>**Population:**<br>**Intervention:**<br>**Comparison:**<br>**Outcome:** |
| Inclusion Criteria for Articles | List any inclusion criteria (i.e., particular study designs, full-text articles, articles published only in English, studies conducted with specific diagnoses or ages, or those occurring in a particular setting). |
| Exclusion Criteria for Articles | List any exclusion criteria (i.e., studies occurring more than 10 years ago; less rigorous research designs, such as qualitative or level V studies; or literature reviews). |
| Review Process | Discuss specifically how the review was conducted, including the following:<br>▪ How was the inquiry question developed?<br>▪ How were the databases, search terms, and criteria determined? |

*Continued*

## Critically Appraised Topic Template—cont'd

- How were the inclusion and exclusion criteria applied? For example, the abstracts of articles returned in the initial search may have been scanned to determine if each study met the inclusion criteria and should be further explored.
- How were individual appraisals completed on each study? In other words, how did you complete the individual critically appraised papers (CAPs)?
- What did you do to ensure quality control in the process? For example, did a mentor or expert in this content area review your analyses, or did you use some other method of peer review?

### Search Results by Level of Evidence (Number of Articles by Category)

| | | |
|---|---|---|
| Quantitative Level I | High-quality randomized controlled trials (RCTs), systematic reviews (SR) of RCTs, and meta-analysis | Insert number of articles by category. |
| Quantitative Level II | Small-scale RCTs, nonrandomized studies *with* a control group such as cohort studies, case-control designs, pretest-posttest designs, and SRs of these studies | |
| Quantitative Level III | Nonrandomized studies *without* a control group, such as one-group pretest-posttest designs, time series/longitudinal studies, repeated measures designs, and cross-sectional studies | |
| Quantitative Level IV | Descriptive studies, including single-subject designs, case studies, case-control designs, and survey studies | |
| Quantitative Level V | Expert opinion, literature reviews, and laboratory research (research not performed on human subjects) | |
| Qualitative Level I | Generalizable studies | |
| Qualitative Level II | Conceptual studies | |
| Qualitative Level III | Descriptive studies | |
| Qualitative Level IV | Case studies | |
| Qualitative Theory | Qualitative theory study | |
| | **Total articles reviewed:** | |

### Main Findings by Level of Evidence (Use bullet points to list the main findings for studies within each level of evidence.)

| |
|---|
| Quantitative Level I |
| Quantitative Level II |
| Quantitative Level III |
| Quantitative Level IV |
| Quantitative Level V |
| Qualitative Level I |
| Qualitative Level II |
| Qualitative Level III |
| Qualitative Level IV |
| Qualitative Theory |

| Critically Appraised Topic Template—cont'd |
|---|
| **Limitations by Level of Evidence (Use bullet points to list the limitations of studies within each level of evidence.)** |
| Quantitative Level I |
| Quantitative Level II |
| Quantitative Level III |
| Quantitative Level IV |
| Quantitative Level V |
| Qualitative Level I |
| Qualitative Level II |
| Qualitative Level III |
| Qualitative Level IV |
| Qualitative Theory |
| **Bottom Line and Recommendations** |
| Use this space to summarize your findings as they relate to clinical practice. Provide a clear and concise answer to your inquiry question. Clearly state your recommendations.<br>Do you recommend:<br>1. Using the intervention (proven effectiveness)<br>2. Using the intervention with caution (conflicting evidence, no evidence, or insufficient evidence)<br>3. Not using the intervention (proven ineffective or the potential for harm) (Glegg & Barrie, 2012) |
| **References of Appraised Articles** |
| Include references for all appraised studies. |
| **References of Other Sources Used to Complete Your Appraisal** |
| Include references for any other sources you consulted to complete your appraisal and make your final recommendations. |
| **Name of Appraiser(s):** **Data Appraisal Completed:** |

Novak, I. (2012). Evidence to practice commentary: The evidence alert traffic light grading system. *Physical & Occupational Therapy in Pediatrics, 32,* 256–259. https://doi.org/10.3109/01942638.2012.698148

| Critically Appraised Topic Template | |
|---|---|
| **Topic Identification** | |
| Inquiry Question | |
| Clinical Scenario | |
| **Search Methods and Review Process** | |
| Databases Searched | |
| Search Terms by PICO Element | **Population:**<br>**Intervention:**<br>**Comparison:**<br>**Outcome:** |
| Inclusion Criteria for Articles | |
| Exclusion Criteria for Articles | |
| Review Process | |
| **Search Results by Level of Evidence (Number of Articles by Category)** | |
| Quantitative Level I | High-quality randomized clinical trials (RCTs), systematic reviews (SRs) of RCTs, and meta-analysis |
| Quantitative Level II | Small-scale RCTs, nonrandomized studies *with* a control group such as cohort studies, case-control designs, pretest-posttest designs, and SRs of these studies |
| Quantitative Level III | Nonrandomized studies *without* a control group, such as one-group pretest-posttest designs, time series/longitudinal studies, repeated measures designs, and cross-sectional studies |
| Quantitative Level IV | Descriptive studies, including single-subject designs, case studies, case-control designs, and survey studies |
| Quantitative Level V | Expert opinion, literature reviews, and laboratory research (research not performed on human subjects) |
| Qualitative Level I | Generalizable studies |
| Qualitative Level II | Conceptual studies |
| Qualitative Level III | Descriptive studies |
| Qualitative Level IV | Case studies |

## Critically Appraised Topic Template—cont'd

| Qualitative Theory | Qualitative theory study |
|---|---|
| | **Total articles reviewed:** |

| Main Findings by Level of Evidence |
|---|
| Quantitative Level I |
| Quantitative Level II |
| Quantitative Level III |
| Quantitative Level IV |
| Quantitative Level V |
| Qualitative Level I |
| Qualitative Level II |
| Qualitative Level III |
| Qualitative Level IV |
| Qualitative Theory |

| Limitations by Level of Evidence |
|---|
| Quantitative Level I |
| Quantitative Level II |
| Quantitative Level III |
| Quantitative Level IV |
| Quantitative Level V |
| Qualitative Level I |
| Qualitative Level II |
| Qualitative Level III |
| Qualitative Level IV |
| Qualitative Theory |

| Bottom Line and Recommendations |
|---|
| |

| References of Appraised Articles |
|---|
| |

| References of Other Sources Used to Complete Your Appraisal |
|---|
| |

**Name of Appraiser(s):** **Data Appraisal Completed:**

# Appendix E

# Professional Journals

This is not intended to be an exhaustive list of journals, but it may be helpful when searching for evidence on your topic or when exploring publication opportunities.

## Aging

*Activities, Adaptation and Aging*

*Age and Ageing*

*Aging and Mental Health*

*American Journal of Geriatric Psychiatry*

*Clinical Gerontologist*

*Clinical Interventions in Ageing*

*International Journal of Aging and Human Development*

*International Journal of Geriatric Psychiatry*

*Journal of Aging and Physical Activity*

*Journal of Aging and Social Policy*

*Journal of Aging Studies*

*Journal of Applied Gerontology*

*Journal of Geriatric Psychiatry and Neurology*

*Journal of Women and Aging*

*Physical and Occupational Therapy in Geriatrics*

*The Aging Male*

*The Gerontologist*

## Education

*Academic Medicine*

*American Journal of Distance Education*

*Computers in the Schools*

*Innovations in Education and Teaching*

*International Journal of Nursing Education*

*Journal of Occupational Therapy Education*

*Journal of Physical Therapy Education*

*Journal of Transformative Learning*

*Online Learning*

*Rehabilitation Research, Policy, and Education*

## Healthcare Administration

*British Journal of Healthcare Management*

*Healthcare Management Forum*

*International Journal of Healthcare Management*

*Journal of Healthcare Management*

*Risk Management and Healthcare Policy*

*Journal of Rehabilitation Administration*

## Healthcare General

*Home Health Care Services Quarterly*

*Home Health Care Management and Practice*

*Internet Journal of Allied Health Sciences and Practice*

*Journal of Allied Health*

*Journal of Interprofessional Care*

*Journal of Women's Health*

*Occupational Therapy in Health Care*

*Public Health Journal*

*The Open Journal of Occupational Therapy*

## Healthcare Technology

*Health and Technology*

*International Journal of Telerehabilitation*

*Journal of Technology in Human Services*

*Journal of Telemedicine and Telecare*

*Technology and Health Care*

*Telemedicine and e-Health*

## Hospice

*American Journal of Hospice and Palliative Medicine*

*Journal of Palliative Care*

*Journal of Hospice and Palliative Care*

*Palliative & Supportive Care*

## Mental Health and Well-Being

*Administration and Policy in Mental Health and Mental Health Services Research*

*Aging and Mental Health*

*American Journal of Health Promotion*

*Canadian Journal of Community Mental Health*

*Community Mental Health Journal*

*International Journal of Qualitative Studies on Health & Well-being*

*Journal of Family Psychotherapy*

*Journal of Health and Social Behavior*

*Journal of Organizational Behavior Management*

*Occupational Therapy in Mental Health*

*Residential Treatment for Children and Youth*

*The Clinical Supervisor*

*Aging and Mental Health*

## Occupational Health

*International Journal of Sports Medicine*

*Journal of Occupational and Environmental Medicine*

*Journal of Occupational Health Psychology*

*Journal of Occupational Rehabilitation*

*Workplace Health & Safety*

## Pediatrics and Early Intervention

*Child Development*

*Frontiers in Pediatrics*

*Infants and Young Children*

*Journal of Early Intervention*

*Journal of Occupational Therapy, Schools, & Early Intervention*

*Journal of Pediatric Psychology*

*Pediatric Physical Therapy*

*Physical and Occupational Therapy in Pediatrics*

*Physical Disabilities: Education and Related Services*

*Topics in Early Childhood Special Education*

## Physical Medicine and Rehabilitation

*American Journal of Physical Medicine and Rehabilitation*

*Clinical Rehabilitation*

*Journal of Occupational Rehabilitation*

*Journal of Orthopaedic & Sports Physical Therapy*

*Journal of Rehabilitation Medicine*

*Physical Medicine and Rehabilitation Clinics of North America*

*Physiotherapy*

*Physiotherapy Theory and Practice*

*Rehabilitation Counseling Bulletin*

*Rehabilitation Research, Policy, and Education*

*Sexuality and Disability*

*Work: A Journal of Prevention, Assessment and Rehabilitation*

## Professional Association Journals

*American Journal of Medical Technology*

*American Journal of Occupational Therapy*

*Art Therapy: Journal of the American Art Therapy Association*

*Australian Occupational Therapy Journal*

*British Journal of Occupational Therapy*

*Clinical Laboratory Science*

*International Journal of Yoga Therapy*

*JAAPA: Journal of the American Academy of Physician Assistants*

*Journal of Allied Health*

*Journal of Athletic Training*

*Journal of Hand Therapy*

*Journal of Laboratory Medicine*

*Journal of Sport Rehabilitation*

*Massage Therapy Journal*

*Physical Therapy & Rehabilitation Journal*
*Physiotherapy Canada*
*Radiologic Technology*
*Respiratory Care*
*World Federation of Occupational Therapists Bulletin*

## Research

*BMC Health Services Research*
*Health Services Research*
*Implementation Science*
*JBI Evidence Implementation*
*Journal of International Medical Research*
*Journal of Medical Internet Research*
*Journal of Multidisciplinary Healthcare*
*OTJR: Occupational Therapy Journal of Research*
*Qualitative Health Research*
*Quality of Life Research*
*Rehabilitation Research, Policy, and Education*
*The American Journal of Medicine*
*The New England Journal of Medicine*
*The Qualitative Report*
*Translational Science in Occupation*

# Glossary

The chapter numbers in parentheses at the end of each definition indicates the chapters where concepts are primarily discussed.

## A

**Abstract:** A short synopsis of a scholarly paper or research study, including the purpose, procedures, outcomes, and conclusions of the work. (Ch 3)

**Acceptance rate:** The percentage of article, grant, or other proposal submissions accepted based on the total number of submissions received. (Ch 16)

**Analysis of covariance (ANCOVA):** An inferential test of comparison used with parametric data to compare mean scores of multiple groups in an inquiry while controlling for initial differences between the groups. (Ch 5)

**Analysis of variance (ANOVA):** An inferential test of comparison used with parametric data to compare the mean scores of three or more groups in one inquiry. (Ch 5)

**Anonymity:** A condition in which data from an inquiry cannot be linked to a participant, even by an investigator. (Ch 12)

**A posteriori coding:** Qualitative data coding in which categories or themes (codes) are extracted from the data after it is collected. Also referred to as emergent coding or in vivo coding. (Ch 8)

**A priori coding:** Qualitative data coding in which categories or themes are named before data collection. Then, during data analysis, the data are organized into these predetermined categories or themes. (Ch 8)

**Artifact review:** A data collection method involving examination of physical materials such as adaptive equipment, medical devices, household items, art, photographs, or films. (Ch 8)

**Assent:** Agreement with inquiry procedures by someone unable to legally provide informed consent. For example, for an inquiry involving children, assent would be obtained from the children, and informed consent would be obtained from the parents or guardians. (Ch 12)

**Asynchronous presentation:** A presentation that is recorded and made available virtually for attendees to access whenever convenient. (Ch 15)

**Attentional bias:** Distortion of inquiry results related to the attention inquiry participants receive while participating in an inquiry. Also known as the Hawthorne effect. (Ch 6)

**Attrition:** The loss of participants during an inquiry. (Ch 4, 6)

**Audit trail:** A record that traces the inquiry process and decision-making to explain the researcher's thought process and increase the dependability of the results. (Ch 9)

**Author guidelines:** Specific requirements for submitting work to a journal or publication. (Ch 16)

## B

**Background:** Relevant information about an inquiry topic and setting, including definitions of key terms, theories, and a summary of prior research to establish context for the current inquiry. (Ch 2)

**Bar graph:** A diagram used to illustrate numerical values of variables using vertically or horizontally placed bars. (Ch 14)

**Boolean operators:** Words that allow you to broaden or narrow a literature search within most databases. The most common Boolean operators are AND, OR, and NOT. (Ch 3)

## C

**Case-control design:** A retrospective nonexperimental research design involving two groups of people—one group with and one group without the condition of interest—to identify risk factors or features of the condition. (Ch 4)

**Case series:** A quasi-experimental research design for studying the effects of a treatment or condition over time. Also may be referred to as a time series design or longitudinal study. (Ch 4)

**Central tendency:** A single average value that describes a set of data. Measures of central tendency include the mean, median, and mode. (Ch 5)

**Chain sampling:** A nonprobability sampling technique involving selecting a small number of participants who meet the participant inclusion criteria and then refer others who also meet the criteria. Also referred to as referral sampling or snowball sampling. (Ch 5)

**Client-centered:** An approach focused on the needs, values, and circumstances of the client, patient, or consumer. In healthcare, this approach involves the client as an active member of the clinical team and the decision-making process. (Ch 14)

**Clinical practice guideline:** Recommendations for practitioners on best practices related to a focused condition or scenario based on a systematic review of the best available research. (Ch 6)

**Clinical significance:** Refers to clinically meaningful inquiry outcomes. Also referred to as practical significance. (Ch 6)

**Closed-access journal:** A traditional subscription-based journal to which individual readers or institutions must pay a subscription fee to access articles within the journal. (Ch 16)

**Closed-ended question:** A survey or interview question that includes predetermined response choices. (Ch 11)

**Cluster sampling:** A probability sampling technique involving division of the population of interest into smaller clusters, often based on geographic location, which are randomly sampled. A variation of this sampling technique is multistage cluster sampling. (Ch 5)

**Code of ethics:** Published ethical standards specific to a professional discipline that outline the core values, principles, and standards of conduct expected of professionals or students of the discipline. (Ch 12)

**Coding:** The process of chunking qualitative data into smaller phrases or words that represent singular ideas, which can then be further processed and interpreted. (Ch 8)

**Coercion:** The use of excessive influence in recruiting and obtaining consent from inquiry participants. (Ch 12)

**Cohort design:** A quasi-experimental research design involving two or more naturally occurring groups, or cohorts, of participants who are followed over time. (Ch 4)

**Co-intervention:** A situation in which inquiry participants inadvertently receive another unplanned intervention during an inquiry that may impact results. (Ch 6)

**Co-investigators:** Other members of an inquiry or grantee group responsible for carrying out various activities associated with an inquiry or a grant. (Ch 13)

**Comprehensive literature search:** An exhaustive search of the literature using well-defined search terms, strategies, and tracking to determine the breadth of information on a topic. A comprehensive literature search, which occurs after the preliminary literature search, supports writing a formal literature review and designing future inquiry procedures. (Ch 2)

**Concurrent design:** A mixed methods design in which the qualitative and quantitative components co-occur and the results are integrated. Also referred to as a convergent design. (Ch 10)

**Confidence interval:** The margin of error or range of values that likely include scores or responses of the population of interest. (Ch 5)

**Confidence level:** The degree of certainty that scores or responses of the population of interest fall within a particular range and are not a chance occurrence. (Ch 5, 6)

**Confidentiality:** Protection of private information disclosed by a participant during an inquiry. (Ch 12)

**Confirmability:** A component of trustworthiness. Confidence that steps were taken in a qualitative inquiry to limit bias. (Ch 9)

**Constant comparative analysis:** A data analysis method used in grounded theory designs that involves coding, sorting, and organizing qualitative data to form a theory. (Ch 8)

**Construct validity:** The degree to which a data collection tool measures the construct it intends to measure. (Ch 6)

**Contamination:** A situation in which participants in a control group accidentally receive the experimental intervention. (Ch 6)

**Content analysis:** A systematic process for identifying, describing, and interpreting qualitative data, which may involve quantifying data by recording the frequency of words, phrases, or themes. (Ch 8)

**Content validity:** The degree to which the items or questions on a data collection tool represent all aspects of the construct being explored. (Ch 6)

**Control:** The researcher's ability to minimize or eliminate interfering or irrelevant influences in an inquiry's design. (Ch 4)

**Convenience sampling:** The process of selecting participants for an inquiry because they are readily available. The most popular type of nonprobability sampling. (Ch 5, 8)

**Convergent design:** A mixed methods design in which the qualitative and quantitative methods co-occur and the results are integrated. Also referred to as a concurrent design. (Ch 10)

**Correlated *t* test:** An inferential statistic used with parametric data to compare the mean scores from one group of participants (i.e., serving as their own control) or to compare individuals after being matched on a particular characteristic, to determine statistically significant differences. Also referred to as a paired samples *t* test. (Ch 5)

**Correlational design:** A nonexperimental research design for comparing two or more variables and looking for a relationship between them. (Ch 4)

**Correlational tests:** Inferential statistics for determining the relationship or association between two or more variables or sets of scores. Examples include Pearson product-moment correlation, Spearman rho, and simple regression analysis. (Ch 5)

**Correlation coefficient:** A number between −1 and +1, representing the relationship between two variables, where −1 indicates a perfect negative relationship, and +1 indicates a perfect positive relationship. (Ch 5)

**Credibility:** A component of trustworthiness. Confidence that the results of a qualitative inquiry are "true" or accurate. (Ch 9)

**Credible sources:** Resources that provide information you can trust. (Ch 2, 3)

**Critical appraisal:** A process used to scrutinize or evaluate the rigor of a research study. (Ch 3, 6, 9)

**Critically appraised paper (CAP):** A concise analysis of an individual research study. (Ch 6)

**Critically appraised topic (CAT):** A summary analysis of multiple research studies on a single topic or intervention. (Ch 6)

**Critical participatory action research (CPAR):** A variation of the qualitative participatory action research design that involves the participants as co-investigators to promote change or action specifically related to issues of inequality. (Ch 7)

**Cross-sectional design:** A nonexperimental research design involving a one-time measurement of participant exposures and outcomes. (Ch 4)

## D

**Data analysis:** The process of organizing and transforming data collected during an inquiry to make meaning of it. (Ch 5, 6, 8)

**Database:** A searchable, electronic collection of information, including citations, abstracts, and, in many cases, full-text articles. (Ch 3)

**Data collection:** The process of gathering or measuring inquiry outcomes. (Ch 5, 6, 8)

**Data saturation:** A condition in qualitative research in which new information or themes cease to emerge with repeated sampling and data collection. Also referred to as theoretical saturation. (Ch 8)

**Deductive reasoning:** A top-down reasoning approach that begins with a general theory, which leads to formulation of a hypothesis, observations to test the hypothesis, and ends with a specific conclusion. (Ch 1, 8)

**Dependability:** A component of trustworthiness. Confidence that the data in a qualitative inquiry are consistent with the results. (Ch 9)

**Dependent variable:** The person, thing, or phenomenon being measured in research. (Ch 4)

**Description of the literature portfolio:** A concise explanation of the body of literature gathered on a topic, including the number of studies, research designs and levels of evidence, and the time frame, setting, and geographic location of studies. (Ch 14)

**Descriptive statistics:** Analysis methods used to describe, organize, and summarize numerical data. (Ch 5)

**Direct costs:** Expenses that are directly related to the provision of a service, product, program, or inquiry. (Ch 13)

**Double-blinded:** Refers to a study design in which the researchers and participants are unaware of the hypothesis being tested or the assignment of participants to experimental and control groups. (Ch 4)

## E

**Effect size:** Refers to the magnitude and direction of the outcome being studied in an inquiry. (Ch 6, 10)

**Emergent coding:** Qualitative data coding in which categories or themes (codes) are extracted from the data after it is collected. Also referred to as a posteriori coding or in vivo coding. (Ch 8)

**Equipment:** Machines or other instruments used to collect data in an inquiry. (Ch 5)

**Ethnography:** A qualitative research design for describing a collective culture or aspects of culture. (Ch 7)

**Evidence-based practice:** Integrating best research evidence, a practitioner's skills and experiences, and a client's unique needs, values, and circumstances to make practice decisions. (Ch 1)

**Evidence-based practice project:** An initiative focused on designing and implementing an evidence-based intervention, program, protocol, or education to address the needs of a specific population or within a specific setting to improve outcomes or processes. May also be referred to as a quality improvement project. (Ch 1)

**Experimental research design:** A quantitative research design that involves the manipulation of at least one independent variable, control of various other phenomena in the methodology, and random selection and random assignment of participants to study groups. (Ch 4)

**Explanatory sequential:** A mixed methods design in which the quantitative methods precede and may inform the later qualitative methods. (Ch 10)

**Exploratory sequential:** A mixed methods design in which the qualitative methods precede and may inform the later quantitative methods. (Ch 10)

**External grants:** Funding offered by outside organizations that seek to support individuals, groups, or other institutions with similar missions to their own. (Ch 13)

**External validity:** The degree to which the results found in inquiry participants can be generalized to similar individuals, groups, or situations. (Ch 4, 6)

## F

**Factorial design:** An experimental research design that investigates two or more independent variables and their interaction with the dependent variable. (Ch 4)

**Feasibility study:** A preliminary investigation used to determine if a full-scale inquiry is viable and practical. Aspects of feasibility explored may include logistical, financial, and organizational factors. (Ch 11)

**Fellowship:** A merit-based training program for individuals to further develop their clinical and/or research skills. Awardees may receive benefits, a stipend/scholarship, or subsidized housing during the fellowship. (Ch 13)

**Field notes:** Detailed annotations made by a researcher during an inquiry, which may include observations, reflections, or contextual information to be considered in the data analysis phase of the inquiry. (Ch 8)

**Fieldwork:** A primary data collection method in ethnography involving the researcher observing and immersing themselves in the study setting. (Ch 7)

**Figure:** A diagram used to illustrate data or information. (Ch 14)

**Flowchart:** A diagram that illustrates a sequence of steps or a process. (Ch 14)

**Focus group:** A data collection method involving an interview or guided discussion on a specific topic with a small group of participants who share similar characteristics or experiences. (Ch 8)

**Forest plot:** A graph used to illustrate each study's effect size and confidence interval and the combined effect size and confidence interval of all studies in a meta-analysis. (Ch 10)

**Frequency:** The number of times a specific variable or response occurs in a data set. (Ch 5)

## G

**Grantee:** A person, group, or organization applying for or receiving a grant. (Ch 13)

**Grantor:** An organization that funds a grant. (Ch 13)

**Grants:** Funds commonly provided by charitable foundations, federal agencies, businesses, individuals, or other entities for a distinct purpose. (Ch 13)

**Grey literature:** Unpublished literature or literature that is neither peer-reviewed nor commercially published. (Ch 3)

**Grounded theory:** A qualitative research design used to construct theories. (Ch 7)

## H

**Handouts:** Paper or electronic information provided to presentation attendees that supplements or supports the presentation. (Ch 15)

**Hawthorne effect:** Distortion of inquiry results related to the attention inquiry participants receive while participating in an inquiry. Named after a series of experiments at Hawthorne Works in the early 1900s, in which worker productivity increased as a result of the extra attention they received from the researchers. Also known as attentional bias. (Ch 6)

**Heterogeneity:** Variability in inquiry outcomes for a group of inquiries in a systematic review. (Ch 10)

**Historical design:** A qualitative research design that uses data from past events or circumstances to better understand current events or make predictions. Also called historiographies. (Ch 7)

## I

**Impact factor:** A method of evaluating the relative importance of a journal based on the average frequency of citations of each article published within a journal over the past 2 years. (Ch 16)

**Incidents:** Manageable chunks of data used in constant comparative analysis to identify similarities and differences. (Ch 8)

**Independent samples *t* test:** An inferential statistic used with parametric data to compare scores from two independent groups (experimental and control groups) to determine statistically significant differences. Also referred to as an unpaired *t* test. (Ch 5)

**Independent variable:** The person, thing, or phenomenon being manipulated in research, which could affect the outcome (or dependent variable). (Ch 4)

**Indirect costs:** Expenses that are not directly related to providing a service, product, program, or inquiry. (Ch 13)

**Inductive reasoning:** A bottom-up reasoning approach that begins with a specific observation, which leads to identification of a pattern, generation of a hypothesis, and ends with establishing a theory. (Ch 1, 8)

**Inferential statistics:** Analysis methods used to test a hypothesis or to make inferences about the population of interest from the sample data. (Ch 5)

**Informants:** A term sometimes used to refer to subjects or participants in qualitative research. (Ch 8)

**Informed consent:** An inquiry participant's agreement to participate, freely given after full disclosure of the inquiry procedures. The informed consent may include written consent, verbal consent, or a waiver of consent, depending on the inquiry topic and logistics. (Ch 12)

**Inquiry:** A term used to collectively refer to a research study or an evidence-based practice project. (Ch 1)

**Inquiry volunteer:** An individual who assists with an inquiry but is not an investigator and does not provide data during the data collection phase. (Ch 12)

**Institutional Review Board (IRB):** An administrative group that reviews inquiry proposals before implementation to ensure ethical procedures and the protection of human subjects or participants. Also called independent ethics committees, ethics review boards, or research review/ethics committees. (Ch 6, 9, 12, 14)

**Instrument validation study:** A nonexperimental research design used to develop, test, refine, and validate data collection tools. These designs involve three phases: item development, tool development, and tool evaluation. (Ch 4)

**Integration:** The explicit combining of quantitative and qualitative components in a mixed methods inquiry. (Ch 10)

**Intercoder reliability:** The degree to which independent coders in qualitative research code data consistently similar to each other. (Ch 8)

**Internal grants:** Funding available within an organization that benefits the organization or its members. (Ch 13)

**Internal validity:** Relates to how well the inquiry methods, data collection, and data analysis were conducted to limit bias. Quality methods increase the chance that observed changes in an inquiry can be attributed to the intervention or treatment provided and not to other possible causes or chance. (Ch 4, 5)

**Interpretative phenomenological analysis (IPA):** A qualitative data analysis method used primarily in phenomenological designs to understand the participants' lived experiences. (Ch 8)

**Interrater reliability:** The degree to which individual raters or evaluators agree or have similar ratings to each other. See also intercoder reliability. (Ch 5, 6, 8)

**Interval data:** Numerical data organized on a continuum or scale on which the distance between numbers is equal, but there is no true zero point. (Ch 5)

**Intervention bias:** Distortion of inquiry results related to differences in how the intervention was provided to study groups or exposure to another intervention that may impact results. (Ch 6)

**Interview:** A data collection method involving verbally asking participants questions. Interviews may be structured, semi-structured, or unstructured. (Ch 5, 8)

**Intrarater reliability:** The degree to which a rater or evaluator is consistent in their ratings. (Ch 5, 6)

**In vivo coding:** Qualitative data coding in which categories or themes (codes) are extracted from the data after it is collected. Also referred to as emergent coding or a posteriori coding. (Ch 8)

## K

**Key argument:** A primary idea supported with evidence. (Ch 16)

**Keywords:** Terms used to describe the population, intervention, outcomes, or problems of interest, which can be used as search terms to locate literature on the topic. (Ch 2)

**Knowledge translation:** A process involving implementing existing research, evaluating the outcomes, identifying supports and challenges in applying research to practice, and disseminating the findings to promote better clinical outcomes. (Ch 1, 11)

**Kruskal-Wallis test:** An inferential test of comparison used with ordinal nonparametric data to compare rankings of scores on the dependent variable for three or more independent inquiry groups. (Ch 5)

## L

**Latent analysis:** Qualitative content analysis involving looking beyond the data at face value and considering the context of the data and its underlying meaning. (Ch 8)

**Lecture:** An oral presentation with little to no interaction between the presenter and the attendees. (Ch 15)

**Likert scale question:** A closed-ended question used to measure perceptions or attitudes related to an inquiry in which respondents are presented with a series of statements and asked to rate their level of agreement with each statement on a five-point or seven-point scale. (Ch 11)

**Line graph:** A diagram composed of lines connecting sequential data points to illustrate changes in a phenomenon over time. (Ch 14)

**Literature matrix:** A comprehensive table for organizing and comparing studies in a literature portfolio by various components, including author, publication date, study purpose, study design or level of evidence, participants, variables, results, and any important points, implications, or themes. (Ch 3)

**Literature portfolio:** The collective body of literature gathered on a topic. (Ch 3, 14)

**Longitudinal study:** A quasi-experimental research design for studying the effects of a treatment or condition over time. Also may be referred to as a case series or time series design. (Ch 4)

**Long-response question:** An open-ended question requiring a lengthier answer, ranging from a few sentences to paragraphs, that is most useful for gathering detailed responses about complex topics. (Ch 11)

## M

**Manifest analysis:** Qualitative content analysis involving looking explicitly at the data at face value without examining deeper or underlying meanings. (Ch 8)

**Manipulation:** Purposeful alteration of one or more variables in a study. (Ch 4)

**Mann-Whitney test:** An inferential statistic used with ordinal nonparametric data to compare the means of two independent samples. (Ch 5)

**Matching:** A process to ensure inquiry participants in different groups (for example, experimental and control groups) are similar at the start of the inquiry to decrease bias in results. (Ch 5)

**Maturation:** Refers to the inquiry participants' growth, development, or changes that occur naturally over time, which may influence inquiry results. See also timing bias. (Ch 6)

**Mean:** A descriptive statistic and measure of central tendency calculated by adding all the scores from a group and dividing by the total number in the group. Also referred to as the average. (Ch 5)

**Measurement bias:** Distortion of inquiry results related to issues with the data collection tools or methods, such as faulty equipment, surveys with biased wording, or participants improving on a measure owing to repeated administration of the same tool. (Ch 6)

**Measures of variation:** Descriptive statistics that describe the spread or variability of scores. Measures of variation include the range and standard deviation. (Ch 5)

**Median:** A descriptive statistic and measure of central tendency representing the midpoint among a set of scores. The score that falls in the center when scores are ranked. (Ch 5)

**Member checking:** The process of asking participants to verify the data and interpretations of it to improve the credibility of the findings. (Ch 9)

**Memorandum of Understanding (MOU):** A written agreement between two parties regarding collaboration on an inquiry or grant. (Ch 13)

**MeSH terms:** Medical Subject Headings or standardized words or phrases used to index articles by topic by grouping similar words to create a hierarchy of terms ranging from very broad to very specific. (Ch 3)

**Meta-analyses:** Statistical procedures used to determine the collective effect size from multiple selected studies in a systematic review. (Ch 10)

**Methodology:** Specific details of an inquiry plan, including when and how participants will be recruited and what procedures and outcomes will be used with participants. (Ch 4)

**Methodology of the literature search:** An in-depth description of a literature search process, including the search terms, criteria, and strategies used. (Ch 14)

**Micro-ethnography:** An ethnographic qualitative research design that involves a narrow focus on a particular aspect of culture rather than the holistic view of culture typical of traditional ethnography. (Ch 7)

**Minimal risk:** The likelihood of harm or discomfort anticipated in an inquiry is no greater than that encountered in daily life or routine physical or psychological testing. (Ch 12)

**Mixed methods designs/research:** Inquiry designs that incorporate both quantitative and qualitative methods into one inquiry for a more holistic understanding of the phenomena of interest. (Ch 7, 10)

**Mode:** A descriptive statistic and measure of central tendency representing the most commonly occurring score or response. (Ch 5)

**Multi-case study:** A quasi-experimental research design used when numerous critical, relevant cases are present to substantiate experimental outcomes. This design includes pretesting, interventions, and posttesting to examine unique cases or situations. In comparison, a single-case study involves only one case. (Ch 4)

**Multiple-choice question:** A closed-ended question that most commonly includes four predetermined response options from which respondents choose their response. (Ch 11)

**Multiple regression analysis:** An inferential test of comparison for exploring the degree to which two or more independent variables can predict future scores for the dependent variable. (Ch 5)

**Multistage cluster sampling:** A probability sampling technique involving sequential stages of cluster sampling (dividing the population of interest into smaller clusters, often based on geographic location, which are then randomly sampled) to narrow a final sample. (Ch 5)

## N

**Needs assessment:** A systematic process for identifying existing supports, challenges, and opportunities for improvement within an organization, setting, or group to guide future decision-making, programming, and resource allocation. The first step in program development. A SWOT analysis is a type of needs assessment. (Ch 2, 13)

**Nominal data:** Numbers applied to nonnumerical variables or descriptive categories that are mutually exclusive but that cannot be ordered or ranked. (Ch 5)

**Nonexperimental research design:** A quantitative research design used to describe or characterize phenomena, to examine relationships among variables, or to determine the reliability and validity of evaluations, tests, or equipment. Also known as a pre-experimental design. (Ch 4)

**Nonparametric data:** Categorical data, including nominal and ordinal data, that is not assumed to be normally distributed. (Ch 5)

**Nonparametric tests:** Statistical tests used with nominal or ordinal data gathered from small samples that were not randomly selected. (Ch 5)

**Non–peer-reviewed:** Refers to content that topic experts have not reviewed before publication. (Ch 16)

**Nonprobability sampling:** The process of nonrandomly selecting participants for an inquiry, for example, selection based on location or convenient access. (Ch 5, 8)

**Nonresponse bias:** Distortion of inquiry results due to systematic differences in inquiry participants who drop out or decline participation. (Ch 5)

**Non-standardized assessment:** A data collection tool that has yet to undergo normalizing or rigorous testing to establish validity and reliability for use with the intended population. (Ch 5)

**Normalizing:** A process used to establish the validity and reliability of standardized assessments. (Ch 5)

**Notice of Award (NoA):** A document informing grant recipients they were selected to receive a grant and describing the terms and conditions of the funding. (Ch 13)

## O

**Observation:** A data collection method involving watching human participants or video recordings of participants or events. (Ch 5, 8)

**One-group pretest-posttest design:** A quasi-experimental research design in which one group of participants receives treatment and a period of no treatment (considered the control period). (Ch 4)

**Open-access journal:** A journal providing free access to its content to readers, institutions, and the public. Also sometimes referred to as pay-to-publish journals. (Ch 16)

**Open-ended question:** A survey or interview question without fixed response choices, which allows respondents to provide detailed answers in their own words. (Ch 11)

**Oral presentation:** A verbal presentation that may include lecture, demonstration, role-playing, question-and-answer periods, or group, interactive, or hands-on activities. (Ch 15)

**Ordinal data:** Numbers applied to nonnumerical variables or descriptive categories that can be ranked or ordered. (Ch 5)

## P

**Paired samples *t* test:** An inferential statistic used with parametric data to compare the mean scores from one group of participants (i.e., they serve as their own control) or to compare individuals after being matched on a particular characteristic, to determine statistically significant differences. Also referred to as a correlated *t* test. (Ch 5)

**Parametric data:** Numerical data, including interval and ratio data, assumed to be normally distributed. (Ch 5)

**Parametric tests:** Statistical tests used with interval or ratio data gathered from randomly selected and assigned or matched samples. (Ch 5)

**Participant bias:** Distortion of inquiry results related to participants responding during data collection in ways that do not accurately represent their views. (Ch 9)

**Participant exclusion criteria:** Characteristics or traits that disqualify participants from engaging in an inquiry. (Ch 5, 8)

**Participant inclusion criteria:** Characteristics or traits that participants must have to qualify for participation in the inquiry. (Ch 5, 8)

**Participants:** Subjects who engage in an inquiry. Also sometimes referred to as informants in qualitative research. (Ch 1, 8, 12)

**Participatory action research (PAR):** A qualitative research design that involves the participants as co-investigators to promote change or action that will positively impact those being studied. See also critical participatory action research. (Ch 7)

**Pay-to-publish journal:** An open-access journal that uses author publication fees to cover costs associated with providing readers free access to the journal's content. (Ch 16)

**Pearson product-moment correlation:** An inferential correlational test used with ratio parametric data to determine the relationship between variables. Also referred to as Pearson *r*. (Ch 5)

**Pearson *r*:** An inferential correlational test used with ratio parametric data to determine the relationship between variables. Also referred to as Pearson product-moment correlation. (Ch 5)

**Pearson's chi-square test:** An inferential statistic used with nonparametric data to determine if differences between observed and expected inquiry results are statistically significant, or if two groups (experimental and control) have similar characteristics. (Ch 5)

**Peer review:** Examination of the inquiry data and results by a researcher not affiliated with an inquiry to determine if that data support the results. (Ch 9)

**Peer-reviewed:** Refers to content evaluated for quality by topic experts before publication. Peer-reviewed publications may also be referred to as scholarly or refereed publications. (Ch 3, 16)

**Percentage:** The frequency of a variable or response divided by the total scores or responses multiplied by 100. (Ch 5)

**Percent change:** The percentage of increase or decrease from one score to another. (Ch 5)

**Phenomenology:** A qualitative research design for describing the lived experiences of individuals related to their condition or experiences from their perspective. (Ch 7)

**Pie chart:** A circular diagram that illustrates numerical values of a variable depicted as sectors of the circle. (Ch 14)

**Pilot study:** A preliminary investigation used to refine the inquiry methods before a full-scale inquiry. (Ch 11)

**Population of interest:** The broader group of people from which a sample is drawn. (Ch 5, 8)

**Poster presentation:** An oral presentation supplemented with an eye-catching vertical or electronic display that combines text and figures. (Ch 15)

**Posttest-only design:** An experimental research design in which participants are randomly assigned and selected, but the pretest is omitted to reduce any potential influence from the test. (Ch 4)

**Pre-experimental design:** A quantitative research design used to describe or characterize phenomena, to examine relationships among variables, or to determine the reliability and validity of evaluations, tests, or equipment. Also known as a nonexperimental research design. (Ch 4)

**Preliminary literature search:** An initial exploration of the literature on a topic, occurring before the more comprehensive literature search, to gain a broad understanding of the relevant research and trends and refine initial inquiry ideas. (Ch 2)

**Presentation:** A method of verbally communicating specific information to an audience to educate, inspire, persuade, or call them to action. (Ch 15)

**Pretest-posttest design:** An experimental research design involving at least two study groups (experimental and control) who are compared during a pretest to evaluate if the groups are similar, provided with an experimental or control condition depending on group assignment, and compared at posttest to assess the impact of the intervention.

This design may also include follow-up testing to determine retention of outcomes. (Ch 4)

**Primary investigator (PI):** The individual primarily responsible for designing and implementing an inquiry, preparing and submitting an Institutional Review Board (IRB) proposal, or preparing a grant proposal and overseeing grant activities if funding is received. (Ch 12)

**Primary source:** First-hand information about a topic, such as an autobiography, an eyewitness account, or an original research article. (Ch 5, 7)

**Privacy:** An individual's control over the timing, setting, and extent of their participation in an inquiry. (Ch 12)

**Probability sampling:** A sampling method that ensures all members of a population of interest have an equal chance of being selected for the sample. (Ch 5)

**Procedural rigor:** Refers to the quality of an inquiry's design and the thoroughness of data collection and analysis methods. (Ch 8)

**Procedures:** The steps or methods implemented with inquiry participants, including any interventions or treatments provided. (Ch 6)

**Program development:** The process of planning, implementing, and evaluating a new program, service, or practice protocol or improving or expanding an existing one. (Ch 11, 13)

**Program evaluation:** The last step in program development, though it usually co-occurs with program implementation. The process involves measuring and comparing program outcomes to the projected outcomes to determine the program's success. (Ch 13)

**Program implementation:** The third step in program development involving carrying out the newly designed or enhanced program. (Ch 13)

**Program planning:** The second step in program development involving a series of tasks to design and secure funding for a program. Tasks include prioritizing needs, identifying supporting literature, setting goals, defining program roles and timelines, designing the program, developing an evaluation plan, and obtaining funding. (Ch 13)

**Prospective study:** A research design in which the study plans are laid out well in advance and the participants are followed moving forward in time. (Ch 4)

**Protected health information (PHI):** Individually identifiable health information in a medical record. (Ch 12)

**Publication aim:** The primary purpose of an article or journal. (Ch 16)

**Purpose:** The aim or objective of an inquiry or program. (Ch 2)

**Purposive sampling:** A nonprobability sampling technique involving selecting participants based on specific attributes, such as a diagnosis, motivational level, or compliance. (Ch 5, 8)

## Q

**Qualitative case study design:** A qualitative research design for exploring naturally occurring contexts, circumstances, and cases. This design involves an in-depth longitudinal analysis of an individual, group, unit, community, institution, or event to answer how or why questions. (Ch 7)

**Qualitative research:** The study of people, events, and social phenomena within natural contexts to determine how or why something happens. Results in rich narrative data. (Ch 7)

**Quality improvement project:** An initiative focused on designing and implementing an evidence-based intervention, program, protocol, or education to address the needs of a specific population or within a specific setting to improve outcomes or processes. May also be called an evidence-based practice project. (Ch 1)

**Quantitative case study design:** A quasi-experimental research design in which an individual, group, unit, community, institution, or event is studied longitudinally. This design includes pretesting, interventions, and posttesting to examine unique cases or situations. (Ch 4)

**Quantitative research:** The objective, systematic process of obtaining numerical data to answer a research question. (Ch 4)

**Quantitative survey design:** A nonexperimental research design involving data collection via self-report surveys from a sample to produce numerical data. The surveys can be cross-sectional (at one point in time) or longitudinal (at multiple points in time). (Ch 4)

**Quasi-experimental research design:** A research design that contains an independent variable manipulated to determine the effect on the dependent variable, but that lacks one or more of the following: a control group, random selection, or random assignment. (Ch 4)

**Quota sampling:** A nonprobability sampling technique involving division of the population of interest into two or more subgroups based on some characteristic. Then, samples are drawn from each subgroup to represent the proportion of the characteristic occurring naturally in the population of interest. (Ch 5, 8)

## R

**Random assignment:** Indiscriminately placing inquiry participants into experimental and control groups to reduce bias. (Ch 4)

**Randomization:** A method of indiscriminately selecting and assigning inquiry participants to experimental and control groups to reduce the risk of bias and increase the ability to generalize results. (Ch 4)

**Randomized controlled trial (RCT):** The most rigorous prospective quantitative study design, which incorporates randomization, control, and manipulation to measure the effectiveness of an intervention. (Ch 4)

**Random selection:** A process of indiscriminately choosing participants for an inquiry in which every participant in the population of interest has an equal chance of being selected. (Ch 4)

**Range:** A descriptive statistic and measure of variation representing the spread of scores in a dataset, calculated by subtracting the lowest score from the highest score. (Ch 5)

**Rating scale:** A closed-ended question requiring respondents to rate or rank items within categories or on a continuum. (Ch 11)

**Ratio data:** Numerical data organized on a continuum or scale on which the distance between numbers is equal, and there is a true zero point. (Ch 5)

**Readability formula:** A method to assess the complexity of text based on the average sentence and word length. (Ch 14)

**Recall bias:** Distortion of inquiry results related to inquiry participants performing better on later repeated inquiry tests because they have learned the material rather than because of an experimental intervention. (Ch 6)

**Record review:** A data collection method involving examination of written records. (Ch 5, 8)

**Recruitment:** The process of finding participants who meet the participant inclusion criteria for an inquiry. (Ch 5, 8, 12)

**Referral sampling:** A nonprobability sampling technique involving selecting a small number of participants who meet the participant inclusion criteria and then refer others who also meet the criteria. Also referred to as snowball sampling or chain sampling. (Ch 5)

**Reliability:** The extent to which inquiry outcomes are consistent or can be replicated in future inquiries. Also refers to the degree to which a data collection tool produces consistent results over time (test-retest reliability), across items (split-half reliability), within an individual rater (intrarater reliability), and among different raters (interrater reliability). (Ch 6, 9)

**Repeated measures design:** A time series design involving various treatment and nontreatment sequences alternated with tests of the same group of participants. (Ch 4)

**Reputation:** The relative prestige of a journal based on factors including the impact factor, publishing history, peer-review process, and credibility within the field. (Ch 16)

**Request for Proposal (RFP):** A document describing a funding opportunity, including the purpose, submission guidelines, and the application deadline. Also referred to as a request for application (RFA), notice of funding opportunity (NOFO), or notice of funding availability (NOFA). (Ch 13)

**Research:** The systematic investigation of a problem, issue, or question to produce *new* knowledge that may be generalized to similar groups or populations. (Ch 1)

**Research design:** A general plan or overall structure of an inquiry. Designs can be quantitative, qualitative, or mixed methods depending on the topic and inquiry aims. (Ch 4)

**Researcher bias:** Distortion of inquiry results because of a researcher's intentional or unintentional influence over inquiry results. (Ch 6, 9)

**Response rate:** The number of surveys completed divided by the total number of surveys distributed to a sample. (Ch 5)

**Retrospective study:** A research design in which participants or phenomena are examined backward in time concerning an outcome that has already occurred. (Ch 4)

## S

**Sample:** A subset of the population of interest who participates in an inquiry. (Ch 5)

**Sampling:** The process of selecting a subset of the population of interest to participate in an inquiry. (Ch 5)

**Sampling bias:** Distortion of inquiry results arising from a sample that does not adequately represent the population of interest. (Ch 5, 6)

**Search criteria:** Parameters defining the desired research characteristics when completing a literature search. For example, the publication date, language of publication, or availability in full text. (Ch 3)

**Search terms:** Keywords derived from a well-constructed inquiry question, which represent a topic, entered into databases to retrieve relevant articles. (Ch 3)

**Secondary source:** Information on a topic at least one step from the original source. An account not based on personal experiences. (Ch 5, 7)

**Semi-structured interview:** A data collection method involving verbally asking participants a series of flexible, guiding questions related to an inquiry topic. The questions need not be covered in the same order or with the same exact wording for each participant, and the interviewer is free to interject additional probing questions as necessary. (Ch 8)

**Short-response question:** An open-ended question that restricts responses to a few words or less and is most useful for gathering straightforward information on topics for which fixed response choices are inappropriate. (Ch 11)

**Simple random sampling:** A probability sampling technique involving indiscriminately choosing participants from the population of interest so that each potential participant has an equal chance of being selected for the inquiry. (Ch 5)

**Simple regression analysis:** An inferential correlational test used after a relationship has been found between two variables to explore the degree to which the independent variable can predict future scores for the dependent variable. (Ch 5)

**Single-blinded:** Refers to an inquiry design where only one group, either the participants or the researchers, is blinded to the treatment. (Ch 4)

**Single-case study:** A quasi-experimental research design involving just one critical, relevant case. This design is used when there are limited cases available, when there are many variables to explore, when using multiple cases is impractical, or when the researcher wants to alter the interventions provided based on the data collected as the study progresses. (Ch 4)

**Significance:** An explanation of why a particular inquiry or program is important or worthy of pursuit. (Ch 2)

**Snowball sampling:** A nonprobability sampling technique involving selecting a small number of participants who meet the participant inclusion criteria and then refer others who also meet the criteria. Also referred to as referral sampling or chain sampling. (Ch 5, 8)

**Solomon four-group design:** An experimental research design involving random assignment of participants to four study groups—two experimental groups (one who receives the pretest and one who does not) and two control groups (one who receives the pretest and one who does not)—to address concerns about the influence of the pretest on the outcomes. (Ch 4)

**Spearman rho:** An inferential correlational test used with ordinal nonparametric data to determine the relationship between two ranked data sets. Also called Spearman's rank correlation coefficient. (Ch 5)

**Spearman's rank correlation coefficient:** An inferential correlational test used with ordinal nonparametric data to determine the relationship between two ranked data sets. Also called Spearman rho. (Ch 5)

**Split-half reliability:** The extent to which a data collection tool produces consistent results across test items. (Ch 6)

**Standard deviation:** A descriptive statistic and measure of variation representing how the scores in a dataset are grouped around the mean. A small standard deviation indicates scores clustered near the mean, whereas a larger standard deviation indicates greater score variability. (Ch 5)

**Standardized assessment:** A data collection tool that has undergone normalizing or rigorous testing to establish validity and reliability for use with the intended population. (Ch 5)

**Statistical significance:** Refers to outcomes attributed to a specific cause or intervention rather than chance alone. Examples of tests of statistical significance include Pearson's chi-square test, *t* test, Wilcoxon rank test, and Mann-Whitney test. (Ch 5, 6)

**Stepwise regression:** A type of multiple regression analysis used to examine the degree to which the independent variables in a study, in various combinations, are most useful for predicting future scores for the dependent variable. (Ch 5)

**Stratified random sampling:** A probability sampling technique involving division of the population of interest into homogeneous subgroups and then indiscriminately sampling each subgroup to ensure each subgroup is adequately represented in the sample. (Ch 5)

**Structured interview:** A data collection method involving verbally asking participants specific, well-designed questions presented in the same order using the same terminology for all participants. (Ch 8)

**Subjects:** Participants in an inquiry. Also sometimes referred to as informants in qualitative research. (Ch 1)

**Survey:** A data collection method that involves participants responding to written questions. (Ch 5, 8, 12)

**SWOT analysis:** A planning tool, or needs assessment, to evaluate the strengths, weaknesses, opportunities, and threats within an organization, setting, or group to develop strategies for viability and improvement. (Ch 2)

**Synchronous presentation:** A presentation in which the presenter and attendees are online or in the same physical location simultaneously. (Ch 15)

**Synthesis:** Integration and collective summary of the findings from multiple research studies rather than discussion of each study individually. (Ch 3, 14)

**Systematic bias:** Inherent flaws in an inquiry's design that may influence or skew results. This may include faulty equipment, untrained inquiry personnel, or biased sampling or testing methods. (Ch 4)

**Systematic random sampling:** A probability sampling technique involving indiscriminately ordering all possible participants and then selecting every nth one for participation. (Ch 5)

**Systematic review (SR):** A study design incorporating precise methods to locate, appraise, synthesize, and disseminate a summary of multiple individual research studies on a focused topic. (Ch 10)

## T

**Table:** An arrangement of rows and columns to organize and present data or information. (Ch 14)

**Test-retest reliability:** The extent to which a data collection tool produces consistent results over time. (Ch 6)

**Tests of comparison:** Inferential statistics used to compare three or more variables or sets of scores at a time. Examples include analysis of variance, analysis of covariance, Kruskal-Wallis test, and multiple regression analysis. (Ch 5)

**Thematic analysis:** A reflective inductive process for identifying and interpreting patterns or themes from qualitative data. (Ch 8)

**Themes:** Central concepts or findings occurring in two or more studies, which strengthens the conclusions and increases the likelihood that results can be generalized to similar situations and populations with the same outcome. Also, recurrent ideas, concepts, or patterns within a qualitative dataset. (Ch 3, 8, 14)

**Theoretical base:** Existing concepts or theories that provide insight into a problem or topic and are used to guide an inquiry. (Ch 3)

**Theoretical saturation:** A condition in qualitative research in which new information or themes cease to emerge with repeated sampling and data collection. Also referred to as data saturation. (Ch 8)

**Time series design:** A quasi-experimental research design for studying the effects of a treatment or condition over time. Also may be referred to as a case series or longitudinal study. (Ch 4)

**Timing bias:** Distortion of inquiry results related to issues with the timing of the intervention or data collection in an inquiry. (Ch 6)

**Transferability:** A component of trustworthiness. Confidence that the results of a qualitative inquiry can be applied to other similar contexts or situations. (Ch 9)

**Triangulation:** Using multiple data sources/perspectives to validate inquiry results, which may include using multiple data collection methods (observation, interviews, focus group), multiple data sources (people from different sites, different points in time, different stakeholders), a team of researchers, or using multiple theories to analyze and interpret the data. (Ch 9, 10)

**Trustworthiness:** The degree of confidence in the qualitative inquiry methods and findings. The four components of trustworthiness are credibility, transferability, dependability, and confirmability. (Ch 9)

***t* test:** An inferential statistic used with interval and ratio data to compare the mean scores of two groups to determine if there is a statistically significant difference. (Ch 5)

## U

**Unpaired *t* test:** An inferential statistic used with parametric data to compare scores from two independent groups (experimental and control groups) to determine statistically significant differences. Also referred to as an independent samples *t* test. (Ch 5)

**Unstructured interview:** A data collection method that involves verbally asking participants questions, but there is no set format, and the questions are not predetermined. (Ch 8)

## V

**Validity:** The extent to which a concept is accurately measured or the results reflect the phenomena of interest in an inquiry. Consistency between data and the findings. (Ch 6, 9)

**Variable:** A person, thing, or phenomenon that is measured or influences another variable in an inquiry. See also independent variable and dependent variable. (Ch 4)

**Vulnerable populations:** Individuals at greater risk of health, financial, or social disparities, which includes children under 18 years of age, pregnant persons, prisoners, individuals who are economically or educationally disadvantaged, and those with impaired decision-making capacity. (Ch 12)

## W

**Waiver of consent:** Eliminating the requirement to have inquiry participants sign an informed consent document. This option may be appropriate if the inquiry involves minimal risk and will not adversely affect the rights or welfare of participants, but this decision ultimately rests with the Institutional Review Board (IRB). (Ch 12)

**Wilcoxon rank sum test:** An inferential statistic used with nonparametric data and particularly small samples to compare the degree and direction of differences between two independent groups (for example, experimental and control groups) to determine if there is a statistically significant difference. (Ch 5)

**Wilcoxon signed rank test:** An inferential statistic used with nonparametric data and particularly small samples to compare the degree and direction of difference from pretest to posttest from one group of participants (i.e., they serve as their own control) or to compare matched pairs of participants to determine if there is a statistically significant difference. (Ch 5)

# Index

References followed by the letter "f" are for figures, "t" are tables, and "b" are boxes.

## Q

## T